THE
MEDICINE
OF THE
ANCIENT
EGYPTIANS

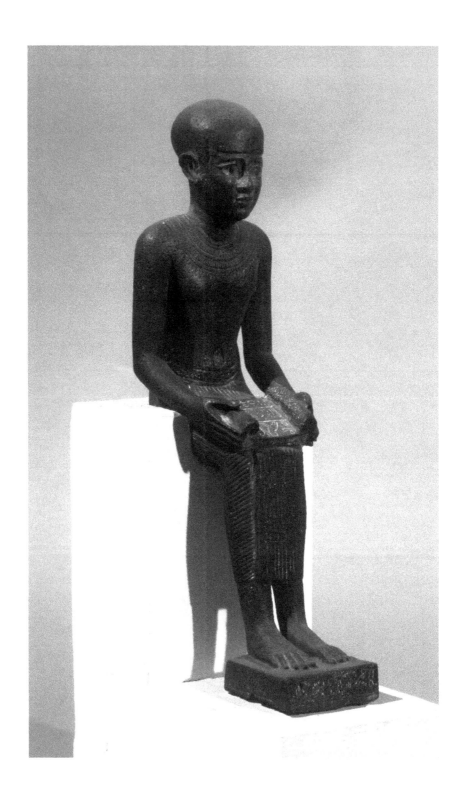

THE
MEDICINE
OF THE
ANCIENT
EGYPTIANS

2: INTERNAL MEDICINE

Eugen Strouhal
Břetislav Vachala
Hana Vymazalová

The American University in Cairo Press
Cairo New York

Page ii: A bronze statue of Imhotep, a famous Egyptian sage and legendary physician, and the architect of the earliest stone pyramid, of King Netjerikhet Djoser of the Third Dynasty, at Saqqara. In later times Imhotep was deified and venerated as the patron of medicine. (Ptolemaic to Roman Period, Egyptian Museum, Cairo [JE 38048], photo © M. Zemima]

Publisher's note: As this book goes to press, some items from the Egyptian Museum in Cairo are being moved to the new Grand Egyptian Museum and the National Museum of Egyptian Civilization.

First published in 2021 by
The American University in Cairo Press
113 Sharia Kasr el Aini, Cairo, Egypt
One Rockefeller Plaza, 10th Floor, New York, NY 10020
www.aucpress.com

Copyright © 2017, 2021 by Charles University, Faculty of Arts

Originally published as *Lékařství starých Egypťanů II. Vnitřní lékařství* in 2017 by Academia, Prague

Translated by Sean Mark Miller

This English edition was supported by the Program for the Development of Fields of Study at Charles University, no. Q11: Complexity and Resilience: Ancient Egyptian Civilisation in Multidisciplinary and Multicultural Perspective.

Dar el Kutub No. 26216/19
ISBN 978 977 416 991 5

Dar el Kutub Cataloging-in-Publication Data

Strouhal, Eugen
        The Medicine of the Ancient Egyptians: Internal Medicine. / Eugen Strouhal, Břetislav Vachala, and Hana Vymazalová.—Cairo: The American University in Cairo Press, 2021.
        p.   cm.
        ISBN 978 977 416 991 5
        1.   Medicine – Egypt — Antiquities
        610.932

1 2 3 4 5   25 24 23 22 21

Designed by Sally Boylan
Printed in the United Kingdom

CONTENTS

4 Internal Diseases and Their Treatment 151

5 Conclusion *(E. Strouhal, H. Vymazalová)* 331

ILLUSTRATIONS

PREFACE

S even years on, the reader has now received the second volume of the three-part compendium *The Medicine of the Ancient Egyptians*, which is devoted to internal medicine. The book contains commented translations of the relevant parts of ten ancient Egyptian medical papyri and ostraca, which after several thousand years make it possible for today's doctors and interested public to approach various internal diseases of the ancient populations of the land on the Nile and the approaches of the physicians then, who, without closer knowledge of the functions of the internal organs, treated the apparent symptoms of the given diseases with the aid of empirically verified and tested means and medicines. However, they also used magical means (Pinch 2010, 133–46), when in their curative performances they, for instance, pronounced various spells and recited formulas, which they certainly knew from both written and oral traditions.

Nevertheless, it is necessary to keep in mind that only a fraction of medical papyri have been preserved to now, which moreover are sometimes incomplete. Our knowledge of Egyptian medicine is thus necessarily quite limited. In terms of the ancient Egyptian written sources, Egyptologists estimate that a mere one one-hundred-thousandth of them has been preserved! The majority of the written records succumbed in antiquity to natural decay or purposeful destruction, culminating in 643 with the definitive ruin and burning of the famous Great Library of Alexandria (el-Abbadi 1992, 145–79), which according to testimony of the period could have contained as many as 700,000 papyrus scrolls and parchments, among which there were certainly also medical papyri represented. Their loss is irreplaceable, but there is still hope that with ongoing archaeological research in Egypt not-yet-known material, iconographic, and written sources will be discovered, including medical texts or at least their fragments.

We may add that the publication of the first volume of this compendium aroused great interest among readers, so the Academia Publishing House prepared a reprint. In the meantime, a slightly modified English version was prepared, which was issued by the American University in Cairo Press (Strouhal et al. 2014). The authors hope that the second volume will also attract readers and arouse a similar response.

The publication of this book was, unfortunately, not shared by our co-author, dear colleague, and friend, Professor Eugen Strouhal, who died in Prague on October 20, 2016, at the age of 85. He was the foremost representative of the fields of physical anthropology and paleopathology, and in him Czech and world science lost one of its great personalities. Nevertheless, Eugen Strouhal will continue to live in our memories and speak to us from the pages of his scientific and popular books and articles. The third volume of *The Medicine of the Ancient Egyptians*, currently being prepared, will also draw from his legacy.

Břetislav Vachala

ACKNOWLEDGMENTS

The authors would like to express their thanks to their colleagues and friends who helped in the preparation of this publication. First of all, thanks go to the Czech Institute of Egyptology of the Faculty of Arts of Charles University, which has supported the project *Medicine of the Ancient Egyptians* in the long term and provided us with invaluable facilities.

For the kind provision of the photography for this volume, we thank Sandro Vannini and Mohammed Megahed. A number of photographs and also valuable advice on the depictions in the Saqqara tombs were kindly provided by the Oxford Expedition in Egypt, and therefore great, cordial thanks go to Yvonne Harpur and Paolo Scremin. It is also necessary to express thanks to the Universitätsbibliothek Leipzig for consent to publish the photographs of the Ebers Papyrus, and to the British Museum and Petrie Museum of Egyptian Archaeology for loaning us the rights to print the photographs of the objects from their collections. Thanks are also owed to the authors of the photographs and drawings from the archives of the Czech Institute of Egyptology, especially Jolana Malátková, Martin Frouz, and Kamil Voděra.

We thank our honored reviewers, Jana Mynářová and Alexandr Ivaškovič, for their stimulating comments. The publication of this book would not have been possible without the cooperation of the American University in Cairo Press; we are grateful particularly to Sally Boylan, Neil Hewison, Mary Ann Marazzi, Ælfwine Mischler, and Nadia Naqib for their invaluable work in processing the manuscript and its conversion into book form.

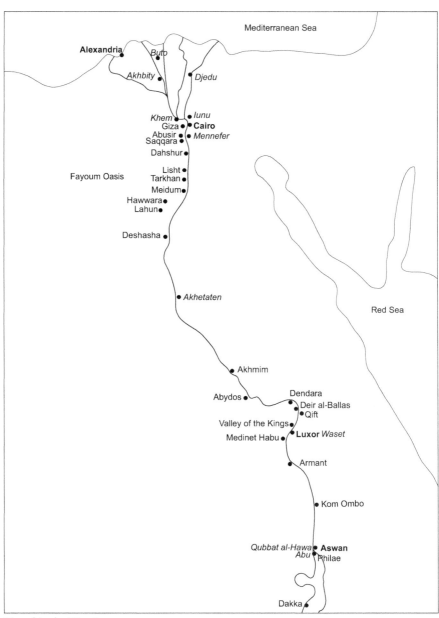

Map of Ancient Egypt.

1

THE ANCIENT EGYPTIAN
INTERNAL MEDICAL WARD

T his second volume of *The Medicine of the Ancient Egyptians* is devoted to the interpretation of internal diseases or symptoms and their treatment from direct translations of the internal medicine parts of ancient Egyptian medical texts. Before you begin, we want to warn you of several differences from the first volume.

Whereas ancient Egyptian surgery, dealing with the treatment of injuries and fractures whose cause was apparent, lay predominantly in rational experiences, the origin of diseases of the internal organs, hidden under the surface of the body, was attributed to the intervention of one of the gods, demons, or a deceased or evil person. The diseases' recognition and treatment was complicated by the then embryonic state of knowledge about human anatomy, physiology, and pathophysiology. This is why physicians, besides empirical knowledge, had recourse much more often than surgeons to treatment with magical means based on religious concepts and mythology. Above all, we find references to the myths about Osiris, Isis, Horus, and Seth, as well as references to other gods of the Egyptian pantheon (see for example Janák 2005 and 2009).

Although it has been passed down for a long time in some popular books on ancient Egypt that physicians drew their knowledge of the human body from mummifiers (for example Krejčí and Magdolen 2005, 335), in fact they had almost nothing in common with them, which is clear already from how the content of their work and their social positions differed. Whereas physicians,

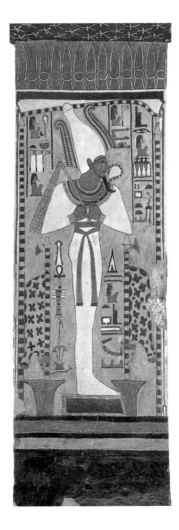

attempting to relieve the course of the diseases of their living patients, were very esteemed in society, embalmers were a low-to-despicable profession, whose task was to preserve the body after death from decay, which was, in the spirit of the faith, then a basic condition of the assurance of eternal life after death (for more, see Strouhal et al. 2014, 4; Vymazalová and Coppens 2011, 182).

The activity of the mummifiers never stood at the root of the scientific autopsy in the course of the millennia of Egyptian civilization: it remained a mere craft, which removed the internal organs from the dead body to avoid putrefaction. It was rough, repelling work, although lector priests generally recited sacred texts during it (Strouhal 1994a, 258). Mummifiers did not have to have a deeper education or even interest in the study, organization, or structure of the internal organs, and they likely did not much consider their function during the life of the mummified person. It was sufficient that they knew the method of the mummification process and during it recognized the main organs: heart, lungs, liver, stomach, and intestines, which played an important role in religious ideas and rituals. These organs were mummified separately.

The heart, which the ancient Egyptians considered correctly to be the center and motor of the organism, was also attributed with other functions and qualities. For example, they deemed it to be the seat of the conscience and human individuality (Janák 2012, 96). During mummification, they left the heart in place within the body and if the mummifiers accidently cut it out when removing the lungs, they were required to return it to the body because the heart played an important

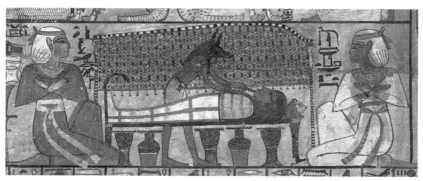

Fig. 2. Mummification of the body was one of the prerequisites of the successful continuation of life after death, and its significance is underlined by the participation of the god Anubis and the protective goddesses Isis and Nephthys (Nineteenth Dynasty, outer coffin of Khonsu from Deir el-Medina, Egyptian Museum in Cairo JE 27302, photo © Sandro Vannini)

role during the judgment after death which every deceased person had to go through in the transition to the next world (Janák 2012, 207–17; Vymazalová and Coppens 2010, 195). The heart was placed in a pan of the scales during the judgment before the gods and showed whether the deceased had lived in accordance with order and was hence worthy of eternal life (Janák 2012, 102). The deceased, sometimes with the help of so-called heart scarabs, amulets shaped like the sacred scarab, and spells from the Book of the Dead, attempted to assure the favorable testimony of their heart (Janák 2012, 102–103).

The remaining removed internal organs were mummified separately and then deposited in four vessels called canopic jars, whose name is derived from the town Canopus on the coast of the Mediterranean Sea near today's Abukir (Verner et al. 2007, 241–42). The four canopic jars were under the patronage of the four sons of the god Horus and also under the protection of four Egyptian goddesses. The lungs were placed in a canopic jar with a lid in the shape of the head of a baboon, depicting the god Hapi, who was protected by the goddess Nephthys. A canopic jar with a lid in the form of a human head of the god Imset, who was under the protection of the goddess Isis, served for the storage of the liver. The stomach belonged in the canopic jar with the lid in the shape of the jackal head of the god Duamutef, protected by the goddess Neith, while the intestines were deposited in the canopic jar with a lid in the shape of the head of a falcon of the god Qebehsenuf, under the protection of the goddess Selket. In some periods, instead of canopic jars, the organs were placed back into the abdominal cavity in the form of mummified packages (Strouhal 1994b, 15–23, and 1995).

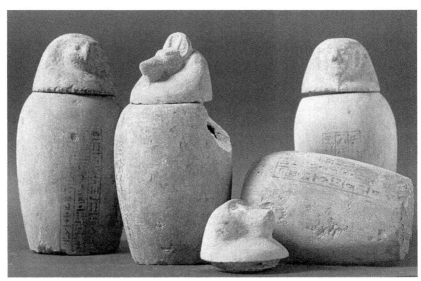

Fig. 3. Four canopic jars with lids in the shape of heads of protective deities, the so-called four sons of Horus (Twenty-seventh Dynasty, the tomb of Imakhetkheretresnet in Abusir, photo © Archive of the Czech Institute of Egyptology, Faculty of Arts, Charles University, Kamil Voděra)

The other organs, such as the brain, the kidney, and the bladder, became part of the mummification waste, which was often preserved for reverential reasons. For example, a hidden deposit of the items from mummification was discovered by Czech Egyptologists in Abusir at Menekhibnekau's tomb from the sixth century BC (Bareš et al. 2011, 69; Smoláriková 2009, 84–87, and 2010, 33–35) and recently also in a tomb from the end of the Old Kingdom (Arias 2017, 188–93).

On the contrary, Egyptian physicians acquired their anatomical knowledge, like butchers, cooks, and everyday Egyptians, during the disembowelment of animals and preparation of food, but moreover also in the study of medical papyrus scrolls in the libraries of the Houses of Life (Vymazalová and Coppens 2011, 174; more in the forthcoming third volume of *The Medicine of the Ancient Egyptians*).

The transfer of knowledge was already possible in the pre-Pharaonic period around 3300 BC through the invention of writing (Dreyer 1998, 113–45, 183–87, pls. 27–35), which also served for recording experiences from the everyday practice of physicians and writing of specialized texts. From prehistoric medicine, the independent medical profession gradually developed, working from the experience of many generations (Strouhal et al. 2014, 19).

It is characteristic of ancient Egyptian that anatomical names and hieroglyphic symbols in the form of human body parts include almost exclusively shapes on the surface of the body. (For ancient Egyptian anatomy, consult Weeks 1970.) Meanwhile, of the fifty-one symbols depicting the internal organs or parts of the bodies of mammals, a full nineteen (37.3 percent) were used also for human anatomy (Nunn 1996, 52–53; for the list of hieroglyphic signs, see Gardiner 1957, 442–548; Hannig 1995, 1025–82), which seems to show that they do not come from observation of human viscera during mummification but from disembowelment of domesticated animals.

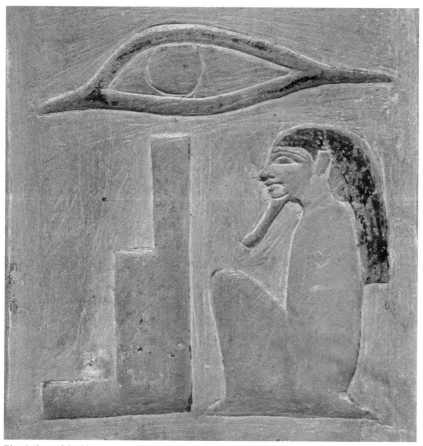

Fig. 4. One of the hieroglyphic characters depicting a part of the human body, the human eye, representing the sound *ir*, here as part of the name of the god of the underworld Osiris (Fifth Dynasty, tomb of Ptahhotep in Saqqara, photo © Hana Vymazalová)

2

PAPYRUS SCROLLS OF EGYPTIAN "INTERNISTS"

The authors of ancient Egyptian medical papyri do not present themselves by their names or even mention the names of the authors of earlier books from which they often adopt shorter or longer parts. They usually do not address their medical instructions to the ill but to the physicians themselves. The profession of a pharmacist is not proven, so the physician himself had to prepare or obtain the medicines, apparently from homemade supplies (see page 170, also e.g., Westendorf 1999, 489–90).

Ancient Egyptian Texts on Internal Medicine

The most significant written source for the study of ancient Egyptian internal medicine is the Ebers Papyrus (Eb), which is also the longest of the medical papyri found so far. It contains 421 cases related to internal diseases. Unlike the Smith Surgical Papyrus (see Strouhal et al. 2014, 19–95) individual cases are not organized in the Ebers Papyrus according to the anatomical principles valid to this day, for example, from head to toe, because this text was not created through systematic accumulation and categorization of cases, but through compilation, that is gradual addition of excerpts from unpreserved specialized scrolls (e.g., on the heart, veins, or stomach) and insertion of other cases by other authors. The result is an unsynoptic conglomeration whose individual themes are often scattered in various places of the papyrus so that it would be necessary to connect them on the basis of the symptoms of the illnesses. The reader can find the original order of the internal cases of Ebers and other

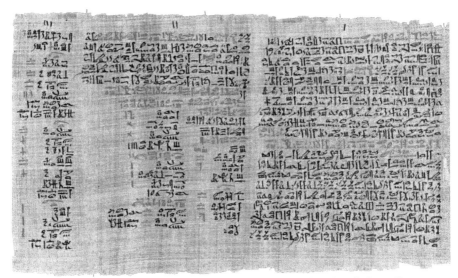

Fig. 5. Beginning of the Ebers Papyrus with spells for the application of medical remedies
(Eighteenth Dynasty, photo © Papyrus and Ostraca Collection of the University Library of Leipzig)

papyri in the translations labeled with the internationally used numbers of their paragraphs (pages 13–149).

Other than the Ebers Papyrus, the greatest number of original, thematically relevant cases are in Papyrus Berlin 3038 (Bln). Besides the original cases, however, the papyrus also contains a series of cases which represent an analogy to the cases from the Ebers Papyrus. One of the cases (Bln 163a), which is the introduction to the entire group of cases and prescriptions devoted to veins *(metu)*, refers to the ancient origin of Papyrus Berlin 3038. The text mentions that the scroll was found in the Archaic Period under the statue of the god Anubis, which was most likely to increase its credibility. We find a very similar reference also in the Ebers Papyrus in case Eb 856a. Both relevant passages prove that the cases were copied from much earlier templates.

The Hearst Papyrus (H) has often been considered as an extract of the most important cases and prescriptions from the Ebers Papyrus, intended for common everyday medical practice. However, this opinion is imprecise, because of the total of 260 cases in this papyrus only 90 of them comprise parallels to the Ebers Papyrus (Westendorf 1999, 35). Roughly one-third of the cases are devoted to internal medicine, whereas the other two-thirds of the cases from the Hearst Papyrus, included in this volume, do not appear in other texts. It is thus not possible to consider it to be only an *excerpt* from the Ebers Papyrus.

In contrast, Papyrus Chester Beatty VI (CB VI), focused on the diseases of the rectum, appears to be distinctly specialized. Of its forty-six internal cases, twenty-four (hence more than half) directly or indirectly concern the problems of this organ. Among the papyri from the Ramesseum (Ram), the papyri Ram III.A, Ram III.B and Ram V provided twenty-six internal cases, whereas only six come from Papyrus London BM 10053 (L).

Besides these texts, we have sporadically drawn also from the Leiden Papyrus (Leid), the Edwin Smith Papyrus (Sm), and from Papyrus Louvre E 4864 (Lvr). It is also possible to find cases related to internal medicine on ostraca, limestone shards covered with writing, coming from the village of Deir el-Medina (DeM).

Cases described in more detail alternate with the more concise in the papyri. The headings given are usually more demonstrative, revealing the symptom of the disease which is to be cured. After them, there often follows a small group of cases containing prescriptions without detailed labeling which are related to the indications defined in the last, more detailed case. Natural thematic groups thus emerge, which likely correspond to the same template of the medical text, or the scribe copying the text purposefully simplified them.

Overview of the Ancient Egyptian Texts on Internal Medicine

In the first volume of this series, the medical texts which contain cases related to surgery and the medical examination of women and children were presented more closely. The most important role was played there by the surgical papyrus of Edwin Smith and the gynecological Papyrus Kahun, which supplemented the less numerous cases from the other preserved texts (Strouhal et al. 2014, 11–18).

Other texts, which were named in more detail in the previous volume, have great significance for investigating ancient Egyptian internal medicine. We present here their place of discovery, approximate date, and also the most important editions, translations, and annotated analyses. Besides the texts mentioned in this and the previous volume of this series, further texts of a medical (and medico-magical) concentration are also known from ancient Egypt, not only the papyrus scrolls or their fragments, but also limestone ostraca from Deir el-Medina, Amarna, and such (for a synopsis see e.g., Bardinet 1995, 13–20; Westendorf 1999, 4–79; or the website of the project of the German Academy of Sciences Science in Ancient Egypt (Wissenschaft im Alten Ägypten; briefly also Vymazalová and Coppens 2011, 180–81).

The most essential collective work dealing with ancient Egyptian medicine is undoubtedly *Grundriss der Medizin der alten Ägypter I–VIII* (Deines and Grapow 1959; Deines and Westendorf 1957, 1961, 1962; Grapow 1958; Deines et al. 1958). Recently issued summary publications, which definitely deserve attention, include also the complete translations of all the texts presented, in the French translation by Bardinet (1995) and the German translation by Westendorf (1999).

The following overview briefly presents the individual texts that are relevant to the study of ancient Egyptian internal medicine. We present the most important of them first, the Ebers Papyrus, followed by other texts arranged by age.

Papyrus Ebers

Provenance: Luxor, perhaps a tomb in Asasif
Date: Seventeenth–Eighteenth Dynasty
Collection: Universitätsbibliothek Leipzig
Publication: Ebers 1875; Joachim 1890; Wreszinski 1913; Bryan 1930; Ebbell 1937; Deines et al. 1958; Ghalioungui 1987; Bardinet 1995, 251–373, 443–51; Westendorf 1999, 547–710; Strouhal et al. 2014, 48–52, 116–23; Pommerening 2010

Papyri from the Ramesseum

Provenance: Luxor, Ramesseum, found in a shaft tomb from the Middle Kingdom, which was under the storerooms of the later memorial temple of Ramesses II.
Date: Twelfth–Thirteenth Dynasty
Collection: The British Museum in London
Publication: Gardiner 1955; Barns 1956; Deines et al. 1958; Bardinet 1995, 446, 451, 454, 466–75; Strouhal et al. 2014, 112–15

Papyrus Edwin Smith

Provenance: Luxor, perhaps found in the tomb along with the Ebers Papyrus (?)
Date: Sixteenth–Seventeenth or Seventeenth–Eighteenth Dynasty
Collection: The New York Academy of Medicine
Publication: Breasted 1930; Meyerhof 1931; Ebbell 1939; Lexa and Jirásek 1941; Deines, Grapow, and Westendorf 1958; Westendorf 1966; Bardinet 1995, 493–522, 453; Westendorf 1999, 711–48; Allen 2005; Strouhal et al. 2014, 27–48, 115–16; Kosack 2011; Sanchez and Meltzer 2012

Papyrus Hearst

Provenance: Deir el-Ballas
Date: Seventeenth–Eighteenth Dynasty
Collection: The Bancroft Library, University of California, Berkeley
Publication: Reisner 1905; Wreszinski 1912; Deines et al. 1958; Bardinet 1995, 375–408; Leake 1952

Papyrus Louvre E.4864
Provenance: Luxor (?)
Date: Eighteenth Dynasty
Collection: Musée du Louvre in Paris
Publication: Posener 1976; Bardinet 1995, 464–65

Papyrus London BM 10059
Provenance: unknown
Date: Eighteenth Dynasty
Collection: The British Museum in London
Publication: Birch 1871; Wreszinski 1912; Deines et al. 1958; Bardinet 1995, 483–92; Leitz 1999; Strouhal et al. 2014, 123–24

Papyrus Berlin 3038
Provenance: Saqqara
Date: Nineteenth Dynasty
Collection: Staatliche Museen zu Berlin
Publication: Brugsch 1863; Erman 1899; Wreszinski 1909; Bardinet 1995, 409–35, 451–54; Strouhal et al. 2014, 125–28

Chester Beatty Papyri
Provenance: Deir el-Medina
Date: Nineteenth Dynasty
Collection: The British Museum in London (BM 10685–10688, 10695)
Publication: Gardiner 1935; Jonckheere 1947; Deines et al. 1958; Bardinet 1995, 455–61, 478–79

Papyrus Leiden I 343 + I 345 (magical papyrus)
Provenance: Memphis
Date: Nineteenth–Twentieth Dynasty
Collection: Rijksmuseum van Oudheden, Leiden
Publication: Massart 1954; Bardinet 1995, 475–77

Cairo Ostracon O.DeM 1091
Provenance: Deir el-Medina
Date: Nineteenth–Twentieth Dynasty
Collection: Egyptian Museum in Cairo (inv. No. 2087)
Publication: Posener 1938; Jonckheere 1954; Deines et al. 1958; Bardinet 1995, 479; Westendorf 1999, 118, 314, 317

Cairo Ostracon O.DeM 1216

Provenance: Deir el-Medina
Date: Nineteenth–Twentieth Dynasty
Collection: Egyptian Museum in Cairo (inv. No. 2271)
Publication: Posener 1938, 29, pl. 49, 49a

3

TRANSLATION OF INTERNAL CASES AND ASSOCIATED PRESCRIPTIONS

T he translation of the Ebers Papyrus is presented first here because this text is the most important and the most extensive of the preserved medical papyri, even though it is not the oldest one. The numbering and division of the individual cases correspond with the standard in Egyptological literature and are based on the original editions of the texts.

Editorial note: Round brackets ( ) mark contemporary additions for better comprehension of the texts. Square brackets [ ] mark restorations of the parts of the texts that are not preserved. The translations try to keep the variety of ancient Egyptian terminology and also reflect the use of red ink, which in the original texts served to mark headings and important parts of the cases, with boldface type.

Ebers Papyrus
Case Ebers 1: 1.1–1.11
The beginning of an incantation on the application of a remedy on any place of the human body. I have come from Heliopolis along with the Great (gods) of the temple, Lords of Protection and Rulers of Eternity, and I have also come from Sais with the Mother

of the Gods (= Neith). They have provided me with their protection. Incantations belong to me that were composed by the Lord of All to prevent the (undesired) activity

of a god, goddess, dead male, dead female, **and so on,** who are in my head, throat, shoulder, meat (or) limb, and to punish the originator,

the highest of those who cause the disease of my meat and the decline of my limbs—something that penetrates

into my meat, head, shoulders, body (or) limbs. I belong

to Re! (And he) said: "I am he who protects the (sick) from enemies!" The ruler (of the sick) is Thoth: he leaves the script to speak,

writes the (medical) books, and gives power to the knowers and physicians, who are in his retinue

to save the one that god wishes to leave alive. And I am the one, whom god wants to leave alive! **Recite**

when applying the remedy on whatever place of the human body which is sick. Really effective, a million times (proven).

Case Ebers 2: 1.12–2.1

Another incantation on freeing any kind of bond. He was freed, he was freed by Isis. Horus was freed by Isis

of the evil, which was done to him by his brother Seth, when he murdered his father Osiris. O Isis,

Great of Magic, release (also) me and free me of all bad, evil, and dangerous,

(unfavorable) activity of a god and goddess, a dead male and dead female, male adversary and female adversary,

who place me in resistance, just like you were freed and released your son Horus! Because I have entered

the fire and stepped out of the water. I will not fall into the trap this day! (This) I have said and I am (re)born

and young. O Re, speak of yourself! (O) Osiris, wail over what came out of you!

Re speaks of himself and Osiris wails over what came out of him. Now you have saved me before all bad,

evil and dangerous, before (unfavorable) activity of a god and goddess, a dead male and dead female. **Incantation, really effective, a million times (proven).**

Case Ebers 3: 2.1–2.6

Incantation on drinking a remedy.

A remedy is coming! It comes that it expels (bad) things from my heart and my limbs. Strong is the magical power (in connection)

with the medicine **and vice versa.** If you remember how Horus was taken

with Seth to the Great Hall in Heliopolis, when it was to be discussed Seth's

two testicles with Horus? (Horus) was then (again)
fresh as he was on the earth. And now (again) does all that he wants just like those gods,
who are (in the next world). **Recite when drinking the remedy. Really effective, a million times (proven).**

Case Ebers 4: 2a.7–2a.10
The beginning of the collection of remedies
(for) driving away diseases of the abdomen:
peas to mix with beer;
drunk by the (sick) person.

Case Ebers 5: 2a.11–2a.15
Another (remedy) for the abdomen, when it aches:
cumin **1/64**,
goose oil **1/8**,
milk **1/16** (a measure);
cook, press, drink up.

Case Ebers 6: 2a.16–2a.20
Another:
figs **1/8**,
the *ished* fruits **1/8**,
sweet beer **1/16** (a measure);
equally.

Case Ebers 7: 2b.7–2b.11
Medicine for purging the abdomen:
milk **1/16 1/64**,
cracked sycomore fruits **1/4**,
honey **1/4**;
cook, press, drink for four days.

Case Ebers 8: 2b.12–2b.16
Another (remedy for) facilitating passing:
honey **1**,
carob flour **1**,
powder of wormwood **1**;
make a suppository.

Case Ebers 9: 2b.17–3.2
Remedy for passing:
the *sheny-ta* seeds **1/8**,
honey **1/8**;
mix together, eat
and wash it down with **1/32** (a measure) of beer
or **1/64** (a measure) of wine.

Case Ebers 10: 3.3–3.9
Another:
the *aamu* plant **1/8**,
carob pod **1/8**,
the *sheny-ta* seeds **1/8**,
honey **1/32**;
mix together.
Eaten by the (sick) person for one day.

Case Ebers 11: 3.10–3.17
Another:
honey **1/8**,
the *sheny-ta* seeds **1/64** (a measure),
date juice **1/64** (a measure),
arugula **1/8**,
oil **1/64** (a measure);
cook. Eaten by the (sick) person
for one day.

Case Ebers 12: 3.18–3.22
Another:
wine **1**,
honey **1**,
the *sheny-ta* seeds **1**;
press, eat for one day.

Case Ebers 13: 4.1–4.11
Another:
fresh dates **1**,
Lower Egyptian salt **1**,
grape juice **1**;

mix with water, place into
a bowl, add to that powder of
arugula, cook
together, place into
an *aperet* jug or a *ba* jug.
Eaten by the (sick) person (as) warm (as is) a finger
and washed down with sweet beer.

Case Ebers 14: 4.12–4.16
Another:
the *sheny-ta* seeds **1/8**,
honey **1/4**;
grind finely. Eaten by the person
and washed down with sweet beer.

Case Ebers 15: 4.17–4.21
Another:
malachite **1**;
grind finely, place into a flat bread,
make (from this) three pills. To be swallowed by the (sick) person
and washed down with sweet beer.

Case Ebers 16: 4.22–5.7
Another remedy for purging the abdomen:
the *wam* fruits **1**,
the *ineb* plant **1**,
the *Avicennia* fruit **1**,
honey **1**,
the *shenfet* fruits **1**;
mix together,
eat for four days.

Case Ebers 17: 5.8–5.16
Another:
the *tiam* plant **1**,
carob pod **1**,
cumin **1**,
figs **1**,
the *ished* fruits **1**,

oil **1**;
mix together.
To be eaten by the (sick) person.

Case Ebers 18: 5.17–6.1
Another (remedy)
for emptying the abdomen:
cow milk **1**,
cracked sycomore fruits **1**,
honey **1**;
grind finely, drink for four days.

Case Ebers 19: 6.2–6.9
Another (remedy) for the abdomen:
hemu of *Ricinus* **1/4**,
squeezed dates
half 1/64 (a measure), yellow nutsedge **1/16**,
roots of bryony **1/16**,
coriander **1/16**,
soured beer **1/32**;
leave overnight (exposed) to the dew, press, drink for four days.

Case Ebers 20: 6.10–6.16
Another (remedy) for driving away impurities
from the abdomen:
thyme (?) **1**;
cook with cow's milk
or sweet beer.
To be drunk by the (sick) person until he passes
the impurities which he has in the abdomen.

Case Ebers 21: 6.17–7.1
Another (remedy) for treating
the lungs:
carob pod **1/64** (a measure),
sweet beer **2/3** (a measure);
leave overnight (exposed) to the dew. To be drunk by the (sick) person
for four days.

Case Ebers 22: 7.2–7.10

Another (remedy) for emptying the abdomen
and passing all the bad things
which are in the body of a person:
the *sheny-ta* seeds **1/8**,
honey **1/8**,
dates **1/64** (a measure),
earth almonds **1/64** (a measure);
mix together,
use for one day.

Case Ebers 23: 7.11–8.2

Another remedy:
herbal decoction **1/2**,
chaste tree **1/32**,
the *aam* plant **1/32**,
the *tiam* plant **1/32**,
pine nuts **1/16**,
yellow nutsedge **1/32**,
juniper berries **1/16**,
incense **1/64**,
Lower Egyptian salt **1/32**;
cook until thickened to **1/32 1/64** (a measure).
Add
honey before you remove it (from the fire).
Cook to the temperature of a finger, drink for one day.

Case Ebers 24: 8.3–8.11

Another remedy for the abdomen:
the *sheny-ta* seeds **1/4**,
arugula **1/4**,
wormwood **1/4**,
sweet beer **1/32 1/64** (a measure);
mix together,
cook, press, drink for one day.
This makes the person evacuate
everything that he has accumulated in the abdomen.

Case Ebers 25: 8.12–8.16
Another (remedy for) emptying the abdomen and driving away putrefaction in the abdomen of a person:
the *shena* seeds, the *Ricinus* seeds
chew up, wash down
with beer until everything comes out that he has in the abdomen.

Case Ebers 26: 8.17–9.9
Remedy for cases
(to ease) urination:
honey **1**,
the *shasha* fruits **1**,
wormwood **1**,
pine nuts **1**,
the *shena* seeds **1**,
inside of a freshwater mussel **1**,
cumin **1**,
the *aam* plant **1**,
the *tiam* plant **1**,
Lower Egyptian salt **1**;
make a suppository, place
into the rectum.

Case Ebers 27: 9.10–9.15
Another (remedy) for correction of urine
and facilitation of excretion:
goose fat **1/64** (a measure),
(the stone) great protection **1/32**;
cook, (remove) at the temperature of a finger,
wash it down with wine.

Case Ebers 28: 9.16–10.2
Another (remedy) for the facilitation of defecation:
arugula **6**,
(which) is like beans
(from) Crete,
the *menuh* plant, which is called *sheny-ta*;
grind finely, add to honey. Eaten by the person
and washed down with **1/64** (a measure) of sweet date beer.

Case Ebers 29: 10.3–10.8

Another:

pine nuts **1/8**,

honey **1/8**;

cook, (remove) at the temperature of a finger,

wash it down with one-third

diluted boiling beer.

Case Ebers 30: 10.9–10.14

Another (remedy) for drawing away of the aching feces from the abdomen of a person:

white gum **1**,

red ink **1**,

human milk; mix

together.

Drunk by the (sick) person.

Case Ebers 31: 10.15–11.2

Another:

wheat flour **1**,

the *tiam* plant **1**,

juniper berries **1**,

the *sheny-ta* seeds **1**,

arugula **1**,

barley **1**;

grind together, make into

(the form) of the *shenes* cake. Eaten by the (sick) person.

Case Ebers 32: 11.3–11.6

Another (remedy) for emptying the abdomen and the extermination of feces:

bitter almonds (?); grind finely,

place into four *feka* cakes, dip

into honey. To be swallowed by the (sick) person.

Case Ebers 33: 11.7–11.9

Another:

malachite **1/64**,

honey; **equally**.

Case Ebers 34: 11.10–11.17
Remedy for purging of the abdomen:
the *sheny-ta* seeds **1**,
the *shena* seeds **1**,
goose fat **1**,
honey **1**,
sweet beer; **mix**
together,
drink for four days.

Case Ebers 35: 11.18–12.3
Another (remedy) for driving away any kind of pains of the abdomen
(and for) treatment of a lung:
sweet diluted beer,
carob pod **1/32** (a measure);
place into the *des* pot and mix, until it dissolves.
You will constantly
warm the mixture.

Case Ebers 36: 12.4–12.9
Another (remedy) for facilitation of defecation:
sweet beer **1/16 1/64** (a measure),
the *shenfet* fruits **1/16**,
Lower Egyptian salt **1/16**,
the *ished* fruits **1/8**;
leave overnight (exposed) to the dew, drink for four days.

Case Ebers 37: 12.10–12.16
Another:
hin of barley;
roast, completely
roast, make
into (the shape) of the *feka* cake, place into
oil. Eaten by the person
who cannot defecate.

Case Ebers 38: 12.17–13.1
Another (remedy) for correction of the abdomen:
the *shasha* fruits **1**,

Anacyclus **1**,
the *djaa* fruits **1**,
malachite **a bit**,
honey **1**;
stir and eat before sleeping.

Case Ebers 39: 13.2–13.11
Another (remedy) for driving away swelling in the abdomen:
figs **1/8**,
the *ished* fruits **1/8**,
raisins **1/8**,
milk **1/8**,
cracked sycomore fruits **1/8**,
the *shena* fruits, bryony **1/8**,
ocher **1/8**,
incense **1/64**,
water; leave overnight (exposed) to the dew, eat for four days.

Case Ebers 40: 13.12–13.15
**Another (remedy) for driving away any disease in the (right) half
of the abdomen:** *Melilotus* **1**,
date juice **1**;
cook in oil, apply.

Case Ebers 41: 13.16–13.21
Another (remedy) for driving away any disease of the abdomen:
roasted figs soak in
fresh oil of the *Moringa* tree, raisins **equally**,
pine nuts **equally**; mix
together. Eaten by the person who has
any disease in the abdomen and make him drink.

Case Ebers 42: 14.1–14.6
Another: roasted figs soak
in fresh oil of the *Moringa* tree, raisins **equally**,
pine nuts **equally**, the *pa-ib* drink
a *hin*, wine a *hin*;
mix together. To be drunk
by the one who has disease in the abdomen.

Case Ebers 43: 14.7–14.10
Another (remedy) for driving away disease of the abdomen:
oil, earth almonds, chaste tree,
a pearl crushed in honey;
mix together, eat for one day.

Case Ebers 44: 14.11–14.17
Remedy for halting evacuation:
fresh carob pod **1/8**,
fresh mash **1/8**,
oil, honey **1/4**,
wax **1/16**,
water **1/16 1/64** (a measure);
cook, eat for four days.

Case Ebers 45: 14.18–14.22
Another: the *shenes* cake (in the form) of a flat cake **1/16**,
ocher **1/32**,
sekhet of *djiu* jug **1/16**,
water **1/16 1/64** (a measure);
drink for four days.

Case Ebers 46: 15.1–15.9
Another:
the *shenfet* fruits **1/8**,
the *ished* fruits **1/8**,
raisins **1/16**,
anise **1/16**,
juniper berries **1/16**,
honey **1/16**,
water **1/16 1/64** (a measure);
leave overnight (exposed) to the dew, equally.

Case Ebers 47: 15.10–15.15
Another:
the *shenes* cake (in the form) of a flat cake **1/16**,
sekhet of *djiu* jug **1/8**,
carob pod **1/32**,
water **1/16 1/64** (a measure);
drink for four days.

Case Ebers 48: 15.16–16.6
Another:
figs **1/8**,
grapes **1/8**,
cracked sycomore fruits **1/32**,
gum **1/32**,
ocher **1/64**,
carob pod **1/32**,
pine nuts **1/8**.
Then recite: "O male baboon,
o female baboon—**and vice versa**—o demon of the disease,
o female demon of the disease—**and vice versa**!" At the same time,
add **1/64** (a measure) of water, leave overnight (exposed) to the dew, drink for
    four days.

Case Ebers 49: 16.7–16.14
Another (remedy) for driving away the urination
of blood which is excessive:
fresh mash **1/8**,
beaten earth almonds **1/64** (a measure),
oil **1/8**,
honey **1/8**;
press, drink for four days. Any kind of (other) remedy
is less effective.

Case Ebers 50: 16.15–16.18
Extermination of a tapeworm:
root of the pomegranate tree
1/64 (a measure), water **1/32** (a measure);
leave overnight (exposed) to the dew, press, drink for one day.

Case Ebers 51: 16.19–16.20
Another: Upper Egyptian barley **1/64** (a measure), Lower Egyptian salt **half**
    1/64 (a measure),
water **1/32** (a measure); equally.

Case Ebers 52: 16.21–17.1
Another:
acacia leaves **1/64** (a measure),

water **1/32** (a measure); leave overnight (exposed) to the dew, press, drink for one day.

Case Ebers 53: 17.2–17.5
Driving away of a tapeworm from the abdomen:
malachite, four pieces; place into
four *feka* cakes. To be washed down by the (sick) person.

Case Ebers 54: 17.5–17.8
Another: the *Avicennia* fruit **1/64** (a measure),
date purée **1/64** (a measure),
water 1/32 **1/64** (a measure);
leave overnight (exposed) to the dew, press, drink for one day.

Case Ebers 55: 17.9–17.13
Remedy for the extermination of a tapeworm:
date seeds **1/8**,
carob pod **1/8**,
sweet beer **1/16 1/64** (a measure);
cook, press, drink up.

Case Ebers 56: 17.14–17.18
Another:
small leaves of the *Potamogeton* **1/64** (a measure),
chaste tree **1/64** (a measure),
sweet beer **1/16** (a measure);
grind, strain, drink up.

Case Ebers 57: 17.19–18.2
Another:
the *kher* of *Avicennia*; leave
for four days to lie,
(then) overnight (expose) to the dew, strain into
the *mehet* bowl the fifth day, place [. . .] **found blank** (place when copying), leave
in the summer overnight (exposed) to the dew, drink up in the morning.

Case Ebers 58: 18.3–18.6
Another: tubers (?) of yellow nutsedge **1/32**,

malachite **1/32**,
water **1/64** (a measure);
cook, drink for four days.

Case Ebers 59: 18.7–18.15
Another:
the *wam* plant **1/4**,
the *shenfet* fruits **1/4**,
kher of *Avicennia* **1/8**,
honey **1/8**,
beer **1/64** (a measure);
grind, leave overnight in honey.
Get up early in the morning and pulp it
in **1/64** (a measure) of beer. To be drunk by the (sick) person.

Case Ebers 60: 18.16–18.20
Another:
the *wam* plant **1/64** (a measure),
water **1/32** (a measure);
leave overnight (exposed) to the dew, drink for four days.
Or with beer (instead of water).

Case Ebers 61: 18.21–19.10
Another:
reed **1/64** (a measure),
Anacyclus **1/4**;
cook with honey,
eat. **Let them enchant:**
"Be freed of the burden,
away with the weakness (caused) in
my abdomen by the residing tapeworm,
created by a god, created by an enemy!
Be cursed, be rid of that which a god created
in this my body!"

Case Ebers 62: 19.11–19.19
Another beneficial remedy
prepared for the abdomen:
reed **1**,

Anacyclus **1**;
grind finely, cook with honey.
Eaten by the person if there are worms in his abdomen.
It is caused by a poisonous seed.
It cannot be killed with any
remedy.

Case Ebers 63: 19.19–19.22
Another: root of the pomegranate tree,
dissolve in beer **1/64** (a measure),
leave overnight in the *hin* vessel in water **1/32 1/64** (a measure). Get up early,
strain through a cloth. Drunk by the (sick) person.

Case Ebers 64: 20.1–20.8
Another (remedy) for driving away of a tapeworm from the abdomen:
the *aba* plant **1**,
wormwood **1**,
natron **1**;
blend to-
gether, eat.
Then (only) evacuates
every tape worm which is in the abdomen.

Case Ebers 65: 20.9–20.15
Another (remedy) for extermination of a tapeworm:
dry fruits of
sycomore **1**,
sweet ("maternal") dates **1**;
thoroughly mash,
place into thick beer.
Drunk by the (sick) person.

Case Ebers 66: 20.16–20.22
**Another (remedy) for driving away the disease
caused by a tapeworm (and/or) the *pened* worm:**
powder from the *pesedj* fruits **1**,
the best *amau* fruits **1**,
goose oil **1**;

mix together,
press, drink for four days.

Case Ebers 67: 20.23-21.7
**Driving away the disease caused
by the *pened* worm:** acacia leaf **1**,
offshoots of the *niaia* plant **1**,
Melilotus **1**,
wild rue **1**;
mix together,
apply it on the abdomen of a woman,
or a man.

Case Ebers 68: 21.8-21.14
Remedy for the extermination of a tapeworm:
acacia leaves; place into water in
the *niu* vessel, leave overnight covered by a cloth.
Get up early in the morning and pound it in
a stone mortar entirely fine.
His nose will be rubbed with reed when
he drinks it all.

Case Ebers 69: 21.14-21.20
**Another (remedy for) driving away the disease caused
by the worm *pened*:**
thyme (?) **1**,
the *ineb* plant **1**,
tjeset of the *Juncus* **1**,
honey **1**;
consume for four days.

Case Ebers 70: 21.21-21.23
Another (remedy) for the extermination of a tapeworm:
the *wam* fruits **1/8**, the *shenfet* fruits **1/16**, Lower Egyptian salt **1/32**,
honey **1/8**; mix together, consume for one day.

Case Ebers 71: 22.1-22.2
Another remedy: dried bark (?) of the sycamore tree **1**, fresh dates **1**; mash
in beer, drink for four days.

Case Ebers 72: 22.2–22.3

Another remedy for the extermination of the *pened* worm: *kher* of *Avicennia*
1/64 (a measure),
beer *djesret* 1/64 (a measure); boil, press, and immediately drink up.

Case Ebers 73: 22.3–22.5

Another: the *wam* fruits 1/8, Lower Egyptian salt 1/32, the *shenfet* fruits
1/32, honey 1/8, sweet beer **half 1/64** (a measure); make (from that) four pills.
To be swallowed by the person
and washed down with beer **half 1/64** (a measure).

Case Ebers 74: 22.5–22.6

Another **remedy:** the *wam* fruits 1/4, the *shenfet* fruits 1/32, beer *djesret* 1/64
(a measure); grind
finely, drink for one day.

Case Ebers 75: 22.6–22.7

Another: the *sheny-ta* seeds 1, cedar oil 1, fat 1, red
natron 1, bull bile 1; make into (the form) of the *feka* cake, eat for one day.

Case Ebers 76: 22.7–22.9

Another: red ocher 1,
the *qesentet* plant (1), starch (1), soft bread 1, asphalt 1, sweet beer; grind
finely, press, drink for one day.

Case Ebers 77: 22.9–22.10

Another: the *sheny-ta* seeds 1, red natron 1, cedar oil 1; make
(into the form) of the *feka* cake, eat for one day.

Case Ebers 78: 22.10–22.11

Another: thorny *bages* bush seeds 1/8, wine 1/64 (a measure), the *amau* fruits
1/64 (a measure);
heat, drink for four days.

Case Ebers 79: 22.11–22.12

Another: beer *djesret* 1, cumin 1, wild rue 1,
Potentilla 1, the *amau* fruits 1, the *tiam* plant 1, the *ished* fruits 1, sweet beer;
cook, drink for one day.

Case Ebers 80: 22.13-22.14

Another: the carob tree fruit **1**, milk **1**, honey **1**, the *sheny-ta* seeds **1**, wine; cook, press, drink for four days. It empties the abdomen!

Case Ebers 81: 22.14-22.15

Another: the *sheny-ta* seeds **1**, hearts of *mesha* bird **1**,
honey **1**, wine **1**, thyme (?) **1**, sweet beer **1**; make into (the form) of the *feka* cake, eat for one day.

Case Ebers 82: 22.16-22.17

Another (remedy for) treating the *pened* worm: the *niaia* plant **1**, the *kemu* stone **1**, the *newa* plant **1**, the *amau* fruits **1**;
cook, press, drink for one day.

Case Ebers 83: 22.17-22.19

Another: date seeds **1/16**, wormwood **1/8**, yellow nutsedge **1/16**,
(the stone) great protection **1/64**, the *shenfet* fruits **1/32**, bindweed **half 1/64** (a measure), the *amau* fruits **1/64** (a measure), cumin
1/64, sweet beer **1/16** (a measure); boil, press, drink for four days.

Case Ebers 84: 22.19-23.1

Another: carob pod **1/8**, red ocher **1/64**,
fermented herbal decoction **half 1/64** (a measure), white oil **1/8**, sweet beer **1/16 1/64** (a measure);
cook, drink it. It is extermination of the *pened* worm!

Case Ebers 85: 23.1-23.2

Another: juniper berries **1/64** (a measure), white oil **1/64** (a measure);
drink for one day.

Case Ebers 86: 23.2-23.4

Remedy for overcoming the painful substances in the abdomen: fresh beef meat **1/64** (a measure), incense **1/64**,
Melilotus **1/8**, juniper berries **1/16**, fresh bread **1/8**, sweet beer **1/16 1/64** (a measure);
press, drink for four days.

Case Ebers 87: 23.4-23.5

Another (remedy) for protection against the painful substances in the abdomen: the *tiam* plant **1/8**, the *ished* fruits **1/8**, the *sekhpet* drink **1/64** (a measure), sweet beer **1/32** (a measure); press, boil, drink for four days.

Case Ebers 88: 23.5–23.7
Another: garden cress **1/64**, the *ished* fruits
1/8, acacia leaf **1/32**, goose fat **1/16**, juniper berries
1/16, sweet beer **1/16 1/64** (a measure); equally.

Case Ebers 89: 23.7–23.9
Another: cracked sycomore fruits **1/8**, grapes **1/16**,
the *ished* fruits **1/8**, figs **1/8**, incense **1/64**, cumin **1/64**,
juniper berries **1/16**, goose fat **1/16**, sweet beer **1/16 1/64** (a measure); equally.

Case Ebers 97: 24.9–24.12
Another (remedy)
for overcoming the painful substances in the abdomen: the *sheny-ta* seeds
    1/8, the *tiam* plant **1/16**, figs **1/8**, carob pod
1/32, the *ished* fruits **1/8**, cumin **1/64**, the *aam* plant **1/32**, goose fat **1/8**,
sweet beer **1/16 1/64** (a measure); equally.

Case Ebers 98: 24.12–24.13
Another (remedy) for extermination of the painful substances in the abdomen:
    the *pesedj* fruits **1/16**, dates **1/64** (a measure), flat (?) beer **1/32** (a measure),
cracked sycomore fruits **1/8**, wine **1/64** (a measure), donkey's milk **1/16** (a measure); cook, press, drink for four days.

Case Ebers 99: 24.14–24.18
Another (remedy) for extermination of the painful substances (and for) driving away the poison of a dead male or dead female from the abdomen of a man or woman:
acacia leaf **1/64** (a measure), its *kheru* part **1/64** (a measure), its *kaa* part **1/64** (a measure), leaves of the *aru* tree **1/64** (a measure),
its *kheru* part **1/64** (a measure), its *kaa* part **1/64** (a measure), chaste tree **1/4**, indigo **1/4**, the *tia* plant **1/4**,
thyme (?) **1/4**, raisins **1/4**, the *niaia* plant **1/4**; combine, prepare for swallowing, eat for four days.

Case Ebers 100: 24.18–24.20
Another (remedy) for extermination the painful substances in the abdomen:

wheat semolina **1/64** (a measure), barley semolina
1/64 (a measure), *wedja* of dates **1/4**, the *shenfet* fruits **1/8**, date seeds **1/4**,
both parts of the *pesedj* fruits **1/4**, wormwood **1/8**; cook, leave overnight
(exposed) to the dew, drink for four days.

Case Ebers 101: 24.20–25.3
Another: tubers (?)
of yellow nutsedge **1/16**, yellow nutsedge from the garden **1/16**, yellow nutsedge **1/16**, juniper berries **1/16**,
pine nuts **1/16**, gum **1/32**, goose fat **1/4**, honey **1/4**, water **1/8 1/4** (a measure);
equally.

Case Ebers 102: 25.3–25.8
**When you observe someone, who has mucuses and cutting pain, with the
consequence of that a stiff abdomen,**
and his stomach hurts: the mucus is in his abdomen and cannot find a way
out. In fact, there is no route by which it could leave. It is putrefying in the
abdomen, it cannot leave
and will (eventually) transform into worms. It does not transform into worms
(however) until it is destroyed.
Then he (the person) passes it out and immediately gets better. When he does
not pass it out in the form
of worms, then you prepare for him the medicine for passing so that he gets
well.

Case Ebers 103: 25.8–25.11
Another (remedy) for
**extermination of the painful substances in the abdomen (and for) exter-
mination of the painful places of a rash on the body of a man**
or woman: flour of earth almonds, cooked **1/4**, the *sheny-ta* seeds **1/8**, sweet
flour **1/8**, date flour **1/8**,
goose fat **1/4**, honey **1/4**; grind together, eat for one day.

Case Ebers 121: 27.5–27.7
Another (remedy) for driving away the painful substances: balsam **1**, red
ocher **1**,
ocher **1**, honey **1**, the substance (?) *seska* **1**, sorghum **1**, gum **1**, resin **1**, laudanum **1**,
fat **1**; mix together, place on it.

Case Ebers 124: 27.14–27.16
Another (remedy) for driving away painful substances:
tortoise shell **1**, natron **1**, fresh *Moringa* oil **1**, cedar oil **1**; mix together, heat, smear with it.

Case Ebers 126: 27.17–27.19
Another (remedy) for driving away
the manifestations of the painful substances: figs **1/8**, wheat flat cake **1/32**, the *ished* fruits **1/8**, ocher **1/32**, water **1/16 1/64** (a measure); leave overnight (exposed) to the dew, drink for four days.

Case Ebers 127: 27.19–27.21
Another remedy for driving away of the manifestations
of the painful substances: the *shenfet* fruits **1**, the pulp of carob pod **1**, ocher **1**, the *shasha* fruits **1**, acacia leaf **1**,
aru tree leaf **1**, cow's milk **1**; cook together, drink for four days.

Case Ebers 128: 27.21–30.2
Another remedy
for an (injury) of the tibial bone: *amem* of a catfish, which is found in its head. It is to be soaked in honey and applied on it that he recovers quickly.

Case Ebers 129: 30.2–30.4
Another (remedy)
for overcoming the painful substances: wheat flour **1**, barley flour **1**, sorghum flour **1**, myrtle **1**,
honey **1**; apply on it.

Case Ebers 130: 30.4–30.6
Another (remedy) for recuperation of a wound when painful substances appeared: sorghum flour
1, sweet beer **1**, plant pigment **1**, acacia leaf **1**, piece of fine cloth **1**,
myrrh **1**, sediment from sweet beer **1**; apply on it.

Case Ebers 131: 30.6–30.17
Incantation of the painful substances.
The painful substances came out of bloating. Two times (recite).—The scroll, whose text
is not (modified) by my hands.—I crush Busiris under foot, I destroy Mendes,

I ascend to heaven
to see what has happened there. They will not conduct offering rituals in Abydos,
until the (undesired) activity of
a god, the activity of a goddess, the activity of a male demon of the disease, the
activity of a female demon of the disease,
the activity of a dead male, activity of a dead female is stopped **and so on**, the activity
of all evil things, which are in this my body, in this my meat, in these my limbs.
When, however, passes the (undesired) activity of the god, the activity of the goddess, the activity of the male demon
of the disease, the activity of the female demon of the disease, the activity of the
dead male, (activity) of the dead female **and so on**,
the activity of all evil things, which are in this my body, in this my meat, in these my
limbs, then I will not say, then I will never say again: "Vomit it! Retch! Disappear
as you appeared!"
**Recite four times. Spit on the affected place of the person. Really effective, a
million times (proven).**

Case Ebers 132: 30.18–31.19
Remedy for the treatment of the abdomen (and) treatment of the rectum:
milk **1/32** (a measure) **1/4**, goose fat **1/8**,
flour from earth almonds **1/64** (a measure), the *sheny-ta* seeds **1/4**, raisins **1/4**;
press, drink for one day.

Case Ebers 133: 30.19–31.1
Another: cracked sycomore fruits **1/2**,
barley flour **1/4**, date flour **1/4**, honey **1/16**, the *sheny-ta* seeds **1/4**,
goose fat **1/8**; press, drink for one day.

Case Ebers 134: 31.1–31.2
Another: goose fat **1/16**, honey **1/16**, the *sheny-ta* seeds **1/4**,
fresh bread **1/4**; press, drink for one day.

Case Ebers 135: 31.2–31.2a
Another: carob juice **1/32** (a measure),
honey **1/8**; press, drink for four days.

Case Ebers 136: 31.2a–31.4
Another: wine **1/64** (a measure), honey **1/32**, the *sheny-ta* seeds **1/8**,
carob juice **1/4**, dough for the *shayt* cakes **1/4**,

goose fat **1/4**; cook, make (into the form) of the *shayt* cake. Eat every day, wash
   it down with diluted
beer.

Case Ebers 137: 31.4–31.6

Another: the *sheny-ta* seeds **1/8**, sweet beer **1/4**, honey **1/16**,
incense **1/64**, juniper berries **1/16**, raisins **1/64** (a measure), figs **1/8**; leave
   overnight (exposed) to the dew,
press, drink for one day.

Case Ebers 138: 31.6–31.8

**Another (remedy) for driving away of poisonous substances from a per-
   son, extermination of the painful substances, driving away of harmful
   substances,**
**which occurred in a person, (and for) treatment of the rectum (and) its
   cooling:** wormwood **1/8**, juniper berries
1/16, honey **1/32**, sweet beer **1/32** (a measure); press, drink for four days.

Case Ebers 139: 31.8–31.11

Another remedy for driving away heat
**in the rectum (and) in the urinary bladder (of a person), who releases
   many winds, without being able (to prevent it):**
the *ibu* plant **1**, salt **1**, watermelon **1**, honey **1**; grind together, form
a suppository, place into the rectum.

Case Ebers 140: 31.11–31.13

Another suppository for cooling of the rectum: wild carrot **1**,
pine nuts **1**, juniper berries **1**, incense **1**, ocher **1**, *nis* part of a tortoise **1**,
cumin **1**, honey **1**, myrrh **1**, camphor **1**; make a suppository, place into the rectum.

Case Ebers 141: 31.13–31.15

Another (remedy) for
driving away the painful substances in the rectum: figs **1**, Lower Egyptian
   salt **1**, incense **1**, marrow of a cattle **1**;
make a suppository, place into the rectum.

Case Ebers 142: 31.15–31.16

Another (remedy) for removal of **heat in the rectum:** antelope
fat **1**, cumin **1**; equally.

Case Ebers 143: 31.16–31.17
Remedy for cooling of the rectum: *Moringa* oil **1**,
carob juice **1**, oil **1**, honey **1/64** (a measure); pour into the rectum.

Case Ebers 144: 31.17–31.20
**Another remedy for calming
the rectum:** incense **1**, amber **1**, balsam **1**, juniper (berries) **1**, cumin **1**,
galenite **1**, carob pod **1**, the *sia* stone **1**, *Moringa* oil **1**, fat **1**, oil **1**, Lower
 Egyptian salt **1**; grind
finely, make (from that) a pill, place into the rectum for four days.

Case Ebers 145: 31.20–32.3
Another (remedy) for movement in the rectum: myrrh **1**,
incense **1**, yellow nutsedge from the garden **1**, Lower Egyptian (yellow nutsedge) from the coast **1**, celery **1**,
coriander **1**, oil **1**, salt **1**; cook, form a fibrous wad,
place into the rectum.

Case Ebers 146: 32.3–32.4
Another remedy: goose yolk **1**, *amem* of a goose **1**;
place into the rectum.

Case Ebers 147: 32.4–32.5
Another (remedy) for the treatment of the rectum: milk **1/64** (a measure),
 goose
fat **1/8**, flour from earth almonds **1/4**, the *sheny-ta* seeds **1/4**, raisins **1/4**;
 press, drink for one day.

Case Ebers 148: 32.6–32.7
Another: barley flour **1/4**, date flour **1/4**, wheat flour **1/4**, honey
1/16, the *sheny-ta* seeds **1/4**, fat **1/8**; (press), drink for one day.

Case Ebers 149: 32.8–32.9
Another: goose fat **1/16**, honey **1/16**, the *sheny-ta* seeds **1/4**, fresh bread
 1/4;
(press), drink for one day.

Case Ebers 150: 32.9
Another: carob juice **1**, honey **1/8**; (press), drink for four days.

Another remedy: wine **1/64** (a measure), honey **1/32**, the *sheny-ta* seeds **1/8**, carob juice

1/4, dough for the *shayt* cakes **1/4**, goose fat **1/4**; cook, make (into the form) of the *shayt* cake.

Eat every day, wash it down with one-third diluted beer.

Another: the *sheny-ta* seeds **1/8**, sweet beer **1/4**, honey **1/16**, incense **1/64**, juniper berries **1/16**, raisins **1/64** (a measure), figs **1/8**, the *ished* fruits **1/8**; leave overnight (exposed) to the dew, drink for four days.

What to do against constipation from heat in the rectum,

when (the person also) suffers stiffness of the leg: the pulp of carob pod **1/32**, fresh mash **1/8**,

wax **1/16**, goose fat **1/8**, water **1/16 1/64** (a measure); leave overnight (exposed) to the dew, drink for four days.

Another (remedy)

for driving away heat in the rectum: the *shasha* fruits **1**,

the *iuhu* fruits **1**, carob pod **1**, pine nuts **1**, wormwood **1**, tubers (?) of

Astragalus **1**, ocher **1**, seeds (?) of sycomore **1**, onion **1**,

"virgin" dates **1**; grind, combine. Drunk by the man or woman who suffers from heat.

Another (remedy) for driving away heat in the rectum:

flour from beans **1**, carob flour **1**,

myrrh **1**, resin **1**, galenite **1**; form a suppository,

place into the rectum.

Remedy for cooling (the rectum from the treatise) "Art of a Physician": onion

1/64, wine **1/64** (a measure), the brain of a sacrificial cattle **1/2**, the *sedjer*

drink **1/32 1/64** (a measure), honey; press, pour into the rectum.

Case Ebers 157: 33.6–33.8
Another: the brain of
a sacrificial cattle **1/64** (a measure), boiled milk **half 1/64** (a measure), honey
  1/64 (a measure), milk fat **1/2**;
press, pour into the rectum for (the whole) day.

Case Ebers 158: 33.8–33.9
Another: carob pod **1**, thyme (?) **1**, water;
pour into the rectum.

Case Ebers 159: 33.9–33.10
Another: carob juice **1**, acacia leaf **1**, leaf
of jujube **1**, milk fat; pour into the rectum.

Case Ebers 160: 33.10–33.12
**Another (remedy for) cooling
the rectum:** carob flour **1/32**, mallow **1/32**, honey **1/4**,
water **1/64** (a measure); press, drink for four days.

Case Ebers 161: 33.12–33.13
Another (remedy for) calming the blood vessels of the rectum: fat
1/64, acacia leaf **1/64**; apply on it.

Case Ebers 162: 33.13–33.15
**Another (remedy) for healing the rectum,
when it aches:** marrow of beef **1**, a coating (?) from dried oil **1**,
wine sediment (**1**); form a suppository for a man or a woman.

Case Ebers 163: 33.16–33.19
Another cooling suppository for the rectum: the *shasha* fruits **1**,
carob flour **1**, wine sediment **1**, wild carrot **1**,
Lower Egyptian salt **1**, barley flour **1**, date flour **1**, honey **1**;
make a suppository, place into the rectum.

Case Ebers 164: 33.19–34.2
**Calming the rectum and calming
the pubic area:** flour from beans **1**, natron **1**, mix
into myrrh **1**, balsam from (the land) of the Medjay **1**,
pine nuts **1**, juniper berries **1**, incense **1**, carob flour **1**,

cumin **1**, honey **1**; blend

together with this honey. Make of this a pill, place it into the rectum for four
days.

Case Ebers 165: 34.3–34.5

Driving away magical (powers) from the abdomen: the pulp of the *hemem*
plant **1**, insides of a freshwater mussel **1**,

incense **1**, *sheny-ta* seeds **1**, sweet beer; pulp together.

Drunk by the (sick) person.

Case Ebers 166: 34.5–34.6

Another: the plant "my hand seizes, my hand grasps" **1**; leave overnight in
1/16 (a measure) of water (exposed)

to the dew and (then) drink up a *hin* (of the) liquid in each of the (following)
four days.

Case Ebers 167: 34.7–34.10

**Another (remedy) for driving away magical (powers) from the abdomen
of a man or woman:**

wild rue **1**, pine nuts **1**, a product of honey fermentation **1**,

natron (**1**); mix together. Consumed by

the (sick) man or woman.

Case Ebers 168: 34.10–34.13

**Another (remedy for) driving away magical (powers and) poisonous sub-
stances (created) by a god**

(or) a dead person from the abdomen of a person: *nehep* of yellow nutsedge
1/8,

the *shasha* fruits **1/8**, peas **1/64**, the *ibu* plant **1/8**;

make flour, place in beer. Drink up before sleeping.

Case Ebers 170: 34.16–34.17

Another: the *ibu* plant **1/64**, *Anacyclus* **1/16**, peas **1/64**,

coriander **1/8**; cook together, eat before sleeping.

Case Ebers 171: 34.18–34.19

Another: *Anacyclus* **1/16**, the *shasha* fruits **1/8**, the *qesenty* stone
1/64, honey **half 1/64** (a measure); mix together, eat before sleeping.

Case Ebers 172: 34.19-34.21
Another:
grapes **1/8**, gum **1/16**, *Anacyclus* **1/8**,
honey **1/16**, the *shasha* fruits **1/16**; grind, eat before sleeping.

Case Ebers 173: 35.1-35.2
Another: the *pesedj* fruits **1/16**, thyme (?) **1/16**, pine nuts **1/16**, sorghum **1/8**,
chaste tree **1/8**, honey **1/64** (a measure); eat before sleeping.

Case Ebers 175: 35.4-35.5
Remedy for driving away heat in the lower abdomen: sorghum **1**, cooked
  wheat **1**,
wheat flour **1**, barley flour **1**, myrtle **1**, honey **1**; apply on the lower abdomen.

Case Ebers 176: 35.5-35.6
Another:
figs **1**, cumin **1**, flour from earth almonds **1**, honey **1**, (beer) sediment **1**; apply
  on the lower abdomen.

Case Ebers 177: 35.7-35.8
Another: juniper berries **1**; incense **1**, the *ished* fruits **1**, dates **1**, oil **1**,
date purée **1**; apply this on lower abdomen.

Case Ebers 178: 35.8-35.9
Another: ground earth almonds **1**, honey **1**, oil **1**,
the *niaia* plant **1**, myrtle **1**; apply this on lower abdomen.

Case Ebers 179: 35.9-35.10
Another: flax seeds **1**,
herbal decoction; place on the lower abdomen of the person who has the aching.

Case Ebers 180: 35.10-35.11
Another: oil from the top
of the vessel *des*; place on the lower abdomen of the person.

Case Ebers 181: 35.11-35.12
Another: mud (from a pond); grate and dissolve in
mesta drink. Place on the lower abdomen of the person.

Case Ebers 182: 35.12–35.14

Another (remedy) for driving away (the activity) of a dead person in the abdomen of a person: the fruits

of the pea **1**, the celery fruit **1**, the *kaa* of the *aru* tree **1**, insides of a freshwater mussel **1**,

the *shasha* fruits **1**; grind finely. Consumed with honey by the person.

Case Ebers 183: 35.14–35.15

Remedy for the treatment

of the chest: carob pod **1/16**, cumin **1/4**, wine; cook, drink for four days.

Case Ebers 184: 35.15–35.18

Another: ground barley

1/4, tubers (?) of yellow nutsedge **1/4**, the *netjer* plant **1/32**, the pulp of carob pod **1/32**, *wetyt*

of a sycamore tree **1/32**, juniper berries **1/16**, the *tiam* plant **1/8**, water;

consume for four days.

Case Ebers 185: 35.18–35.21

Another (remedy) for the treatment of the chest, (for) driving away any disease in the abdomen (and for) treatment of the

lungs: diluted sweet beer, carob pod **1/32** (a measure); place into the *des* pot and mix,

until it dissolves. Rub the solution and constantly warm

it. Drink a *hin* of this every day.

Case Ebers 186: 35.21–36.2

Another (remedy) for driving away fever

(caused) by the painful substances in the chest: figs **1**, grape seeds **1**, the *ished* fruits **1**, the juniper

berries **1**, incense **1**, garden cress **1**, cumin **1**, *wedja*

of dates **1**, sweet beer; cook, press, drink for four days.

Case Ebers 187: 36.2–36.3

Another (remedy) for protection from the painful substances in the chest:

acacia leaf **1/8**, sweet beer **1/16 1/64** (a measure); grind, leave overnight (exposed) to the dew, press, drink for four days.

Case Ebers 188: 36.4–36.17

Examination of pain of the stomach. When you examine someone who has constipation of the stomach, feels aversion to food, his body is emaciated and his heart goes weakly like a person suffering from heat of the rectum, then you must look at him stretched out (on his back). If you discover that his abdomen is hot and he has constipation of the stomach, then you say on this: "It is a case of (a disease) of the liver." **You prepare a secret herbal medicine, which the physician makes:** the *pakh-serit* plant, date seeds; **combine, press with water. Drunk by the sick person for four mornings, until his abdomen empties.** When that happens and you find (= palpate) both canals (= halves) of his abdomen, of the right half **hot** (and) the left half cold, **then you say on this:** "It is the (case when) the sign of the disease manifests its gluttony." **Then you look at him again,** and if you find that he has an entirely cool abdomen, **you will say:** "His liver is open, is soaked with the liquid. (The patient) accepted the medicine."

Case Ebers 189: 36.17–37.4

When you examine someone who is suffering in his stomach and all the places of his body feel strained, like when exhaustion falls (on him), you place your hand on his stomach. When you find that his stomach moves (?)—leaves and comes under your fingers, **then you say on this:** "It is fatigue from food, which prevents him from eating further." **You prepare for him his purgative:** date seeds; press in settled beer. His appetite returns to him. **When you examine him after this** and you discover that the area of his ribs is hot and his abdomen is cool, **then you say:** "The fatigue (from food) has receded." (But) you must force him to protect his mouth from any roasted meat (= that he avoids it).

Case Ebers 190: 37.4–37.10

When you examine someone who has constipation, convulses (just like) in a fit of coughing and the sign of the disease is under the area of the ribs like a clod of feces, **(then you say on this:)** "It is an accumulation on both sides of the rib area. His stomach has reduced." **You**

prepare for him a strong effective medicine to drink: fresh mash cooked with oil and

honey, wormwood **1/32**, pine nuts **1/16**, the *shasha* fruits **1/8**; place on it (the mash), cook

together, drink for four days. **When you examine him afterwards** and you discover that the sign of his disease is

like in the first case (i.e., in the case Ebers 188), he is recovered.

Case Ebers 191: 37.10–37.17

When you examine someone who is suffering in his stomach,

his arms and breast hurt on the side of his stomach, and it is said of him that his face is green,

then you say on this: "It is what came through the mouth. It is a dead person who has passed around him." **You prepare for him an invigorating**

herbal medicine: peas **1**, bryony **1**, the *niaia* plant **1**,

thyme (?) **1**, six-row barley flour **1**; cook in oil. To be drunk by the (sick) person.

Then you place on him your bent hand **on (the stomach); his arms have calmed and the pain has left. Then you say:**

"This ailment descended into the intestines and rectum. I will never repeat this medicine again."

Case Ebers 192: 37.17–38.3

When you examine someone who suffers in his stomach and often vomits, and you

immediately find also on his face that his eyes are sore and his nose is

running, **then you say on this:** "It is freeing of his mucuses. The mucuses (however) cannot descend to the pelvis."

You prepare for him the wheat *shenes* cake and a lot of wormwood, add to it a *debeh* measure

of onion. You must intoxicate him with beer. (Add) **fatty beef meat.**

Eaten by the (sick) person and washed down with offering beer, until his eyes open

and the runny nose retreats, which leaves in the mucuses.

Case Ebers 193: 38.3–38.10

When you examine someone

who has constipation of the stomach, you must place your hand on it. When you discover

that the sign of his disease is distention, which trembles at the touch with deft fingers, **then you say on this:** "It is an accumulation of feces that has not yet solidified."

You prepare for him an herbal medicine:

mendji fruit seeds **1/64** (a measure) **1/2**, cooked in oil and honey, the *tiam* plant **1/16**, pine nuts **1/16**, the *shasha* fruits **1/8**, yellow nutsedge

from the coast **1/16**, yellow nutsedge from the garden **1/16**, wine, milk. **To be eaten, washed down with sweet beer,**

until he quickly **recovers.**

Case Ebers 194: 38.10–38.17

When you examine someone who suffers in his stomach, his arm and breast

hurt on the side of his stomach, and it is said of him that his face is green, **then you say on this:** "It is what came through the mouth. It is a dead person who has passed around him." **You prepare for him an**

invigorating herbal medicine: peas **1**, bryony **1**, the *niaia* plant **1**,

thyme (?) **1**, flour of barley **1**; cook in beer. To be drunk by the (sick) person.

Then you place on him your bent hand on (the stomach); his arms have calmed and the pain has left.

Then you say: "This ailment descended into the intestines and rectum. I will never repeat this medicine again."

Case Ebers 195: 38.17–39.2

When you examine someone who is suffering in his stomach and often vomits, and you immediately find also on his face that his eyes are sore and his nose is running,

then you say on this: "The mucuses are dissolving for him. It is freeing of his mucuses. His mucuses cannot descend

to the pelvis." **You prepare for him** the wheat *shenes* cake and a lot of wormwood, add to that a *debeh* measure of onion. You must intoxicate him with beer. (Add) **fatty beef**

meat. To be eaten by the (sick) person and washed down with offering beer, until his eyes open

and the runny nose retreats, which leaves in the mucuses.

Case Ebers 196: 39.2–39.7

When you examine

someone who suffers immediately (constipation of the stomach) like gluttons of (possibly even) feces and is flaccid

like one who pants (after) running, **then you say:** "It is a closing of the accumulation, which cannot get up.

(The patient) is not amiable because of (his) bad condition. Pustule appeared:
it is the result of putrefaction. The sign of the disease has manifested itself."
You prepare for him
medicine, which will smash (the symptom of the disease).

Case Ebers 197: 39.7–39.12

When you examine someone who is suffering in his stomach and his body is
all strangely shriveled. When you examine him and do not find any sign
of a disease on the abdomen besides wrinkles on the body, what are on pips,
then you say on this:
"It is a disquiet of your home (= of the heart)." **You prepare for him a medi-**
cine against that: hematite from Elephantine grind, flax
seed, carob; cook in oil and honey. Eaten by the (sick) person for four
mornings
to quench his thirst and to drive away the disquiet of his heart.

Case Ebers 198: 39.12–39.21

When you examine
a (patient's) constipation in the stomach, and you discover that being
enclosed and constricted caused it, (the patient) is depressed and
his stomach is dry, **then you say on this:** "It is a nest (= accumulation) of
blood, which has not yet settled." You make (it) to
leave with a remedy. **You prepare for him:** wormwood **1/8**, pine nuts **1/16**,
the *ished* fruits
1/8, the *shasha* fruits **1/8**; cook in offering beer, press together.
Drunk by the (sick) person. **This comes out of his mouth or rectum as**
the blood of a pig, when it is boiled. In the meantime, you prepare a
bandage for him.
(The blood) flows out, before you prepare this medicine. Then you prepare
for him a real best
ointment from beef fat, celery seeds, of the *shawyt* plant, myrrh
and resin. **Grind it and apply on it.**

Case Ebers 199: 39.21–40.5

When you examine someone who is suffering from constipation in his
stomach, and you discover that it leaves and comes under your fingers like
oil inside

a bladder, **then you say on this:** "It leaves by his mouth thanks to an herbal decoction." **You prepare for him:**

sorghum **1/64** (a measure) **1/2**, date seeds **1/64** (a measure) **1/2**; combine, press in the male herbal decoction. Grind, cook in oil

and honey. Eaten by the (sick) person (for) four mornings. Before, it must be applied with the *mikat* stone; dry,

grind, blend.

Case Ebers 200: 40.5–40.10

When you examine someone suffering in his stomach, and you discover it (the symptom of his disease) on his back,

like someone stung by a scorpion, **then you say on this:** "These are the painful substances, which have passed to his

back. A disease, which I will attend to with the supplemental medicines." Perform against it, do not run from it! **You prepare**

for him: the *khemtu* from *djesfu* and give (the patient) a supplemental remedy: myrtle **1**, the *niaia* plant **1**,

acacia leaf **1**, mason's gypsum **1**; **grind, cook** in the sediment of sweet beer. Apply on it for four days, until he quickly recovers.

Case Ebers 201: 40.10–40.14

When you examine constipation in his stomach

and you discover that (the stomach) is very bitter, **then you say on this:** "It is constipation (caused by) the female demon Hayt."

You must destroy (the constipation). It is the female demon Nesyt, who has settled in the abdomen. **You prepare for him:** the *tiam* plant **1**,

the *shasha* fruits **1**, yellow nutsedge from the coast **1**, yellow nutsedge from the garden **1**, carob pod **1**;

cook in sweet beer. Thus, you destroy this case (caused) by the female demon Hayt.

Case Ebers 202: 40.14–40.18

When you examine someone

who has constipation in his stomach, he vomits very painfully and suffers

like with the *sekhet* disease, **then you say:** "It is the accumulation of feces, which have not yet settled." **You prepare**

for him a beverage: figs **1/8**, milk **1/16**, cracked sycomore fruits **1/8**;

overnight leave to stand in sweet beer **1/32** (a measure), press, drink very often, so that he recovers quickly.

Case Ebers 203: 40.18–41.5

When you examine

someone suffering in his stomach, place your hand on him (his stomach). When you discover that (the constipation) has settled

in the right half (of the abdomen), **then you say:** "It accumulated and formed a nub." **You prepare for him**

a medicine acting immediately: sorghum; press, drink for four days. **When you examine him**

after doing this and you discover that this sign of his disease is like at the beginning,

then you prepare for him strong medicine so that it (the constipation) comes out and he recovers: peas **1/64,**

bitter almonds (?); grind, cook in sweet beer. **Then you must prepare for him strong remedies from oil, so that the (constipation) comes down:** the *aat* stone, barley; **grind,** cook **in oil and honey.** Eaten

by the (sick) person for four days.

Case Ebers 204: 41.5–41.13

When you examine someone who has constipation in his left half (of the abdomen, constipation) it is under the area

of the ribs and not across, then you say on this: "It made a bank, it created a sand bar."

You prepare for him a medicine for its initial state: the *pesedj* fruits **1/4** grind, the *tiam* plant **1/8,** pine nuts

1/16, the *shasha* fruits **1/8;** cook together in oil **2/3** (a measure) and honey **1/3.**

Eaten by the (sick) person for four days. **When you examine the patient after doing this** and you discover that (the constipation) has expanded and

continued downwards, **then you prepare:** powder (from) the *pesedj* fruits entirely cook until soft. Eaten

by the (sick) person for four days, in order to fill his abdomen and his intestine writhes like a centipede. **Then place your hand**

on him (on the stomach), and when you discover that it is scattered and pounded like grains, **then you prepare for him an immediately acting drink**

for cooling: sorghum **1,** the *iuhu* fruits **1,** water; press, drink for four days.

Case Ebers 205: 41.13–41.21

When you examine someone suffering in his sto-

mach, and you discover (constipation) placed across, (the patient) has pain on both sides, his abdomen has aversion to bread and his heart is affected, (then) do not act against it (the disease). It is (incurable) and you get out of its way. **(When however . . ., then) you fight with it with the effective**

medicine containing drink of barley. When it (the stomach) moves again under your fingers, **you prepare for him**

four morning (remedies), such as the *djesfu* is, which enters into him (the patient) and renews his internal strengths: earth almonds **1/2**, balls

of gum **1/8**, ocher **1/16**; cook in oil and honey. Eaten by the person for four days.

When afterwards (the stomach) moves under your fingers like grains of sand, all his limbs burn

as the consequence of the "bitterness" disease, **(then you serve him)** moldy bread, impurities and a dish from poultry. Act

against it, do not run away from it!

Case Ebers 206: 41.1–42.8

When you examine someone who has constipation of the stomach, he is in fear, it is difficult to

approach his (stomach), when he has eaten something, the stomach shriveled (?) and his legs and hip joint (?) hurt, but not his thighs. **When you examine**

him and you discover that his stomach is stuffed like a woman who beats a child,

and his face is withered, **then you say on this:** "It is constipation caused by mucuses."

Act against it, do not run away from it! **You prepare for him medicine, which is a secret**

for a physician's assistant, besides your own offspring: green barley; do not dry it, cook in

water, do not bring it to a boil, remove from the fire and blend it with

date seeds, press, and to be drunk for four days, until he quickly recovers.

Case Ebers 207: 42.8–43.2

When you examine someone

who has constipation, he trembles (like) in fear, his face is pale and his heart

is pounding. **When you examine him and you discover that his heart is in heat and his abdomen is distended, (then you say on this:)**

"It is a deeply (placed) accumulation. He ate roasted meat." You prepare for him a medicine for

cleaning away the roasted meat and purging the intestines with beverage drink:

sweet beer; leave to stand overnight with cracked sycomore fruits. Eat and drink for four days. You get up early every day because of that, to see what comes from his rectum. **When feces come from him like the black *arut* substances,** then you say on this: "This roasted meat descended to his stomach. His abdomen, which is (entirely) affected, is worse in this." **When you examine him after doing this** (and you discover that) what comes from his rectum is like ground beans and there is dew on it, which rise like the secretion of *tepaut*, **then you say** on that which is in his stomach: "It has left." **Then you make for him a cooling medicine and place it on the fire (?). It acts that it pushes out everything cooked.**

Case Ebers 208: 43.2–43.4

Another **remedy for driving away constipation in the stomach:** bread from jujube **1**, watermelon **1**, crocodile dung **1**, sweet beer **1**, wine **1**; mix together, apply on it.

Case Ebers 209: 43.4–43.8

Another (remedy) for the treatment of constipation in the right half (of the abdomen), when the female demon Nesyt affected it:
the *shenfet* fruits **1/16** (a measure), white barley **1/8**, green barley **1/8**, offshoots of bryony
1/16, juniper berries **1/16**, mountain celery **1/8**, Lower Egyptian celery **1/8**, leaves of the lotus
1/8, myrrh **1/16**, myrtle **1/8**, ship verdigris **1/8**, cedar oil **1/16**, the *tjun* plant
1/8, honey **1/32**, beer **1/64** (a measure), **duck oil 1/8**; leave overnight (exposed) to the dew, press, drink for four days.

Case Ebers 210: 43.8–43.13

Another (remedy)
for driving away constipation in the right half (of the abdomen) when calming: figs **1/8**, the *ished* fruits **1/8**,
the *qesenty* stone **1/16**, raisins **1/16**, anise **1/16**, juniper berries **1/16**,
milk **1/8**, honey **1/8**, pure incense **1/8**, white gum **1/32**, cracked
sycomore fruits **1/16**, ocher **1/32**, acacia leaf **1/32**, wine **1/64** (a measure), leaves of jujube **1/32**,
leaves of the sycomore tree **1/32**, beer **1/16 1/64** (a measure); leave overnight (exposed) to the dew, press, drink for four days.

Case Ebers 211: 43.13–43.15
Another (remedy) for driving away constipation
and "bloodshed" in the stomach: grape juice **1**, fermented herbal decoction
1, *Moringa* oil **1**; mix together, apply on it.

Case Ebers 212: 43.15–43.19
Another remedy for stomach: earth almonds **1/64** (a measure), raisins
    1/64 (a measure),
the *sheny-ta* seeds **1/4**, figs **few**, cracked fruits of the sycomore or carob
    pod from an oasis;
grind finely, place into sweet offering beer, leave overnight (exposed) to
    the dew, without it seeing the
sun, cover. Add to that honey **1/64** (a measure) and goose fat **1/64** (a mea-
    sure), mix together.
Drunk by the man or woman.

Case Ebers 213: 43.19–43.21
Another (remedy) for driving away constipation in the stomach: bread
    from jujube **1**,
tomcat feces **1**, red ocher **1**, watermelon **1**, sweet beer **1**, wine **1**; mix
    together,
apply on it.

Case Ebers 214: 43.21–44.1
Another remedy for the stomach: honey **1**, *Moringa* oil **1**, incense **1**,
    wine **1**;
mix together, cook, eat.

Case Ebers 215: 44.1–44.3
Another: honey **2**, sorghum flour **2**,
the *sheny-ta* seeds **1**; make into four *feka* cakes for four days (this way):
    once the honey is warm,
add (to it) the sorghum flour and the *sheny-ta* seeds. Eat for four days.

Case Ebers 216: 44.4–44.5
Another (remedy) for the stomach: incense **1/64**, pine nuts **1/64** (a mea-
    sure), the *sheny-ta* seeds **1/4**, honey
1/4, wine **1/64** (a measure), goose oil **1/64** (a measure); cook, eat for one
    day.

Case Ebers 217: 44.5–44.7
Another (remedy) for driving away disease of heart:
date flour **1/4**, carob pod **1/32**, the *amau* fruits **1/64** (a measure), sweet beer
    1/16 1/64 (a measure); cook, press,
drink for four days. Thickening up to **1/32** (a measure).

Case Ebers 218: 44.7–44.8
Another: milk **1/64** (a measure), honey **1/16**, water **1/32** (a measure); cook,
press, drink
for four days.

Case Ebers 219: 44.8–44.10
Remedy for driving away a rush of heat in the heart: anise **1**,
the *ished* fruits **1/8**, wheat semolina **1/8**, gum **1/32**, leaves of a muskmelon
1/32, the *qesenty* stone **1/32**, honey **1/4**, water **1/16** (a measure); leave over-
    night (exposed) to the dew, drink for four days.

Case Ebers 220: 44.11–44.12
Another (remedy) for treatment of the heart: muskmelon **1/32**, cracked
    sycomore fruits **1/64** (a measure), ocher **1/32**, fresh
dates **1/64** (a measure), honey **1/64** (a measure), water **1/16** (a measure); leave
    overnight (exposed) to the dew, press, drink for one day.

Case Ebers 221: 44.13–44.15
**Beginning (of a collection) of remedies for driving away poisonous sub-
    stances from the abdomen and heart:** *Anacyclus*
fruits **1/16**, the *shasha* fruits **1/8**, ocher **1/64**, honey **2** (?) **1/2**; mix
together, eat before sleeping.

Case Ebers 222: 44.15–44.17
Another: yellow nutsedge **1/8**, the *shasha* fruits **1/8**,
pine nuts **1/16**, malachite **1/64**, amber **1/32**, the *pesedj* fruits **1/32**, honey
2 (?) **1/2**; mix together, eat before sleeping.

Case Ebers 223: 44.17–44.19
Another: gum **1/32**,
grapes **1/16**, the *shasha* fruits **1/8**, *Anacyclus* **1/16**, honey
2 (?) **1/2**; mix together, eat before sleeping.

Case Ebers 224: 44.19–44.22
Another remedy: earth almonds
grind **1/64** (a measure), *hemu* of *Ricinus* **1/8**, the *khesau* of the sycomore tree
1/8, fresh dates **1/8**,
leaves of the lotus **1/8**, fresh mash **1/32** (a measure), water **1/16** (a measure);
press, drink up immediately.

Case Ebers 225: 44.22–45.4
**Another (remedy) for driving away poisonous substances of a god and a
dead person from the abdomen of a person:** leaves
of acacia **1/32**, *aru* tree leaf **1/32**, *qaa* of the *aru* tree **1/32**,
carob pod **1/8**, salt **1/32**, grapes **1/8**, insides of a freshwater mussel **1/32**, the *shasha*
fruits **1/8**, *Anacyclus* **1/16**, honey **2** (?) **1/2**; mix together, eat
before sleeping.

Case Ebers 226: 45.4–45.6
Another: anise **1/8**, figs **1/8**, Lower Egyptian celery **1/32**, the *qesenty* stone **1/32**,
honey **1/16** (a measure), grapes **1/32**, earth almonds **1/16**, bread from jujube
1/16, the *ibu* plant **1/32**,
coriander **1/16**; press, eat before sleeping.

Case Ebers 227: 45.6–45.8
**Another (remedy) for driving away poisonous substances from the heart
and driving away heart weakness, fainting, and shooting pain in the heart:**
anise **1/8**, figs
1/8, celery **1/16**, ocher **1/32**, the *shasha* fruits **1/8**, honey **1/32**, water **1/32** (a
measure); equally.

Case Ebers 228: 45.9–45.10
Another: grapes **1/16**, earth almonds **1/8**, bread from jujube **1/16**, the *ibu* plant
1/16, celery **1/32**,
anise **1/16**, water **1/32** (a measure); equally.

Case Ebers 229: 45.10–45.12
**Immediately acting drink for driving away the poisonous substances of a
god and a dead person and (for) defeating of all (evil)
things:** figs **1/8**, the *ished* fruits **1/8**, wheat semolina **1/32**, ocher
1/32, water **1/64** (a measure); equally.

Case Ebers 230: 45.12–45.13

Another (remedy), an immediately acting drink for the real treatment of the heart: figs **1/8**, ocher

1/16, gum **1/32**, water **1/32 1/64** (a measure); equally.

Case Ebers 231: 45.13–45.16

An immediately acting drink for driving away (the activity of) a dead person in the abdomen and (for) driving away

poisonous substances of a god and a dead person, painful substances, and (for) defeating all evil things: Lower Egyptian celery

1/32, earth almonds **1/4**, cracked sycomore fruits **1/8**, figs **1/8**, sorghum **1/64**, the *shasha* fruits

1/64, honey **1/32**, water **1/32** (a measure); equally.

Case Ebers 232: 45.16–45.18

Another: flour from earth almonds **1/8**, figs **1/8**, grapes

1/8, anise **1/16**, pine nuts **1/16**, yellow nutsedge **1/32**, cumin **1/64**, honey

1/8, water **1/32** (a measure); equally.

Case Ebers 233: 45.18–45.20

Another (remedy) for treatment of the heart and (for) the expulsion of the painful substances: ocher **1/32**,

gum **1/32**, figs **1/8**, raisins **half 1/64** (a measure), the *ished* fruits **1/8**, wheat

semolina **half 1/64** (a measure), water **1/32** (a measure); cook, consume for four days.

Case Ebers 234: 45.20–45.21

Another: figs **1/8**, wheat semolina **1/8**, honey

1/8, ocher **1/32**, water **1/16 1/64** (a measure); equally.

Case Ebers 235: 45.21–45.22

Another (remedy), immediately acting drink for cooling the heart:

figs **1/8**, anise **1/8**, ocher **1/8**, honey **1/32,** water **1/32** (a measure); equally.

Case Ebers 236: 45.23

Another (remedy) for driving away poisonous substances from the heart: celery **1/16**, the *ibu* plant **1/32**, sweet beer **1/16 1/64** (a measure); cook, drink for four days.

Case Ebers 237: 46.1

Another: the *ibu* plant **1/64**, celery **1/32**, peas **1/64**, sweet beer **1/32** (a measure); cook, leave overnight (exposed) to the dew, press, drink for four days.

Case Ebers 238: 46.2–46.3

Another (remedy), an immediately acting drink for driving away poisonous substances from the abdomen and from the heart, which is real: powder from the *ibu* plant
1/64, coriander powder **1/16**, sweet beer **1/64** (a measure); drink before sleeping.

Case Ebers 239: 46.4–46.5

Another: the *ibu* plant **1/64**, coriander **1/16**, peas **1/64**, *Anacyclus* **1/16**, sorghum **1/16**, the *shasha* fruits **1/8**, honey **1/2**; cook, eat before sleeping.

Case Ebers 240: 46.6–46.8

Another: decoction from barley with removed inside (thus from) crushed and cooked barley **1/64** (a measure), the *qesentet* plant **1/16**, carob pod **1/32**, honey **1/16**, *mut* of *Astragalus* **1/32**, [. . .] of the sycamore tree **1/32**; cook, press, leave overnight (exposed) to the dew, drink for four days.

Case Ebers 241: 46.8–46.9

Another (remedy) for protection from a poisonous substance: offshoots of the twigs cook until soft in oil, place on it.

Case Ebers 242: 46.10–46.16

Beginning (of a collection) of remedies, which Re prepared for himself: lukewarm honey **1**, wax **1**, incense pellets **1**, the *sar* plant fruit **1**, carob pod **1**, the *shasha* fruits **1**, tubers (?) of yellow nutsedge **1**, wild rue seeds **1**, the *ibu* plant **1**, bryony **1**, quality (?) incense **1**, red clay **1**, coriander seeds **1**, juniper pellets **1**, cedar pellets **1**, fresh mash; mix together, apply it on the painful place.
It stops the (harmful) activity of a god, a dead male, a dead female, demons male and female (causing) pain on any place of the body of a person; so that he quickly recovers.

Case Ebers 243: 46.16–46.19

Another, second remedy, **which** Shu **prepared for himself:** wheat flour **1**, Lower Egyptian salt **1**, oil **1**, coriander powder **1**, soot from the wall **1**, carob flour **1**, flour from beans **1**, incense **1**, the *qesentet* plant **1**, ocher **1**, herbal decoction **1**; mix together, apply it on the affected place.

Case Ebers 244: 46.19–46.22

Another, third remedy,

which Tefnut prepared for Re himself: flour from the *amaa* grain **1**, the *shenfet* fruits **1**, goose oil **1**;

knead together, apply it on any painful place, any place (of the harmful) activity of a god and goddess, so that

he recovers quickly.

Case Ebers 245: 46.22–47.1

Fourth remedy, which Geb prepared for Re himself: carob flour **1**,

pea flour **1**, myrtle powder **1**; grind it finely in the product of the fermentation of date juice,

apply on any painful place, place (affected by the harmful) activity of a god and any kind of evil things, so that he quickly recovers.

Case Ebers 246: 47.2–47.5

Fifth remedy, which Nut prepared for Re himself: a brick from the wall **1**, *Cynodon* roots **1**,

a stone from the coast **1**, natron **1**, Lower Egyptian salt **1**, fresh mash **1**, oil **1**, honey **1**, cedar oil **1**, flat cake (in the form) of the *shenes* cake **1**; cook, mix together, apply it on any painful place, (affected) by

male and female demons (causing) pain and the (harmful) activity of any kind of (evil) thing.

Case Ebers 247: 47.5–47.10

Another, sixth (remedy), which Isis prepared for Re

himself to drive away the pain of his head: coriander seeds **1**, bryony fruits **1**, chaste tree **1**, *Anacyclus* fruits **1**, pine nuts **1**, honey **1**; mix

together, blend that with honey, apply on it until he quickly recovers. If the one for whom

this remedy is made has any pain of the head, in any bad and evil things, he recovers quickly.

Case Ebers 248: 47.10–47.12
Remedy for driving away the activity (of demons) in the head: the pulp of carob pod **1**, *khesau* of
the *ima* tree **1**, natron **1**, mud **1**, cooked bones of the Nile perch **1**,
cooked (bones) of a red Nile perch **1**, cooked skull of a *Synodontis* **1**, honey **1**, laudanum **1**; grease the head with that for four days.

Case Ebers 249: 47.13–47.14
Another: dill seeds **1**, bryony fruits **1**, coriander seeds **1**, thyme (?) **1**, myrtle **1**, donkey's fat **1**; grease the head with it.

Case Ebers 250: 47.14–47.15
Another (remedy) for pain in half of the head: the skull
of the *Clarias* catfish; cook until soft in oil. Smear the head with that for four days.

Case Ebers 251: 47.15–48.3
Knowledge of what can be prepared from
***Ricinus* for the benefit of people; as was found in the old treatises.**
Grate its roots in water; place on the head of one who is aching and he will recover immediately like
one who is not aching. Also it can be chewed, (namely) a bit of its seeds with beer,
by a man who has diarrhea. **It is to drive away the *hayt* disease from a person's abdomen.** Also
hair of women can be grown from its seeds. **Grind, mix together, place in oil,**
then the woman smears her head with it. Also, oil can be prepared from its seeds for smearing the one who has a rash with symptoms of bad rash. The manifestations (of the disease) appear like
with one for whom they (never) appeared. He will (nevertheless) equally be refreshed with ointments
smearing on ten days (in) early mornings to drive them away. **Really effective, a million**
times (proven).

Case Ebers 252: 48.3–48.5
Another (remedy) for **driving away quivering in the head:** when the head of a person quivers,
you lay a hand on his head, without him feeling pain. **Then you prepare for him:** natron ground in
oil, honey, wax. Mix together, apply on it.

Case Ebers 253: 48.5–48.7
Another remedy for
the head, when it aches, and (for) retreat of the painful substances: incense
   1, pulp (?) of the *ibu* plant **1**, laudanum **1**,
reed **1**, fat **1**; grind, cook, grease with it.

Case Ebers 254: 48.7–48.9
Another (remedy) for the head, when it aches, and (for) the retreat
of the painful substances: incense **1**, cumin **1**, juniper berries **1**, goose oil **1**;
cook, grease with it.

Case Ebers 255: 48.9–48.10
Another (remedy) for the treatment of the head: camphor **1**, wild mint **1**,
   soft part
of balsam **1**, incense **1**; grease with it every day. It is a treatment of the head.

Case Ebers 256: 48.10–48.11
Another: quality (?)
incense **1**; grease the head with that very often.

Case Ebers 257: 48.11–48.13
Another (remedy) for recovering the head, when it aches:
reed **1**, juniper **1**, cedar resin **1**, laurel fruits **1**, incense **1**,
fat **1**; grind, place on the head.

Case Ebers 258: 48.13–48.14
Another: cumin **1**, resinous gum **1**, the *tentem* plant fruit **1**,
myrrh **1**, *Moringa* **1**, juniper berries **1**, lotus (**1**); grind, place on the head.

Case Ebers 259: 48.14–48.17
Another (remedy) for
cooling the head, when it aches: ocher **1**, incense **1**, petrified wood **1**, the
   waneb
plant **1**, camphor **1**, fallow deer's antler **1**, gum **1**, the *netjerit* stone **1**,
stonemason's clay **1**, carob pod **1**, water **1**; grind, place on the head.

Case Ebers 260: 48.17–48.20
Another (remedy) for the head and for
the temple: incense **1/64**, resin **1/64**, the *netjerit* stone **1/32**, the *senen* resin **1/32**,

malachite **1/16**, galenite **1/32**, hematite from Qus **1/32**, the *wah-nehbet* stone **1/64**, water **half 1/64** (a measure); grind, place on the temple.

Case Ebers 261: 48.21–48.22

Beginning (of a collection) of remedies for driving away accumulation of urine, when the pubic area aches: wheat **1/8**,
dates **1/4**, earth almonds, cooked **1/4**, water **1/2 1/4**; grind, press, drink for four days.

Case Ebers 263: 49.2–49.4

Another (remedy) for the correction of urination: inflorescence of
reed **1/8**, fresh dates **1/4**, roots of bryony **1/4**, honey **half 1/64** (a measure), juniper
berries **1/4**, water **1/16** (a measure); press, drink for four days.

Case Ebers 264: 49.4–49.6

Another (remedy) for rectification of frequent urination: yellow nutsedge **1**,
pine nuts **1**, root of the *beheh* plant **1**; pound together, leave overnight in sweet beer.
Drink up including its sediment.

Case Ebers 265: 49.6–49.8

**Another (remedy) for driving away heat in the urinary bladder,
when he (the patient) suffers from retention of urine:** Lower Egyptian salt **1/64**, milk fat **1/64** (a measure), *Moringa* oil **1**, honey **1**,
sweet beer **1**; pour into the rectum.

Case Ebers 266: 49.8–49.10

Another (remedy for the) correction of urination, when it is not in order: juniper
berries **1/16**, the *shasha* fruits **1/8**, goose fat **1/8**, honey **1/64** (a measure), earth almonds **1/32**, date
seeds **1/16**, fresh dates **1/32**; leave overnight (exposed) to the dew, press, drink for four days.

Case Ebers 267: 49.10–49.11

**Another remedy prepared for one
who suffers accumulation of the urine:** beef skin (leather) **1**, anise **1**; make into (the form) of the *pat* cake. Eaten by the (sick) person.

Case Ebers 268: 49.12–49.13

Another: flax seeds **1/8**, the pulp of carob pod **1/32**, wheat, crushed **1/4**, goose fat **1/8**, honey
1/8, the *ihu* plant **1/8**, water **1/32** (a measure); cook, press, drink for four days.

Case Ebers 269: 49.13–49.14

Another (remedy) for the correction of urination: myrtle **1**; grate
with an herbal decoction. Place on the glans (of the penis).

Case Ebers 270: 49.14–49.15

Another: the stalk of *Juncus* **1**, beans,
roasted **1**; place in oil. Smear the glans (of the penis) with it.

Case Ebers 271: 49.15–49.17

Another: the *hin* vessel full of water from
a pond **1**, pine nuts **1**, twigs of bryony **1**, herbal decoction **1**, beer foam **1**,
leaves of a muskmelon **1**, fresh dates **1**; mix together, press, drink for four days.

Case Ebers 272: 49.17–49.18

Another: wood of
the jujube; grate into a one-third diluted *mesta* drink. Smear the glans (of the penis) with it.

Case Ebers 274: 50.2–50.3

Another remedy for driving away of urine, when it is excessive: wheat
semolina **1/8**, the *ished* fruits **1/8**, ocher **1/32**, water **1/64** (a measure); leave overnight (exposed) to the dew, press, drink for four days.

Case Ebers 275: 50.4

Another: gum **1/4**, wheat semolina **1/4**, fresh mash **1/4**; press, drink for four days.

Case Ebers 276: 50.5–5.6

Another (remedy) for driving away of leakage of urine: pine nuts **1**, yellow nutsedge **1**, beer
(1) *hin*; cook, press, drink for four days.

Case Ebers 277: 50.6–50.8

Another (remedy) for driving away urine, when it is excessive: gum **1/4**, wheat semolina **1/4**, fresh mash **1/4**, ocher **1/32**, water and honey **1/32 1/64** (a measure);

leave to stand overnight, press, drink for four days.

Case Ebers 278: 50.8-50.9

Another: *Cynodon* roots **1/4**, grapes **1/8**, honey

1/4, juniper berries **1/32**, sweet beer **1/64 half 1/64** (a measure); cook, press, drink for four days.

Case Ebers 279: 50.10-50.11

Another: the *ished* fruits **1/8**, wheat semolina **1/8**, ocher **1/32**, gum **1/32**, water **1/32** (a measure); equally.

Case Ebers 280: 50.11

Another: gum **1/8**, honey **1/32**, water **1/64** (a measure); press, drink for one day.

Case Ebers 281: 50.11-5.13

Another (remedy)

for driving away leakage of urine: pine nuts **1**, yellow nutsedge **1**, beer (**1**) *hin*;

cook, press, drink for one day.

Case Ebers 282: 50.13-50.15

Remedy for holding of urine: mountain celery **1/4**,

Lower Egyptian celery **1/8**, the Upper Egyptian *ibu* plant **1/16**, juniper berries **1/16**, fresh mash **1/8**,

the Lower Egyptian *ibu* plant **1/16**, the *peshnet* stone **1/16**, the *wam* plant **1/16**, the *duat* plant **1/16**, water **1/16**; leave overnight (exposed) to the dew, press, drink for four days.

Case Ebers 283: 50.16-50.21

(Another remedy) for the correction of urination, when the pubic region aches, at the first (appearance) of pain: honey

1, incense **1**, pine nuts **1**, yellow nutsedge **1**, baker's yeast **1**, the *khesau* of the sycamore tree **1**, roots of *Ricinus* **1**, ocher **1**, fresh dates **1**,

root of bryony **1**, mash; warm up, press, place in the *tjab* vessel.

To be made at sunrise before the time of breakfast appears and to be drunk so that he quickly recovers.

Beginning (of a collection) of remedies for making the heart accept food: fatty

meat **1/16**, red (?) ocher **1/32**, figs **1/8**, juniper berries **1/16**, incense

1/64, cumin **1/64**, garden cress **1/64**, the *tiam* plant **1/16**, goose fat **1/8**, the *ished* fruits **1/8**,

djesret beer **1/64** (a measure), sweet beer **1/16 1/64** (a measure); drink up.

Another: sweet beer **1/64** (a measure), the *sekhpet* drink **1/64** (a measure), *djesret* beer

1/64 (a measure), date flour **1/8**, wheat flour **1/8**, juniper berries **1/16**, incense **1/64**,

garden cress **1/64**, raisins **1/8**, figs **1/8**, goose fat **1/8**; cook, press, drink for four days.

Another: the *shenfet* fruits **1/32**, sweet beer **half 1/64** (a measure); cook, press, drink for one day.

Another: wine **half 1/64** (a measure), wheat

semolina **1/8**; leave overnight (exposed) to the dew, press, drink for one day.

Another: the *tiam* plant **1/8**, earth almonds **1/8**, incense **1/64**,

marrow (of beef) **1/8**, ocher **1/16**, wine **1/16** (a measure); cook, press, drink for four days.

Another: bread dried by roasting

half 1/64 (a measure), earth almonds **1/4**, the *qesenty* stone **1/32**, honey **1/32**, water **1/32** (a measure); press, drink for four days.

Another: roasted bread **1/8**, earth almonds

1/8, honey **1/32**, water **1/64** (a measure) **1/2**; grind, press, drink for four days.

Case Ebers 291: 51.10–51.11
Another: fatty meat **1/16**, wine

1/64 (a measure), raisins **1/16**, figs **1/16**, celery **1/16**, sweet beer **1/16 1/64** (a measure); cook, press, drink for four days.

Case Ebers 292: 51.12–51.13
Another: *wetiu* cake (?) **1/8**, *heken* cake (?) **1/8**, *wedja* of dates **1/8**, honey **1/32**, wine

1/64 (a measure); cook, press, drink for one day.

Case Ebers 293: 51.13–51.14
Another: figs **1/8**, earth almonds **1/8**, incense **1/64**, *wedja* of dates **1/32**,

onion **1/32**, sweet beer **1/16 1/64** (a measure), fatty meat **1/4**, [. . .] from willow **1/8**; cook, press, drink for four days.

Case Ebers 294: 51.15–51.19
Beginning (of a collection) of remedies for leaving of mucuses from the pelvic area: the *sem* herb, bindweed

is its name. It grows on its stomach like *Cynodon*, forms its blossom like the lotus,

and its leaves can be found like white wood. It should be brought and smeared on the

pelvic area. Then the mucuses quickly leave. Its fruits can also be placed on the food of the one suffering

from painful substances to make (them) leave the pelvic area.

Case Ebers 295: 51.19–52.1
Another. When you observe someone who has mucuses in
his throat, it hurts him to move with his neck, his head hurts, he has a stiff
neck, his neck is heavy and he cannot even
look at his abdomen, because it is hard for him, then you say (on that): "Mucuses in his throat."
Then you make him grease himself (with ointments) and embellish (with makeup), until he gets well quickly.

Case Ebers 296: 52.1–52.7
Another. When you observe
someone who has mucuses and cutting pain, with the consequence of that
a stiff abdomen, and his stomach

hurts. The mucus is in his abdomen and cannot find a way out, there is no route
by which it could leave. It is putrefying in his abdomen, it cannot leave and will
(eventually) transform into
worms. It does not transform into worms until it is destroyed. Then he (the sick person)
passes it out and immediately gets better. When he does not pass it out in the form of
worms, **then prepare for him** the medicine for passing so that he gets well quickly.

Case Ebers 297: 52.7–52.10
Another (remedy) for
driving away of mucuses from the abdomen: figs **1/8**, the *ished* fruits **1/8**, raisins **1/16**,
cumin **1/64**, acacia leaf **1/32**, red (?) ocher **1/64**, the *niaia* plant **1/32**, arugula **1/8**,
sweet beer; leave overnight (exposed) to the dew, drink for four days.

Case Ebers 298: 52.10–52.13
Another. What to do for a person, who has pain in his forehead
and mucuses in his throat: laudanum **1**, balsam **1**, a twig of juniper
1, incense **1**, galenite **1**, ocher **1**, ibex fat **1**; grind, mix
together, place on the head.

Case Ebers 299: 52.13–52.15
Another remedy: *Potentilla* **1**, the *nehdet* stone **1**, cumin **1**, juniper
berries 1, myrrh **1**, cedar resin **1**, ibex fat **1**, laudanum **1**; mix
together, leave overnight (exposed) to the dew, press, drink for four days.

Case Ebers 300: 52.15–52.17
Another (remedy) for driving away mucuses from the abdomen
of a man or woman: figs **1/8**, the *ished* fruits **1/8**, raisins **1/16**, incense **1/64**,
cumin **1/64**, the *sheny-ta* seeds **1/8**, honey **1/8**, sweet beer **1/16 1/64** (a measure); press, drink up.

Case Ebers 301: 52.17–52.19
Another
remedy for expulsion of a disease from any place of the human body: a
scalded herbal decoction;
grind finely, blend with a fermented herbal decoction, apply on it.

Case Ebers 302: 52.19–52.20
Another (remedy)
for driving away the bitter disease: carob pod; grind in honey, eat with
beer.

Case Ebers 303: 52.21–52.22
Another (remedy) for protection from an inflammation: frog; cook until
soft in oil, smear
with it.

Case Ebers 304: 52.22
Another: head of the *djedeb* fish; cook until soft in oil, apply on the person's
meat (= the body).

Case Ebers 305: 53.1–53.2
Beginning (of a collection) of remedies for driving away a cough: fresh
carob pod; place into water into a new *hin*
vessel, drink for four days.

Case Ebers 306: 53.2–53.3
Another: carob pod; cook in sweet beer;
drink **1/64** (a measure) for four days.

Case Ebers 307: 53.3–53.6
Another: You fill a steam vessel half with water and half with
carob pod, set it aside for four days—during the day in the sun and overnight
exposed to the dew.
Then you pour off **a quarter of the 1/64** (a measure) from this steam vessel.
Have (the one), who has a cough,
drink it for four days, until he quickly recovers.

Case Ebers 308: 53.6–53.9
Another: *hin* of date flour; make
a flat cake, place into two *mehet* bowls, place on the fire, heat this flat cake.
Then take it (from the fire)
after doing this, and blend it with fat and *Moringa* oil. Eaten by the (sick)
person
warmed up, until he quickly recovers.

Case Ebers 309: 53.9–53.10

Another: carob pod **1**, squeezed dates **1**,
hin of milk; drink up.

Case Ebers 310: 53.10–53.12

Another: cow's milk boil until it
dissolves milk fat, add to that sour milk. To be sipped by the (sick) person and washed down with boiled
milk for four days.

Case Ebers 311: 53.12–53.15

Another: date seeds; pound, place into a linen
pouch. Place this pouch in grape juice for one day and then it should be placed on fire. Take the (created) mash,
empty the pouch, place (its contents) into the *hin* pot, add to it water and press as is done with
beer. Drink for four days.

Case Ebers 312: 53.15–53.18

Another: fermented herbal decoction **1/4**,
oil **1/4**, beer **1/4**; place into a pot and cook. Then grind *Melilotus*
1, myrtle **1**, add to the pot. After cooking and pressing, you give it (to the sick person)
to drink it for four days.

Case Ebers 313: 53.18–53.21

Another: date flour **1/64** (a measure); place in water, make the dough, blend it.
Then you place two *pega* bowls on the fire and heat them, place this dough in them
and make a flat cake. Once it is baked, you finish it with honey
and beef fat; eat for one day.

Case Ebers 314: 53.21–54.1

Another: cow's milk, earth almonds; place into a steam vessel and
place on the fire like when you cook beans. When cooked,
the person chews up these earth almonds and washes it down with this milk for four days.

Case Ebers 315: 54.1–54.3
Another:
honey, sour milk; mix together, eat and wash down with beer,
one-third of which is diluted, for four days.

Case Ebers 316: 54.3–54.4
Another: tooth of a pig; grind finely, place into
four *feka* cakes; eat for four days.

Case Ebers 317: 54.4–54.5
Another: juice from date purée,
honey, sour milk; **cook,** eat with the *feka* cake for four days.

Case Ebers 318: 54.5–54.6
Another: sorghum flour **1/64** (a measure), goose
oil 1/64 (a measure), honey **1/64** (a measure); cook, eat for four days.

Case Ebers 319: 54.6–54.8
Another: date flour **1/32**,
the *shenfet* fruits **1/32**, the *tiam* plant **1/8**, the *sheny-ta* seeds **1/8**; grind finely, mix
together, add to beer **1/16** (a measure). Leave overnight (exposed) to the dew,
press, drink for four days.

Case Ebers 320: 54.8–54.9
Another: the *tiam* plant **1/32**, the *amau*
plant **1/32**; grind finely, place on the fire, swallow its smoke through a reed
straw for one day.

Case Ebers 321: 54.10–54.12
Another immediate (remedy) for driving away a cough from the abdomen:
figs **1/8**, the *ished* fruits **1/8**,
raisins **1/16**, cumin **1/64**, leaves of the acacia **1/32**, red (?) ocher **1/64**,
the *niaia* plant **1/32**, arugula **1/8**, sweet beer; leave overnight (exposed) to the
dew, drink for four days.

Case Ebers 322: 54.12–54.14
Another:
sorghum; roast and blend with beer. Heat up the *bedja* mold,
make a flat cake, eat for two days.

Case Ebers 323: 54.14–54.17

Another: honey *hin*, beef fat
hin, juice from date purée **2** *hin*, roasted sorghum
hin, gum of the acacia; grind together, cook, eat as warm
as your finger.

Case Ebers 324: 54.17–54.18

Another: fresh carob pod; place into a steam vessel (filled) half with water
and half with carob pod.
Drink *hin* of this every day for four days.

Case Ebers 325: 54.18–55.1

Another: red glass **1**,
red chalk **1**, the *aam* plant **1**; grind together. **Then you bring** seven stones
and heat them up on the fire. Take one of them, place
on it this (remedy) and cover it with a new pot, whose bottom has been drilled
through.
Then you place a reed straw into this opening.
Place your mouth to the straw and swallow its smoke. Equally with each
stone.
Eat something fatty—fatty meat or oil.

Case Ebers 326: 55.2–55.4

**Beginning (of a collection) of remedies for extermination of the *gehu*
disease:** the substance (?) "divine falcon" **1/16**, insides of a freshwater
mussel
1/16, the *hemut* stone **1/16**, droppings of the *idu* birds **1/16**, *Moringa* oil **1/8**,
sweet beer
1/64 (a measure); mix together, press, drink for four days.

Case Ebers 327: 55.4–55.7

Another: figs **1/8**, the *ished*
fruits **1/8**, grapes **1/8**, cracked sycomore fruits **1/8**, incense **1/64**, cumin **1/64**,
juniper berries **1/16**, wine **half 1/64** (a measure), goose fat **1/8**, sweet beer
1/64 (a measure); grind
finely, mix together, press, drink for four days.

Case Ebers 328: 55.7–55.9

Another: the *amau* fruits **1/64** (a measure), fresh

bread **half 1/64** (a measure), ocher **1/32**, juniper berries **1/8**, oil **1/64** (a measure), Lower Egyptian salt **1/4**;

mix together, press, drink for four days.

Case Ebers 329: 55.9–55.10

Another: incense **1/64**, fresh *Juncus*

1/8, carob pod **1/32**, wine **1/64** (a measure); boil, press, drink for four days.

Case Ebers 330: 55.10–55.12

Another: the *sheny-ta* seeds **1/8**, onion

1/8, the *hemut* stone **1/8**, the *tia* plant **1/8**, rotting meat **1/64** (a measure), goose

oil **1/8**, beer *djesret* **1/16**; cook, press, drink for four days.

Case Ebers 331: 55.12–55.13

Another: incense **1/64**, fresh *Juncus*

1/8, carob pod **1/32**, wine **1/4**; cook, press, eat for one day.

Case Ebers 332: 55.13–55.14

Another: Lower Egyptian salt **1/16**, (the stone) "great

protection" **1/16**, ocher **1/16**, wine **1/16**, beer *djesret* **1/64** (a measure); press, drink for four days.

Case Ebers 333: 55.14–55.16

Another:

crocodile dung **1/64** (a measure), *wedja* of dates **1/64** (a measure), sweet beer **1/64** (a measure); grind, mix together,

eat for one day.

Case Ebers 334: 55.16–55.19

Another: green reed **1/16**, fresh bread **1/16**, the *sheny-ta* seeds

1/8, the *pekhet-aa* fruits **1/8**, celery **1/8**, juniper berries

1/16, cumin **1/64**, figs **1/16**, grapes **1/16**, wine **half 1/64** (a measure), *djesret* beer

1/16 1/64 (a measure); press, drink for four days.

Case Ebers 335: 55.19–55.20

Another: honey **1/32**, *djesret* beer **1/4**, wine **1/64** (a measure); press, drink for one day.

Case Ebers 477: 67.7–67.9

Beginning (of a collection) of remedies for the treatment of the liver: figs
   1/8, the *ished* fruits

1/8, grape seeds **1/16**, cracked sycomore fruits **1/8**, bryony fruits **1/16**,

gum **1/32**, incense **1/64**, garden cress **1/64**, water **1/32 1/64** (a measure); leave
   overnight (exposed) to the dew, press, drink for four days.

Case Ebers 478: 67.9–67.11

Another:

figs **1/8**, raisins **1/8**, pine nuts **1/16**, reed **1/16**, incense **1/64**, ocher **1/32**,
water **1/32**; equally.

Case Ebers 479: 67.11–67.13

Another: leaves of the lotus **1/8**, wine **1/16** (a measure), jujube flour **1/8**, figs **1/8**,
milk **1/16**, juniper berries **1/16**, incense **1/64**, sweet beer **1/16** (a measure);
   leave overnight (exposed) to the dew, press, drink

for four days.

Case Ebers 480: 67.13–67.15

Another: figs **1/8**, the *ished* fruits **1/8**, anise **1/4**, jujube bread **1/8**, carob pod

1/32, cracked sycomore fruits **1/16**, grape seeds **1/16**, garden cress **1/64**,
   incense **1/64**,

sweet beer **1/16** (a measure); leave overnight (exposed) to the dew, press, drink
   for four days.

Case Ebers 481: 67.15–67.16

Another: figs **1/8**, cracked sycomore fruits **1/8**, juniper

berries **1/16**, the Upper Egyptian *sia* stone **1/8**, water **1/16** (a measure); leave
   overnight (exposed) to the dew, press, drink for four days.

Case Ebers 561: 73.2–73.3

Another. What to do against painfully swollen legs:

red natron **1** blend with fermented date juice; apply on it.

Case Ebers 584: 75.4–75.5

**Another (remedy) for driving away the painful substances developed in all
   the limbs of a person:** sediments *shamu*,

tomcat feces, dog feces, the myrtle fruit; apply on it. This is to drive away the
   swelling.

Case Ebers 603: 76.19–76.21

**Beginning (of a collection) of remedies for easing
the knee:** the *git* plant **1**, fatty meat **1**, wheat flour **1**, honey **1**;
grind together, apply it on the knee.

Case Ebers 604: 76.21–77.1

Another (remedy) for the knee when it dropped: straw;
sieve, stir into water, apply on it and he will recover quickly. To be done for
    every limb you want (to cure).

Case Ebers 605: 77.2–77.3

Another (remedy) for driving away pain in the knee: flour from the *qaat*
    fruits **1**, wild rue **1**; mash in sweet
beer; cook, apply on it.

Case Ebers 606: 77.3–77.4

Another: the swamp hen *(sehihet)* **1**; crush in a mortar, all which
belongs to it is **present**; apply on it.

Case Ebers 607: 77.4–77.5

Another (remedy for) driving away limping: the *qenet* plant **1**, the pea fruit **1**,
flour from the threshing floor **1**; blend with the product of the fermentation of
    date juice; apply it on both knees.

Case Ebers 608: 77.5–77.9

**Another (remedy)
for easing the knee:** substance *seska* **1**, product of the fermentation of date
    juice **1**, the
pea fruit **1**, Lower Egyptian salt **1**, beef fat **1**, beef marrow **1**, beef meat **1**, beef
spleen **1**, sediment of sweet beer **1**, honey **1**, *Melilotus* **1**, myrtle
1; knead together, apply on it.

Case Ebers 609: 77.9–77.12

Another (remedy) for the treatment of a disease in the knee:
the greasy substance *djat* **1**, flour from the threshing floor **1**, Lower Egyptian
    salt **1**, red natron **1**,
wild rue **1**, the *iagut* fruits **1**, sediment of sweet beer **1**, *Melilotus* **1**; cook
    together, apply on it.

Case Ebers 610: 77.12–77.14

Another (remedy) for easing the knee: oil **1**, honey **1**, red clay **1**, the fruits of bryony **1**, the pea fruit **1**, celery seeds **1**, *Anacyclus* seeds **1**; grind, apply on it.

Case Ebers 611: 77.14–77.15

Another (remedy) for driving away a swollen blister on (the foot) of a person: the *wadu* plant from the field, a tadpole from the canal; cook until soft in oil, smear both legs with it.

Case Ebers 612: 77.15–77.17

What to do with a kneecap, when it aches: the *shasha* fruits; grind finely, blend with the water diluted *mesta* drink; apply on it until he recovers.

Case Ebers 613: 77.17–77.18

Another (remedy) for recovering the aching calf: fat **1**, honey **1**, incense **1**, malachite pellets **1**, dried myrrh **1**; cook, apply on it.

Case Ebers 614: 77.18–78.2

Another: fennel **1**, acacia leaf **1**, *mafet* tree leaf **1**, bryony **1**, wax **1**, gum of the acacia **1**, incense **1**, fresh *Moringa* oil **1**, balsam **1**, camphor **1**, yellow nutsedge **1**, cedar pellets **1**, juniper pellets **1**, water of the heavenly dew, dried myrrh **1**, chaste tree **1**, juniper berries **1**, pine nuts **1**; grind finely, apply it to the calves for four days.

Case Ebers 615: 78.2–78.3

Another (remedy) for driving away the tremor in both legs: pine nuts **1**, the pea fruit **1**, the *Anacyclus* fruit **1**, beef fat **1**; cook, apply on it for four days.

Case Ebers 616: 78.4–78.6

Beginning (of a collection) of remedies for fingers, when they ache, or for the toes. After that make for him a remedy (for) cooling: acacia leaf **1/4**, jujube leaf **1/4**, ocher **1/32**, pigment of malachite **1/32**, insides of a freshwater mussel **1/8**; grind, apply on it.

Case Ebers 617: 78.6–78.10

When you find the fingers or toes aching, liquid issues from them, they smell

badly, they look like worms,

then you say on that: "A disease that I will treat."

You prepare for him a medicine for extermination of the worm: the Upper Egyptian *sia* stone **1/32**,

the Lower Egyptian *sia* stone **1/32**, cedar oil **1/8**; grind, apply on it.

Case Ebers 618: 78.10–78.11

Another (remedy) for a nail on a toe: honey **1/4**, ocher **1/64**, hemp **1/32**, resin **1/32**, the *ibu* plant **1/32**; equally, apply on it.

Case Ebers 619: 78.11–78.12

Another:

honey **1/8**, ocher **1/64**, oil **1/32**; equally.

Case Ebers 620: 78.12–78.16

Another (remedy) for the treatment of a toe

aching: ocher **1**, natron **1**, (the stone) great protection **1**, red ocher **1**, the *khenenu* stone from

the courtyard **1**, flax seed **1**, starch **1**; cook, make into powder. **After**

you make a powder of this, you prepare an ointment from marrow, fat, honey and oil. Grind together, place on it.

Case Ebers 621: 78.16–78.18

Another remedy for the toes:

red ocher **1**, a shard of a new *hin* vessel **1**, product of honey fermentation **1**; apply on it.

Case Ebers 622: 78.18–78.19

Another (remedy for) the treatment of a nail, when it falls off. You prepare for him (the patient): natron **1**, incense **1**,

oil **1**, ocher **1**; and sprinkle natron on it.

Case Ebers 623: 78.19–78.21

Another (remedy) for driving away

trembling in the fingers: the *tjun* plant fruit (**1**), beef fat **1**, *seska* **1**, milk **1**, Lower Egyptian salt **1**, sycomore (fruits) **1**; cook, mix together, apply on it.

Case Ebers 624: 78.21–79.2

Another: incense 1, cumin 1,

wax 1, red ocher 1, the *netjerit* stone 1, honey 1, figs 1, ocher 1;
cook together, apply on it.

Case Ebers 625: 79.2–79.4

Another (remedy) for driving away quivering on any limb of a person's body: sorghum 1,

resin 1, honey 1, verdigris 1; place a greyhound's feces on it, do not
place a hand on it.

Case Ebers 626: 79.4–79.5

Another: sorghum 1, carob pod 1, malachite 1; cook, place on it. Do not place
a hand on it.

Case Ebers 627: 79.5–79.7

Beginning (of the collection) of ointments for strengthening of the blood vessels and remedies for the calming of the blood vessels: tomcat

oil 1, petrified wood 1, resin of the *ikeru* tree 1; mix together,
smear with it.

Case Ebers 628: 79.7–79.8

Another: coriander seeds 1, leather from the sandal producer 1, the substance (?) *seska* 1;

grind together, smear with it.

Case Ebers 629: 79.8

Another: snake fat 1; smear with it.

Case Ebers 630: 79.8–79.10

Another (remedy) for setting

in motion everything (= limb): flat cake of barley bread 1, the pea fruit 1, wild rue 1; apply

to it.

Case Ebers 631: 79.10–79.14

Another (remedy) for the treatment of the blood vessels in the left half (of the abdomen): figs 1/8, the *ished* fruits 1/8, grapes

1/8, reed 1/32, wine 1/64 (a measure), anise 1/8, juniper berries 1/32, *Potentilla*

1/32, incense **1/64**, cumin **1/64**, carob pod **1/64**, ocher **1/32**, jujube

bread **1/8**, leaves of a muskmelon **1/8**, sweet beer **1/16** (a measure); leave overnight (exposed) to the dew, press, drink

for four days.

Case Ebers 632: 79.14–79.17

Another remedy for the left half (of the abdomen): figs **1/8**, the *ished* fruits
1/8, raisins

1/8, carob pod **1/32**, anise **1/8**, ocher **1/32**, gum **1/32**, garden

cress **1/64**, incense **1/64**, cumin **1/64**, cracked sycomore fruits **1/8**, wine **1/64**
(a measure), the *sekhpet*

drink **1/64** (a measure), *djesret* beer **1/64** (a measure); leave overnight (exposed)
to the dew, press, drink for four days.

Case Ebers 633: 79.17–79.19

Another: figs **1/8**, the *ished* fruits **1/64**,

grapes **half 1/64** (a measure), anise **half 1/64** (a measure), carob pod **1/8**, gum **1/32**,

ocher **1/32**, water **1/16** (a measure); leave overnight (exposed) to the dew, drink
for four days.

Case Ebers 634: 79.19–79.22

Another (remedy) for easing the blood vessels in the knee:

Lower Egyptian salt **1**, the *nehdet* stone **1**, ibex fat **1**, honey **1**,

incense **1**, celery **1**, the *heny-ta* plant **1**, zinc **1**, onion **1**, a grain of copper **1**,

beef fat **1**, cumin **1**, oil **1**, natron **1**; grind, apply on it.

Case Ebers 635: 79.22–80.2

Another (remedy) for setting loose
the stiffness in every limb: fatty beef meat; apply on the affected
place.

Case Ebers 636: 80.2–80.4

Another (remedy): ointment for recovering the bone in any limb of a
person's body; really effective:

natron **1**, pumice **1**, fat **1**, black flint **1**, honey **1**;
mix together, apply on it.

Case Ebers 637: 80.4–80.6

Ointment for easing of everything (= every limb):

gum **1**, red clay **1**, myrrh **1**, ocher **1**, beef fat **1**, wax **1**; when the blood vessels are warm (by the sun), apply on it.

Case Ebers 638: 80.6–80.8
Another: red (?) ocher **1**, faïence **1**, grain of copper **1**, incense **1**, honey **1**, natron **1**, Lower Egyptian salt **1**, red ocher **1**, ibex fat **1**; mix together, apply to it for four days.

Case Ebers 639: 80.8–80.9
Another: meat of a *Clarias* catfish **1**, sediment of sweet beer **1**, the *git* plant **1**, honey **1**; apply to it for four days.

Case Ebers 640: 80.9–80.14
Another:
pumice **1**, red clay **1**, grains of copper **1**, sediments of the *sedjer* drink **1**, natron **1**, ibex fat **1**, *Melilotus* **1**, dung of a donkey **1**, fresh seeds (?) [. . .] **1**, the substance (?) *seska* **1**, the *tjun* plant **1**, the *pesedj* fruits **1**, carob pod **1**, beans **1**, white oil **1**; grind, mix together, apply on it.

Case Ebers 641: 80.14–80.15
Another: fresh dates **1**, the fresh *wam* plant **1**, beef fat **1**, honey **1**; apply on it.

Case Ebers 642: 80.15–80.17
Another (remedy) for making the blood vessels accept a remedy: milk (of a woman)
who gave birth to a boy; leave overnight in a new *hin* vessel, until it sours. Smear any painful place with it.

Case Ebers 643: 80.17–80.18
Another: date purée, beer sediment; smear with it.

Case Ebers 644: 80.18–80.19
What to do with a blood vessel which quickly protrudes on any limb: the *khesau* of the *ima* tree **1**, the *tjun* plant **1**, product of the fermentation of honey **1**. Mix together, apply on it.

Case Ebers 645: 80.19-80.21
Another: beef meat **1**,
(beef) spleen **1**, Lower Egyptian salt **1**, wheat semolina **1**, hematite **1**, ibex
fat **1**, beef brain **1**; apply on it.

Case Ebers 646: 80.21-81.1
Another: *Moringa* oil **1**, incense **1**, Lower Egyptian salt **1**,
substance (?) *seska* **1**, laudanum **1**, honey **1**, beef meat **1**; apply on it.

Case Ebers 647: 81.1-81.4
Another (remedy for)
calming of the blood vessels of the toes: wax **1**, beef fat **1**, acacia leaf **1**,
powder from the *tjun* plant **1**, roots of the *Cynodon* **1**, amber **1**, powder from
gum **1**, carob flour **1**, honey **1**; cook, apply on it.

Case Ebers 648: 81.4-81.6
Another (remedy) for easing
the blood vessels of the toes: *amaa* grain of emmer **1**, *amaa* of
barley **1**, oil **1**; cook together, apply on it at the temperature of a finger. Really
    effective.

Case Ebers 649: 81.7-81.10
Another (remedy) for easing the blood vessels: wax **1**, beef fat **1**, pine nuts **1**,
fresh incense **1**, yellow nutsedge **1**, coriander seeds **1**, the bryony fruit **1**,
sar plant seeds **1**, myrtle **1**, galenite **1**; cook, apply on it after smearing
with myrrh.

Case Ebers 650: 81.10-81.14
Another (remedy) for calming of the blood vessels in the shoulder: sweet
    myrrh **1**,
incense **1**, chaste tree **1**, *ibu* plant seeds **1**, dill seeds **1**,
yellow nutsedge **1**, a male (substantial) herbal decoction **1**, cedar sawdust **1**,
    the substance (?)
seska **1**, the *ished* fruits of the sycomore **1**, starch from barley malt **1**; blend
together, apply on it.

Case Ebers 651: 81.14-81.17
Another (remedy for) calming of the blood vessels on any limb:
wax **1**, beef fat **1**, pine nuts **1**, mud **1**, chaste tree **1**, cuttlefish

bone **1**, galenite **1**, honey **1**; mix together, apply on it (after) smearing with myrrh.

Case Ebers 652: 81.17–81.20
Another (remedy) for reviving of the blood vessels and refreshment of the blood vessels:
resin **1**, incense **1**, cedar oil **1**, wax **1**, sawdust of the camphor tree **1**, cedar sawdust **1**, coriander seeds **1**, pork fat **1**, beef fat **1**. Cook, apply on it (after) smearing with myrrh.

Case Ebers 653: 81.20–82.1
Another (remedy): ointment for calming of the blood vessels:
laudanum **1**, the highest quality (?) of incense **1**, the *tenti* plant seeds **1**, coriander seeds **1**; smear with it for many and many days.

Case Ebers 654: 82.1–82.4
Another (remedy) for easing the joints of any limb:
honey **1**, wax **1**, the highest quality incense **1**, laudanum **1**, milk fat **1**, carob flour **1**, the *shasha* fruits **1**, wild rue seeds **1**; grind together, smear with it.

Case Ebers 655: 82.4–82.6
Another: juniper berries **1**, tubers (?) of *Astragalus* **1**, bryony **1**, red clay **1**, celery seeds **1**, incense pellets **1**, juniper seeds (?) **1**; mix together, apply on it.

Case Ebers 656: 82.7–82.10
Another (remedy) for easing the stiffness in any limb of a person's body: natron **1**,
beans **1**, oil of the second day **1**, hippopotamus oil **1**, crocodile oil **1**, oil of a red mullet **1**, oil of a *Clarias* catfish **1**, incense **1**, sweet myrrh **1**, honey **1**; cook, apply on it.

Case Ebers 657: 82.10–82.13
Another (remedy) for easing the blood vessels:
beef fat **1**, wine sediment **1**, onion **1**, soot from the wall **1**, the bryony fruit **1**, the pea fruit **1**, wild rue seeds **1**, Upper Egyptian *sia* stone **1**, incense **1**, myrrh **1**; smear the body (with that) after exposing to the sun.

Case Ebers 658: 82.13–82.16
Another ointment
for easing stiffness: pork fat **1**, snake oil **1**,
oil of the *ibtjersu* animal **1**, mouse oil **1**, tomcat oil **1**; combine
together, apply on it.

Case Ebers 659: 82.16–82.17
Another (remedy) for easing *shut* disease of the blood vessels: myrtle **1**,
fat **1**, beef spleen **1**, incense **1**, beans **1**; apply on it.

Case Ebers 660: 82.18–82.19
Another: onion **1**, watermelon **1**, Lower Egyptian salt **1**, honey **1**, fat
of an ibex **1**, the substance (?) *seska* **1**, beef meat **1**, hematite **1**, carob pod **1**;
apply on it.

Case Ebers 661: 82.19–82.20
Another:
"male" clay **1**, coriander seeds **1**, dates **1**; apply on it.

Case Ebers 662: 82.20–82.22
Another (remedy)
for mitigating the tremor of a blood vessel: the *djat* mussel **1**, dried date juice
1, Lower Egyptian salt **1**,
sediment of sweet beer **1**; apply on it.

Case Ebers 663: 82.22–83.8
Another (remedy) for softening a blood vessel: the *pesedj* fruits **1**,
beans **1**, *amaa* grain **1**, carob pod **1**, cedar sawdust **1**, sawdust of
the Lebanese cedar **1**, willow sawdust **1**, jujube sawdust **1**, sycomore sawdust
1, juniper sawdust **1**,
acacia leaf **1**, jujube leaf **1**, *ima* tree leaf **1**, the sycomore leaf **1**, flax seed **1**, the
fruits of the
ima tree **1**, white oil **1**, goose oil **1**, pig feces **1**, pine nuts
1, myrrh **1**, onion **1**, the *sheny-ta* seeds **1**, offshoot of the *git* plant **1**, watermelon **1**, the
tiu plant **1**, fennel **1**, the Lower Egyptian *ibu* plant **1**, flax seeds **1**, Lower
Egyptian salt **1**,
mountain salt **1**, the *ineb* plant **1**, red ocher (**1**), ocher **1**, natron **1**, beef fat (**1**),
the *shasha* fruits **1**; mix together, apply on it.

Case Ebers 664: 83.8–83.9
**Another (remedy) for setting loose the stiffness in
any limb:** fresh (beef) meat **1**, the fresh *git* plant **1**, honey **1**; grind, apply on it.

Case Ebers 665: 83.9–83.10
Another: beef
spleen **1**, date purée **1**, the substance (?) *seska* **1**, grind together, apply on it.

Case Ebers 666: 83.10–83.12
Another: beef
spleen **1**, bryony **1**, *amaa* grain of emmer wheat **1**, the pea fruit **1**, Lower
  Egyptian salt
1; apply on it.

Case Ebers 667: 83.12–83.13
Another: carob pod **1**, wax **1**, honey **1**, the *sar* plant **1**, Lower Egyptian salt **1**,
date purée **1**; equally.

Case Ebers 668: 83.13–83.14
Another: Lower Egyptian salt **1**, date purée **1**, the substance *djat* **1**, natron **1**,
Melilotus **1**; equally.

Case Ebers 669: 83.14–83.15
Another: Upper Egyptian *Potamogeton* **1**, Lower Egyptian *Potamogeton* **1**,
  papyrus stalk **1**, the *tia* plant **1**,
Potentilla **1**, red (?) ocher **1**; apply on it.

Case Ebers 670: 83.15–83.18
Another (remedy for) easing the stiffness in any limb: the substance *djat* **1**,
date juice **1**, Lower Egyptian salt **1**, sediment of wine **1**, natron **1**, beef fat **1**,
figs **1**, *Melilotus* **1**, honey **1**, donkey dung **1**, fresh seeds (?) [. . .] **1**, the *shenfet*
fruits **1**, the substance (?) *seska* **1**; cook, apply on it.

Case Ebers 671: 83.18–83.19
Another: the *tjun* plant **1**, carob **1**, the *pesedj* fruits **1**, beans **1**,
oil **1**, honey **1**; grind, apply on it.

Case Ebers 672: 83.19–83.20
Another: myrtle **1**, beef fat **1**, beans **1**,

incense **1**; apply on it.

Case Ebers 673: 83.20–83.22
Another: the *pesedj* fruits **1**, beans **1**, the *shepes* plant **1**, black flint **1**,
cuttlefish bone **1**, carob pod **1**, incense **1**, myrtle **1**, gum **1**, red ocher **1**,
   hematite **1**,
Lower Egyptian salt **1**, honey **(1)**; grind, apply on it.

Case Ebers 674: 83.22–84.1
Another: sediment (of sweet beer/wine?) **1**, date juice **1**, Lower Egyptian salt **1**;
cook, apply on it.

Case Ebers 675: 84.1–84.5
Another (remedy for) easing the stiffness in any limb: honey **1**,
wax **1**, carob pod **1**, chaste tree **1**, juniper berries **1**, celery seeds **1**,
tubers (?) of yellow nutsedge **1**, wild mint **1**, oil **1**, the *peshnet* stone **1**, cedar
resin **1**, the *djesret* beer **1**, *Anacyclus* seeds **1**, incense **1**, ocher **1**, flour
from the *amaa* grain **1**; cook, apply on it.

Case Ebers 676: 84.5–84.6
Another: gypsum **1**, Lower Egyptian salt **1**, sweet beer **1**, the fruits
of the sycomore **1**; apply on it.

Case Ebers 677: 84.6–84.8
Another: the *ibu* plant **1**, the *djesret* plant **1**, pigment of malachite **1**,
camphor **1**, the *pesedj* fruits **1**, yellow nutsedge **1**, chaste tree **1**, celery seeds **1**,
   coriander
seeds **1**, hippopotamus oil **1**; apply on it.

Case Ebers 678: 84.8–84.10
Another: the *pesedj* fruits **1**, beans **1**, the *shepes* plant **1**,
herbal decoction **1**, the (sycomore) fruits mashed with the bird/insect (?) *irhen-
net*, mash including its wings;
apply on it.

Case Ebers 679: 84.10–84.12
Another: white oil **1**, goose fat **1**, ibex fat **1**, juniper
pellets **1**, cedar oil **1**, sweet myrrh **1**, the *shasha* fruits **1**, onion **1**, wax **1**; cook,
apply on it.

Another: the *shenfet* fruits **1**, Lower Egyptian salt **1**, honey **1**, date juice **1**, natron **1**, the substance (?) *seska* **1**, beef fat **1**, sediment (of sweet beer/wine?) **1**; cook, apply on it.

Another remedy prepared for

a blood vessel, when it protruded in any limb: fermented herbal decoction **1**, pomace

1; make from that a pellet, warm, apply on it.

Another: the *nehed* stone **1**, incense **1**,

bryony fruit **1**, the *hepapat* plant **1**, substance (?) *seska* **1**, starch of

barley malt **1**, celery **1**, yellow nutsedge **1**, cedar resin **1**; cook, apply on it.

Another:

the sycomore fruits **1**, sediment of sweet beer **1**; cook, apply on it.

Another (remedy) for

driving away the *shepet* disease of a blood vessel: earth almonds **1**. To be chewed up by the (sick) person. Place the yolk of an egg of a pintail into the rectum.

Another: wild carrot **1**, wax **1**, honey **1**; apply on it.

Another (remedy)

for strengthening the blood vessels: beef fat **1**, incense **1**, wax **1**, juniper berries **1**,

the bryony fruit **1**, camphor **1**, cumin **1**; mix together, apply on it for four days.

Another (remedy). Ointment for soothing the blood vessels: galenite **1**, wax **1**, incense **1**, camphor

1, dried myrrh **1**, beef fat **1**, sweet *Moringa* oil **1**; apply on it for four days.

Case Ebers 688: 85.3–85.5
Another (remedy) for easing
the blood vessels: sweet myrrh **1**, cedar sawdust **1**, date flour **1**, oil
of a spinner **1**; cook together, apply on it for four days.

Case Ebers 689: 85.5–85.7
Another (remedy) for the stretching of contortion and
easing of stiffness: date juice **1**, Lower Egyptian salt **1**, mud **1**, oil **1**,
natron **1**, wild rue **1**; mix together, apply on it.

Case Ebers 690: 85.7–85.8
Another (remedy) for easing (stiffness): natron **1**,
Lower Egyptian salt **1**, cedar resin **1**, beer sediment **1**; apply on it.

Case Ebers 691: 85.8–85.9
Another: honey **1**,
Lower Egyptian salt **1**, donkey dung **1**; cook, apply on it.

Case Ebers 692: 85.9–85.10
Another: oil **1**, honey **1**, fresh
tepaut **1**; cook, apply on it.

Case Ebers 693: 85.10–85.12
Another (remedy) for cooling of the blood vessels: beef fat **1**, donkey
fat **1**, ram fat **1**, the *pesedj* fruits **1**, peas **1**, bryony **1**, Lower Egyptian salt **1**; apply
on it.

Case Ebers 694: 85.12
What to do with a blood vessel when it is stiff: the *niaia* plant **1**, *Potamogeton*
1; pound, apply on it.

Case Ebers 695: 85.13–85.14
Another (remedy) for setting everything in motion: sculpting clay **1**, wild
mint **1**, the *shasha* fruits **1**,
oil **1**, wax **1**; cook, press, drink for four days.

Case Ebers 696: 85.14–85.16
Another (remedy) for driving away agglomeration of painful substances
in an arm,

when it trembles: a barley decoction; mold and leave to ferment entirely. Drink 6 *hin* warmed up to (evoke) vomiting for four days.

Case Ebers 705: 86.4–86.5

Beginning (of a collection) of remedies for driving away the *shepen* disease, which affects the body of a man or woman: Lower Egyptian salt 1/4, incense **1/4**, herbal decoction **1/32** (a measure); lay into the rectum. It may be prepared also without the addition of incense.

Case Ebers 706: 86.5–86.6

Another:
urine **1/64** (a measure), carob pod **half 1/64** (a measure), oil **1/64** (a measure); equally.

Case Ebers 707: 86.6–86.8

Another: herbal decoction **1/32 1/64** (a measure), *Moringa* oil **half 1/64** (a measure), a grain of copper **1/16**, galenite **1/16**, honey **1/8**; equally.
It is beneficial also for driving away the painful substances.

Case Ebers 750: 89.16–89.18

Beginning (of a collection) of remedies for driving away the devastating bitter disease: date flour **1/32** (a measure), water **1/2**; cook,
when 2 *hin* are left, drink at the temperature of a finger, then vomit. This is prepared for driving away the devastating bitter disease and its expulsion from every limb.

Case Ebers 752: 89.20–89.22

Another (remedy) for driving away the *nesyt* disease from a person: the *shenfet* fruits **1/16** (a measure),
white six-row barley **1/8**, juniper berries **1/16**, offshoots of bryony **1/16**; mix together, drink up.

Case Ebers 753: 89.22–89.23

Another: bitter almonds (?); cook with an herbal decoction, drink up.

Case Ebers 754: 89.23–90.2

Another: figs **1/4**, the *ished* fruits **1/4**, white oil **1/8**, honey **1/32**, raisins **1/16**, juniper berries **1/16**, sweet beer **1/64** (a measure); cook, press, drink up.

Case Ebers 755: 90.2–90.3

Another: wild mint **1**, dates **1**, carob pod **1**, Lower Egyptian salt **1**, product of the fermentation of date juice **1**, honey **1**, **found empty** (place in copying).

Case Ebers 756: 90.4–90.5

Another: two testicles of a fair (?) donkey; grind finely, place into wine. Drunk by the (sick) person to remove it (the disease) quickly.

Case Ebers 757: 90.6–90.7

Beginning (of a collection) of remedies for the treatment of the right half (of the abdomen, affected) by the *ruyt* disease: fresh mash **1/32**, six-row barley
1/16, the *djesret* beer; apply on it.

Case Ebers 758: 90.7–90.11

Another: incense **1/64**, juniper berries **1/16**, the Lower Egyptian
ibu plant **1/16**, the *ibkhi* drink **1/16**, mountain celery **1/16**, Lower Egyptian celery **1/16**,
the *peshnet* stone **1/16**, the *tiam* plant **1/16**, *Juncus* **1/16**, the *khebu* plant **1/16**, *Potentilla* **1/16**, white six-row
barley **1/16**, green six-row barley **1/16**, cedar resin **1/64** (a measure), the plant *git* **1/16**,
the *pesedj* fruits **1/64** (a measure), the *rudj* stone **1/16**, myrtle **1/8**, honey **1/32**; apply on it.

Case Ebers 759: 90.11–90.13

Another: bind-
weed **1**, raisins **1**, sorghum **1**, mash **1**, fenugreek **1**, the *qesentet* plant **1**, *amaa* grain of barley **1**; mix together, apply on the (right) half (of the abdomen).

Case Ebers 760: 90.13–90.14

Another: the *git* plant **1**, goose oil **1**, honey
1; apply on it.

Case Ebers 854: 99.1

Beginning of the secret of the physician: knowledge of the operation of the heart (meaning) knowledge of the heart.

Case Ebers 854a: 99.2–99.5

There are arteries in every limb (of the human body). With regard to these (places), on which any physician, any "pure" priest of Sakhmet,

any (knowledgeable) guardian places his hands or fingers, (namely) on the head, on the crown of the head, on the hands, on the heart region, on the

arms and on the legs, (then) he measures (directly) the heart, because its arteries (lead) to each limb.

(The heart) speaks in the arteries of every limb.

Case Ebers 854b: 99.5–99.6

There are four arteries in

both nostrils (of a person). **Two** supply mucuses, **two** supply blood.

Case Ebers 854c: 99.6–99.10

There are four arteries

inside both temples, which subsequently pump blood to the eyes and (also) cause all of the eye disease (emerging) in their opening. In regard to

the water, which flows from them, it is the irises that excrete it. **Another interpretation:**

they are the pupils of the eyes that cause it.

Case Ebers 854d: 99.10–99.12

There are four arteries, which split at the head,

empty in the temple of the head and subsequently cause loss (of hair), baldness, and festering. This is what they create on the outside.

Case Ebers 854e: 99.14–99.17

Regarding how the ears go deaf: There are **two** arteries, which cause it and which lead to

the eye root (= muscle). **Another interpretation.** Regarding these (arteries), which cause deafness of the ears,

they are the (arteries), which are on both temples of a person and (containing) earwax in them (by the demon called) Remover of Heads.

(And the person) accepts the (demon's) breath.

Case Ebers 855a: 99.12–99.14

Regarding the air,

which comes into the nose: it enters to the heart and lungs. They get it to the whole body.

Case Ebers 855b: 99.17-99.18
If it is a (disease) of flooding the heart: it is a gastric liquid.
The limbs (of a person) are entirely limp.

Case Ebers 855c: 99.18-99.19
If it is a (disease) of depression of the heart: it is the artery
(called) The Recipient, which causes it. It provides water to the heart.

Case Ebers 854 belongs to c: 99.19-99.21
Another interpretation
to the whole eye (sic!=body). When the (artery) is deaf and the mouth (of the person) does not open, then all
of his limbs are weakened by these (substances), which the heart accepts.

Case Ebers 855d: 99.21-100.2
If it is
a weakness starting in the heart:
it is a diversion (of the heart) until the lungs and liver.
Its arteries become deaf after falling (= stopping to work) due to their temperature. Its diversion
will release.

Case Ebers 854f: 100.2-100.5
There are four arteries (leading) to both ears (of a person), namely **two** on his right shoulder and **two**
on his left shoulder. The breath of life comes into his right ear, the breath of death comes into
his left ear. **Another interpretation:** (the breath of life) comes into the right shoulder, the breath of death comes into
the left shoulder.

Case Ebers 854g: 100.5-100.6
There are six arteries, which lead to both arms: **three** to the right, **three** to the left.
They lead all the way to the fingers (of a person).

Case Ebers 854h: 100.6-100.7
There are six arteries, which lead to both legs: **three** to the right leg, **three** to the left leg.
They reach all the way to the sole of the foot.

Case Ebers 854i: 100.7

There are two arteries (leading) to both testicles (of a man). They create
the semen.

Case Ebers 854k: 100.7–100.8

There are two arteries

(leading) to the buttocks: **one** to (one) buttock, **the second** to (the second)
buttock.

Case Ebers 854l: 100.8–100.10

There are four **arteries (leading) to the liver.** They

provide it with water and air and subsequently (also) they create any kind of
symptoms of a disease because of

blood congestion.

Case Ebers 854m: 100.10

There are four **arteries (leading) to the lungs and to the spleen.** They provide water and air (to both) the same way.

Case Ebers 854n: 100.11

There are two arteries (leading) to the urinary bladder. They provide urine.

Case Ebers 854o: 100.11–100.14

There are four arteries, which open

into the rectum. They give it water and air and (then) take (them) away. The
rectum is also

open to every artery of the right half (of the abdomen), the left half (of the
abdomen), the arm, and leg, when they overflow (= they are clogged)
with feces.

Case Ebers 855e: 100.14–100.16

If it is a flabby heart, the heart or cardiac arteries do not speak,
the heart is mute and its manifestations are not palpable with the hands,
then air fills them.

Case Ebers 855f: 100.16–100.17

If it is a rebelling heart, then it is weakened by the heat
of the rectum. You discover in the (patient) with strong (symptoms) that everything in the stomach turns for him like an iris of the eye.

Case Ebers 855g: 100.17–100.18

If it is an expanding

heart, it means that the cardiac arteries are under (the influence of) feces.

Case Ebers 855h: 100.18–101.2

If it is any kind of bitter disease, it enters

the left eye and leaves (again) through the navel. It is a (magical) wind called by a "pure" priest.

The heart permits the (bitter disease) to enter its arteries. (And the disease) burns and burns the entire body.

At the same time, the heart drops, when it burns thus. The cardiac arteries tremble

as a consequence of that. Although the (arteries) are (thus) affected by it,

they manage to resist the bitter disease. If, however, the (priest caused?) bitter disease persists, then the (arteries) overflow.

Case Ebers 855i: 101.2–101.5

If it is a falling heart, it drowns itself. **Another interpretation.**

The heart itself overflows. It rises and falls, until it reaches the throat, and (has) in itself the liquid *wiat.*

Case Ebers 855k: 101.5–101.8

If it is a kneeling heart, the heart is pulled down, although

it is (as an organ) in its place and filled with blood by the lungs. However, a reduction occurs. The heart radiates

(and as an organ) tires itself. The appetite (of the patient) for food is little

and choosy.

Case Ebers 855l: 101.8

If it is a dry heart (= not filled with blood?), the blood in the heart coagulates.

Case Ebers 855l bis: 101.8–101.10

If it is

a kneeling (affected) by the painful substances, it means that the heart (of the patient) is smaller in his body.

The painful substances are attacking him, (so that) he weakens and kneels.

Case Ebers 855m: 101.11

If it is an old age weakness, the heart (of a person) has been affected by the painful substances.

Case Ebers 855n: 101.11–101.14
If it is
a dance of the heart, it means that it leaves through the left (part) of the chest, collides with its support and becomes distant from its place. It means that its fat on the left side (of the body) has decided to join with the (patient's) shoulder.

Case Ebers 855o: 101.14–101.15
If it is an advanced bitterness
of the heart, it means that the heart is submerged, when it has sunk, and is not in its place.

Case Ebers 855p: 101.15–101.18
If it is a heart
which is in its place, its fat is on the left side (of the body), it does not rise or lower for anything and remains in its place.

Case Ebers 855q: 101.18–101.20
If it is a constantly trembling heart, (although) its fat is in the left (part) of the chest,
it means a lack of its declining movements (= regular pulse), which only aggravates its suffering.

Case Ebers 855r: 101.20
If it is a constricted stomach, the stomach has enlarged.

Case Ebers 855s: 101.20–102.2
If it is
a spicy stomach, until it stings, if it is a stinging (in) the heart, then the heat has penetrated the heart. The heart is red-hot with heat, like when a person gets a stinger.

Case Ebers 855t: 102.2–102.4
If it is a somber heart like with a person who has eaten
cracked sycomore fruits, then his heart is obscured like him who has eaten cracked sycomore fruits.

Case Ebers 855u: 102.4-102.5

If it is a languishing of the heart and forgetfulness of the heart, the breath
of the lector priest causes it.

It enters the lungs in various ways and it comes to the heart being affected.

Case Ebers 855v: 102.6-102.9

If it is an impairment of the heart by constriction, it means that it has been
affected by a tightening through heat.

It means more frequent weakness. The heart is absorbed by the heat of anger.

Filling the heart with blood causes it. It is caused by drinking (bad?) water. It
(also) emerges through eating

spoiled foods in a warm state.

Case Ebers 855w: 102.9-102.11

**If it is a heart hidden by darkness (= insanity?); the heart has
an appetite,** it means that it is anxious, the darkness is in the body as a consequence of the heat of anger.

That is caused by cases of the absorption of the heart.

Case Ebers 855x: 102.11-102.14

**If it is that all of the meat (of a person) is hot, just like
the heart of a person is exhausted, who was worn out by a (long) journey,**
it means that his meat

is tired with this, just like the meat of a person is tired out after a long walk.

Case Ebers 855y: 102.14-102.15

**If it is an intense tremor (= rage?) for something that comes from outside (like
the activity of a demon),** it means that the heart is turning (like a spindle)
as a result of something that entered from outside (like the activity of a demon).

Case Ebers 855z: 102.15-102.16

If it is a flooded heart, it means that the heart (of a person) is forgetful,
just like one who thinks of something else.

Case Ebers 856a: 103.1-103.2

**The beginning of the book on the spread of the painful substances in
any limb of a person, as was found in the writings
under the feet (of the statue) of Anubis in Khem, and were brought
to His Majesty, King of Upper and Lower Egypt Den,** the justified.

Case Ebers 856b: 103.2–103.3
As for a person, there are
in him twenty-two arteries (leading) to his heart. They provide to all the
places of his body (air).

Case Ebers 856c: 103.3–103.5
There are in (the person) two arteries (leading) like a braid in
his chest. They form the heat in the rectum. **What to do against that:**
fresh dates, *hemu* of *Ricinus*,
tepaut of the sycomore; pound together in water, press, give to drink (to
the sick person) for four days.

Case Ebers 856d: 103.5–103.8
There are
in (the person) two arteries (leading) to his thigh. When his thigh hurts
and both legs tremble, **then you say on this:** "It is
an arterial braid in his thigh. He has fallen ill." **What to do against that:**
herbal decoction, chaste tree,
natron; cook together. Drunk by the (sick) person for four days.

Case Ebers 856e: 103.8–103.11
(There are in the person two arteries leading to his throat.) When his
throat hurts and he sees
poorly, then you say on this: "They are the arteries (leading) to the throat.
They have fallen ill." **What to prepare against that:**
myrtle, water of a spinner, pine nuts, *Anacyclus* seeds; blend
with honey, place on his neck, apply on it for four days.

Case Ebers 856f: 103.11–103.13
There are in (the person) two arteries (leading) to his upper arm.
When his shoulder
hurts and his fingers tremble, **then you say on this:** "It is mucuses." **What**
to prepare against that: make him vomit from fish, beer,
and wild rue or meat, and apply a watermelon on his fingers until he
recovers.

Case Ebers 856g: 103.13–103.16
There are two arteries in him (leading) to
the back of his head. **There are two arteries in him** (leading) to his forehead.

There are two arteries in him (leading) to his eye. **There are two arteries in him** (leading) to

his eyebrows. **There are two arteries in him** (leading) to his nose. **There are two arteries in him** (leading) to his right ear; the breath of life comes into them.

There are two arteries in him (leading) to his left ear; the breath of death comes into them.

Case Ebers 856h: 103.16–103.18
All (of these arteries)

lead to the heart (of a person), they divide at the nose and all are joined at the rectum. They cause

the disease of the rectum. The excreted substances evoke the onset (of the disease). The arteries through the leg begin the dying (of a person).

Papyri from the Ramesseum
Case Ramesseum III.A, I. 3–4 = Ebers 604: 76.21–77.1
[... k]nee: straw; sieve,

stir into water and bandage the knee with that [. . .].

Case Ramesseum III.A, I. 10–11 = Ramesseum III.A, I. 26–27 = Ebers 20: 6.10–6.16
Driving away impurities from the abdomen: thyme (?) (?) **1** cook [. . .].

Case Ramesseum III.A, I. 26–27 = Ramesseum III.A, I. 10–11 = Ebers 20: 6.10–6.16
Driving away impurities [. . .]
[. . .] cook with milk of [. . .]. To be drunk by the person.

Case Ramesseum III.A, I. 27
Driving away [painful] substances [. . .].

Case Ramesseum III.A, I. 28–29
[. . .]
[. . .] in any limb. It is the extermination of a tapeworm.

Case Ramesseum III.A, I. 29–30
What is prepared in the case of the difficult excretion from the rectum of a person: [. . .] date seed **1**/[. . .], [. . .]
flat cake. To be eaten by the person and washed down with diluted beer [. . .].

Case Ramesseum III.B, I. 1–2

Driving away the hunger of both knees: the innards

of a Nile tilapia; place on it. A salamander sliced in half, place on it and bandage with this. Bull bile, a swamp hen, mash and [apply on it . . .].

Case Ramesseum III.B, I. 8–10

Driving away *tepau* [. . .]: slice a salamander, cook until soft in oil.

Place a little on one *tepa*; if his body gets hot under it, do not do [it] against it; if [its body] does not [get hot] under it, grease (all of the *tepau*)

many [times]. Then you fumigate him early in the morning.

Case Ramesseum V.1

[. . .] knee: [. . .] mix and apply on it for four days.

Case Ramesseum V.2 = Ebers 656: 82.7–82.10

Remedy for easing any kind of stiffness: natron **1**, beans **1**, the *tjun* plant **1**, white oil **1**, hippopotamus oil **1**, crocodile oil **1**, oil of a *Clarias* catfish **1**, oil of a mullet **1**, incense **1**, wax **1**, myrrh **1**, honey **1**. Cook together and apply on it every day, until he gets well.

Case Ramesseum V.3

Easing stiffness and stretching a contortion: white oil **1**, *Moringa* oil **1**, fat of a centipede **1**, hippopotamus oil **1**, lion's oil **1**, donkey's oil **1**, crocodile oil **1**, mouse oil **1**, lizard's oil **1**, the oil of the animal *pertjersu* **1**, snake oil **1**, earth almonds oil **1**, the *sefer* oil **1**, wax **1**. Cook together and smear with that every day, until he gets well.

Case Ramesseum V.4

[. . .]: wild rue [**1**], beer sediment **1**, Lower Egyptian salt **1**, natron **1**, dates **1**; [. . .].

Case Ramesseum V.5 = Hearst 94: 7.14–7.16 = Ebers 657: 82.10–82.13

[. . .] beef fat [**1**], sweet myrrh **1**, wine sediment **1**, onion **1**, [. . .] *djabut* **1**, [. . .] **1**, [. . .] bryony **1**, [. . .] of the pea **1**, [. . .] **1**, wild rue seeds **1**, the Lower Egyptian *sia* stone **1**. Cook, smear with this and expose to the sun.

Case Ramesseum V.6

[. . .] *Clarias* catfish [. . .] **1**, [. . .] **1**, [. . .] **1**, the *tjun* plant **1**. Grind and apply on it for four days.

Case Ramesseum V.7
[. . .] pieces of clay **1**, *Anacyclus* seeds **1**, dates **1**. Cook and apply on it for four days.

Case Ramesseum V.8
[. . .] beef fat **1**, [. . .] **1**, [. . .] **1**, the *qesenty* stone **1**, [. . .] **1**, the *maa* tree fruit **1**, celery **1**, [. . .] **1**, [. . .] **1**, [. . .] **1**, [. . .] **1**, salt **1**, [. . .] **1**. Cook together and apply on it, until he gets well.

Case Ramesseum V.9
[. . .] the *amaa* of emmer wheat **1**, the pea fruit **1**, [. . .], [. . .] **1**, wax **1**, pumice **1**, hematite **1**. Cook and apply on it.

Case Ramesseum V.10
[. . .] red ocher **1**, hematite **1**, bull's spleen **1**, wax **1**, wheat semolina **1**, [. . .].

Case Ramesseum V.11
[. . .] oil **1**, wax **1**, *khentet* from incense **1**. Cook together and apply on it, until he gets well.

Case Ramesseum V.12
Cooling of the blood vessels and strengthening a weakness: jujube leaves **1**, acacia leaves **1**, honey **1**. Mash in honey and apply on it for four days.

Case Ramesseum V.13
Another remedy: acacia leaves **1**, beef fat **1**, cedar sawdust **1**; apply on it for four days.

Case Ramesseum V.14
Easing the *shut* disease of the blood vessels (*metu*): beef fat **1**, goat fat [**1**], sheep fat **1**, honey **1**, wax **1**, oil **1**, mint **1**, sorghum **1**. Cook and apply on it.

Case Ramesseum V.15
Easing contortion: ocher **1**, sweet myrrh **1**, a grain of copper **1**, honey **1**, natron **1**, Lower Egyptian salt **1**, red ocher **1**, ibex fat **1**. Cook together and apply on it.

Case Ramesseum V.16
Remedy for easing stiffness: white oil **1**, oil [. . .] **1**, hippopotamus oil **1**, donkey

oil **1**, ibex fat **1**, beef fat **1**, pieces of cedar resin **1**, the *anenu* tree fruit [**1**], sweet myrrh **1**, the *sefe*[*r*] oil [**1**]. Cook and apply on it for four days.

Case Ramesseum V.17

Easing a knotted blood vessel (*met*): *pesedj* fruits **1**, beans **1**, gum **1**, red ocher **1**, the *tjun* plant **1**, hematite **1**, black flint **1**, Lower Egyptian salt **1**, honey **1**. Grind and apply on it for four days.

Case Ramesseum V.18

Easing of the blood vessels (*metu*): beef fat **1**, beef tongue **1**, beef spleen **1**, date seeds **1**, incense **1**, emmer wheat **1**, beef marrow **1**. Blend and apply on it for four days.

Case Ramesseum V.19

Easing the *shut* disease of the blood vessels (*metu*): onion **1**, Lower Egyptian salt **1**, [. . .], ibex fat [**1**], goose oil **1**, *khet* of a goose **1**, *wedja* of dates [**1**], incense **1**, the *pesedj* fruits **1**, laudanum **1**, [. . .].

Case Ramesseum V.20

[. . .] black flint **1**, carob pod **1**, incense **1**, a grain of copper **1**, beef fat **1**, wax **1**, honey **1**. Cook and apply on it.

Edwin Smith Papyrus
Case Smith 22: 11–14

When you examine a person having pain (in) the rectum, when he gets up or sits down, he is having pain from an amassing in both of his legs
greatly, you give him a remedy: oil, (the stone) great protection, acacia leaves.
Grind finely, cook together, grease with this a bandage of fine cloth, place into the rectum,
until he recovers quickly.

Hearst Papyrus
Case Hearst 1: 1.1

[. . .] put on a *feka* cake and another on it, soak (it) in honey and to be swallowed by the (sick) person.

Case Hearst 2: 1.1–1.2
Medicine for emptying the abdomen

[. . .] the *shasha* fruits **1/32**, blend with an herbal decoction, make into seven pellets and soak them in honey. To be swallowed by the (sick) person.

Case Hearst 3: 1.2–1.4
Remedy
[. . .] bitter almonds (?) soak in honey. To be swallowed by the (sick) person, chewed up with a finger of honey afterwards [. . .] sweet beer for four days.

Case Hearst 4: 1.4
Remedy for driving away an agglomeration of painful substances in the rectum: myrtle; apply on it.

Case Hearst 7: 1.6
Remedy for the rectum when it aches: fumigate with limestone, sand, an herbal decoction, or beer.

Case Hearst 16: 1.16–2.1 = Ebers 182: 35.12–35.14
Driving away a dead person, which is effective: the
pe[a. . .] fruit **1**, the *kaa* of the *aru* tree **1**, insides of a freshwater mussel **1**, the *shasha* fruits **1**. Grind finely. To be consumed with honey
by the (sick) person.

Case Hearst 18: 2.4–2.5 = Ebers 49: 16.7–16.14
Remedy for driving away blood, when it is excessive: fresh mash **1/8**, beaten earth almonds **1/64** (a measure), oil
1/8, honey **1/8**. Press and drink for four days. Any (other) remedy is less effective.

Case Hearst 19: 2.5
Remedy for diarrhea: cow's blood cook and eat.

Case Hearst 20: 2.5–2.6
Remedy for putting the demon Hayt to sleep: add
pig's blood to wine and drink immediately.

Case Hearst 25: 2.9–2.10
Remedy for driving away constipation: six-row barley made into semolina, wash and leave overnight (exposed) to the dew. In the morning you press (it); add to that honey **1/8**, strain through a cloth and drink for four days. I saw that it is effective.

Case Hearst 26: 2.10–2.11
Remedy for overcoming painful substances in the abdomen: the *shasha* fruits
1/8, the *aamu* plant **1/8**, the *sheny-ta* seeds **1/8**, sweet beer **1/16** (a measure),
date purée **1/64** (a measure). Consume for four days.

Case Hearst 27: 2.11–2.12
Remedy for driving away *henut* of both legs: the dried *ihu* fruits **1/64** (a
measure),
wheat semolina **1/4**, beaten earth almonds **1/64** (a measure), oil **1/8**, honey **1/8**,
water **1/4** (a measure). Grind, press, and eat for four days.

Case Hearst 28: 2.12–2.14
Remedy for the treatment of the left half (of the abdomen):
figs **1/4**, *ished* fruits **1/8**, raisins **1/8**, anise **half 1/64** (a measure), gum **1/32**,
ocher **1/32**, incense **1/64**, garden cress (?) **1/32**, cumin **1/32**, cracked sycomore fruits
[**1/32**], water **1/16** (a measure). Leave for the night (exposed) to the dew, press,
and drink for four days.

Case Hearst 29: 2.14–2.15
Remedy for overcoming painful substances in the abdomen: figs **1/8**, *ished*
fruits **1/8**, the *sheny-ta* seeds **1/8**, oil
1/8, the *aamu* plant **1/4**, carob pod **1/16**, juniper berries **1/4**, sweet beer **1/16** (a
measure). Cook, leave for the night (exposed) to the dew, press, thicken to
half of **1/16** (a measure) and drink for four days.

Case Hearst 30: 2.15–2.17
Driving away of painful substances in the chest: the pea fruit **1/16**, *ished*
fruits **1/8**, milk **half 1/64** (a measure), incense **1/64**, earth almonds **1/8**, figs
1/8, the *shenfet* fruits **1/64**, sweet beer
1/64 (a measure). Equally, thicken to **1/64** (a measure) and reduce to **1/30**.

Case Hearst 35: 3.4–3.6 = Ebers 294: 51.15–51.19
Remedy for making mucuses leave from the pelvic area: the *sem* herb, bindweed is its name. It grows on its stomach
like a *Cynodon*, forms its blossom like a lotus, and its leaves can be found like
white wood. It should be brought and its leaf rubbed
onto the pelvic area. Then (the mucuses) quickly leave.

Case Hearst 36: 3.6-3.7

Driving away magic in the abdomen: the insides of a freshwater mussel, incense, pine

nuts; mix into one. To be eaten by the (sick) person.

Case Hearst 37: 3.7-3.8

What is prepared against the cracking (of the blood vessels) in the limbs: resin crushed with oil, cook until soft,

and place against cracking in all the limbs of a man or woman.

Case Hearst 41: 3.10-3.11 = Ebers 584: 75.4-75.5

Remedy for driving away painful substances developed in all the limbs of a person: sediments *shamu*, tomcat feces,

dog feces, myrtle fruit. Apply on it. This is to drive away swelling.

Case Hearst 42: 3.11-3.13

Remedy for extermination of painful substances

in all limbs: fatty meat **1/32** (a measure), both halves of the *pesedj* fruits **1/64 half 1/64** (a measure), *Melilotus* **1/64** (a measure), thyme (?) **1/16**, juniper berries **1/16**, incense **1/16**, *djeseret* beer **1/32 1/64** (a measure), sweet beer **1/16 1/64** (a measure). Cook, press, and consume for four days, thicken to **1/32** (a measure).

Case Hearst 43: 3.13-3.14

Another: incense **1/64**, cumin **1/64**, fresh bread **1/8**, *merhet-sa* oil **1/16**, honey **1/16**, sweet beer **1/16** (a measure). Cook, press, and consume for four days.

Case Hearst 44: 3.14-3.15

Another: dill **1/32**, dates **1/8**, rai-

sins **1/8**, wine **1/64** (a measure). Cook, press, and consume for four days.

Case Hearst 45: 3.15-3.17

Another: *hemaret* **1/16** (a measure), carob juice **1/16** (a measure), fat **1/4**, honey **1/4**. Pound together, strain through a cloth, press, and consume for four days. You add honey before you take it.

Case Hearst 46: 3.17-4.1

A medicine for extermination of the substances (causing) pain in all limbs: crushed and sorted barley **half 1/64** (a measure), both halves of the *pesedj* fruit **1/64** (a measure), the *tiam* plant **1/8**, yellow nutsedge **1/8**, juniper berries **1/16**, water **1/4 1/8** (a measure). Cook, leave overnight (exposed) to the dew, press, and consume for four days.

Case Hearst 47: 4.1–4.2
Remedy for extermination of the substances (causing) pain in the abdomen:
dates **half 1/64** (a measure), acacia leaves **1/8**, earth almonds **half 1/64** (a measure), milk **1/32** (a measure), goose oil **1/64** (a measure); equally.

Case Hearst 48: 4.2–4.3 = Ebers 217: 44.5–44.7
Remedy for driving away the pain of the heart: date flour **1/4**, carob pod **1/32**,
the *amau* fruits **1/64** (a measure), sweet beer **1/16 1/64** (a measure). Cook, press, and drink for four days. Thickening to **1/32** (a measure).

Case Hearst 49: 4.3 = Ebers 218: 44.7–44.8
Another remedy: milk **1/64** (a measure), honey **1/14**, water **1/32** (a measure). Cook, press, and drink for four days.

Case Hearst 50: 4.4
Remedy for making the heart to accept food: figs **1/8**, anise **1/8**, ocher **1/32**, honey **1/32**, water **1/64** (a measure); equally.

Case Hearst 51: 4.4–4.5
Remedy for treating the heart (*haty*): black
emmer wheat **1/16** (a measure), water **1/2** (a measure). Cook, press, and drink for four days. Thickening to six (times) 1/64 (a measure).

Case Hearst 52: 4.5–4.6
Another: juniper berries **1/16**, earth almonds **1/64** (a measure), milk **1/8**, goose oil **1/16**, water **1/16** (a measure); equally.

Case Hearst 53: 4.6 = Ebers 4: 2a.7–2a.10
Remedy for driving away pain in the abdomen: peas blended with beer. Drink.

Case Hearst 54: 4.6–4.7
Remedy for driving away magic in the abdomen: the insides of bitter almonds (?) **1**, *wedja* of dates **1**, pine nuts **1**, incense **1**. Eat
and wash (it) down with beer.

Case Hearst 55: 4.7–4.8 = Ebers 5: 2a.11–2a.15
Remedy for the abdomen, when it aches: cumin **1/32**,
goose oil **1/8**, milk **1/16** (a measure); equally.

Case Hearst 56: 4.8 = Ebers 6: 2a.16–2a.20
Another: figs **1/8**, *ished* fruits **1/8**, sweet beer **1/16** (a measure); equally.

Case Hearst 57: 4.8–4.9
A liquid medicine for the treatment of the lungs: ocher **1/32**,
gum **1/32**, honey **1/8**, figs **1/8**, water **1/16 1/64** (a measure). Leave for the
   night (exposed) to the dew and drink for four days.

Case Hearst 58: 4.9–4.10 = Ebers 7: 2b.7–2b.11
A medicine for purging of the abdomen: milk **1/16 1/64** (a measure),
   cracked sycomore fruits **1/4**,
honey **1/4**. Cook, press, and drink for four days.

Case Hearst 59: 4.10–4.11
Remedy for making him excrete: juniper berries **1**, honey **1**, sweet beer.
Press and drink for four days.

Case Hearst 60: 4.11
Another: the *khershu-mat* stone **1**, sweet beer. Cook, press, and drink up.

Case Hearst 61: 4.11–4.12
Remedy for driving away a cough: milk **1/16 1/64** (a measure), the *kerek*
   stone **1/16**, the *aam*
plant **1/16**, incense **1/64**, ocher **1/32**, marrow **1/8**. Cook and drink for four days.

Case Hearst 62: 4.12–4.14
The drink with a fast effect (for) treatment of the urinary bladder and
   correction of urination: *hemu* of
Ricinus **1/8**, dates, which began to grow **1/8**, pine nuts **1/32**, pomace **1/16**,
   bryony **1/32**, muskmelon leaves **1/32**, beaten earth almonds
1/4, foam (or water for washing) **1/16 1/64** (a measure). For the night (expose)
   to the dew and drink for four days.

Case Hearst 63: 4.14–4.15 = Ebers 277: 50.6–50.8
A medicine for driving away urine, when it is excessive: gum **1/4**, wheat

semolina **1/4**, fresh mash

1/4, ocher **1/32**, water **1/16 1/64** (a measure) equally.

Another: *Cynodon* roots **1/4**, grapes **1/8**, honey **1/4**, juniper berries **1/32**, sweet beer **1/64 half 1/64** (a measure). Cook,

press, and drink for one day.

Another: gum **1/8**, honey **1/32**, water **1/64** (a measure). Cook, press, and drink for one day.

Another: *ished* fruits **1/8**, wheat semolina **1/8**, ocher **1/32**, gum **1/32**, water **1/32** (a measure); equally.

Correction of the urine: milk **1/4**, honey **1/4**, juniper berries **1/4**, *Cynodon* **1/8**, sweet

beer **1/2 1/8** (a measure). Press and drink for four days.

Remedy for holding the urine: mountain celery **1/2** (a measure), Lower Egyptian celery **1/8**, the Upper Egyptian *ibu* plant **1/16**, juniper

berries **1/16**, fresh mash **1/8**, the Lower Egyptian *ibu* plant **1/16**, the *peshnet* stone **1/16**, the *wam* plant **1/16**, the *duat* plant **1/16**, water **1/16**. For the night (expose) to the dew, press,

and drink for four days.

Treatment for the penetration of heat into his urinary bladder: cooked wheat **half 1/64** (a measure), *ihu* fruits **half 1/64** (a measure), goose oil **1/8**, water **1/16** (a measure). For the night

(expose) to the dew, press, and drink for four days.

Driving away the penetration of heat into the urinary bladder: cooked wheat flour **1/64** (a measure), cooked barley flour **1/64** (a measure), sorghum **1/64** (a measure), figs **1/64** (a measure), juniper berries **1/4**, pine nuts **1/4**, incense **1/64**, cumin **1/64**, goose oil **1/4**, honey **1/4**, earth almonds **1/4**, water **1/4 1/8** (a measure).

For the night (expose) to the dew and drink for four days. Thickening to **three 1/64** (a measure).

Case Hearst 71: 5.7–5.9 = Ebers 243: 46.16–46.19

The second remedy, which Shu prepared for himself: wheat flour **1**, Lower Egyptian salt **1**, oil **1**, coriander

powder 1, soot from the wall **1**, carob flour **1**, beans flour **1**, the *qesentet* plant **1**, incense **1**, ocher **1**, herbal decoction **1**.

Mix together and bandage the painful place with this.

Case Hearst 72: 5.9–5.10 = Ebers 244: 46.19–46.22

The third remedy, which Tefnut **prepared** for Re himself: flour from the *amaa* grain **1**, *shenfet* fruits **1**, oil **1**. Knead together

and bandage any painful place with this to drive away the disease and the (harmful) activity of a dead male or dead female in the limbs of a person, so that he gets well quickly.

Case Hearst 73: 5.10–5.12 = Ebers 245: 46.22–47.1

The fourth

remedy, which Geb **prepared** for himself: carob flour **1**, pea flour **1**, myrrh powder **1**. Grind finely with fermented

date juice and bandage with this any painful place to drive away the disease and the (harmful) activity of a dead male or dead female.

Case Hearst 74: 5.12–5.15 = Ebers 246: 47.2–47.5

The fifth remedy, which Nut **prepared**

for Re himself: brick from the wall **1**, offshoot of the *Cynodon* **1**, scraping stone **1**, natron **1**, salt **1**, fresh mash **1**,

oil **1**, cedar oil **1**, honey **1**, flat *shenes* cake **1**. Cook together and bandage with this any painful place to (drive away) the disease and the (harmful) activity of a dead male or dead female in

the limbs of a person, so that he gets well quickly.

Case Hearst 75: 5.15–6.2 = Ebers 247: 47.5–47.10

The sixth remedy, which Isis **prepared** for Re himself to drive away the pain from his head: coriander seeds **1**,

Anacyclus fruits **1**, bryony fruits **1**, pine nuts **1**, the *aamu* plant **1**, honey **1**. Mix together,

blend honey with that, and bandage with this the head, so he gets well quickly.

About the one for whom this remedy is prepared for any kind of pain: who has pain of the head on the forehead and inside by the (harmful)

activity of a god or goddess, a dead male, or dead female, whatever bad or evil in the head and every limb. He gets well quickly. Really effective!

Case Hearst 76: 6.2–6.4 = Ebers 248: 47.10–47.12

Remedy for

driving away the activity (of demons) in the head and the *seket* disease in the head: the pulp of the carob pod **1**, *khesau* of the *ima* tree **1**, natron **1**, mud **1**, cooked bones of the Nile perch **1**, cooked red tilapia **1**,

cooked skull of *Synodontis* **1**, honey **1**, laudanum **1**. Grease the head with that for four days.

Case Hearst 77: 6.4–6.5 = Ebers 249: 47.13–47.14

Another remedy: dill seeds **1**, bryony fruits **1**,

coriander seeds **1**, the *innek* plant **1**, myrtle **1**, donkey fat **1**. Grease the head with that for four days.

Case Hearst 79: 6.11–6.12 = Ebers 221: 44.13–44.15

Driving away poisonous substance from the abdomen and from the heart (*haty*): *Anacyclus*

1/16, the *shasha* fruits **1/8**, ocher **1/64**, honey **1/2**. Mix together and eat before sleeping.

Case Hearst 80: 6.12–6.14 = Ebers 222: 44.15–44.17

Remedy for driving away poisonous substance from the abdomen and the heart (*haty*):

yellow nutsedge **1/8**, the *shasha* fruits **1/8**, pine nuts **1/16**, malachite **1/64**, amber **1/32**, the *pesedj* fruits **1/16**, honey **1/2**. Mix together and eat before sleeping.

Case Hearst 81: 6.14–6.15 = Ebers 223: 44.17–44.19

Another remedy for driving away poisonous substances from the abdomen and from the heart (*haty*): gum **1/32**, grapes **1/16**, the *shasha* fruits **1/8**, *Anacyclus* **1/16**,

honey **1/2**. Mix together and eat before sleeping.

Case Hearst 82: 6.15–6.16 = Ebers 224: 44.19–44.22

Another remedy: *hemu* of *Ricinus* **1/8**, the *khesau* of the fig tree **1/8**, fresh dates **1/8**, lotus leaves **1/8**, fresh mash **1/8**, water **1/32** (a measure). Press and immediately drink up.

Case Hearst 83: 6.16–7.2

Driving away the poisonous substances of a god and dead person from the abdomen of a man or woman: acacia leaves **1/32**, leaves of the *aru* tree **1/32**, the *kaa* of the *aru* tree **1/32**, carob pod **1/8**, grapes **1/8**, Lower Egyptian salt **1/32**, insides of a freshwater mussel **1/32**, peas **1/8**, galenite **1/64**, the *shasha* fruits **1/4**, the *sheny-ta* seeds **1/8**, honey **1/32**, herbal decoction **1/16 1/64** (a measure). Cook, press, and drink for four days.

Case Hearst 84: 7.2–7.4 = Ebers 226: 45.4–45.6

Another remedy: anise **1/8**, figs **1/8**, salt **1/32**, ocher **1/32**, honey **1/32**, water **1/32** (a measure), grapes **1/16**, earth almonds **1/16**, bread from the jujube **1/16**, the *ibu* plant **1/32**, coriander **1/16**. Overnight (expose) to the dew and drink for four days.

Case Hearst 85: 7.4–7.6

Another remedy: the *abdju* fish, fill the mouth with incense, cook and eat before sleeping.

What is recited against this as an incantation: "O dead male and dead female, hiding, hidden, which you are in this my meat, in these my limbs, leave from this my meat, from these my limbs. Look, I brought feces for you to eat, hidden, crawl away! Hidden, retreat away!"

Case Hearst 86: 7.7–7.9

Another remedy: *Anacyclus* **1/64**, pine nuts **1/32**, yellow nutsedge **1/32**, the *shasha* fruits **1/32**, coriander seeds **1/32**, bryony fruit **1/64**, the *aamu* plant **1/32**, honey **1/8**, peas **1/32**, ocher **1/64**. Mix together and eat before sleeping.

Case Hearst 87: 7.9–7.10

Another remedy: the *ibu* plant **1/8**, coriander seeds **1/32**, peas **1/64**, sweet beer **1/32** (a measure). Press and drink up before sleeping.

Remedy on the pubic area, when it aches: sorghum **1/4**, gum **1/32**, water **1/64** (a measure). For the night (expose) to the dew and drink every day.

Remedy for cooling of the rectum:

beaten earth almonds **1/4**, *wedja* of dates **1/4**, mash **1/8**, sorghum **1/4**, water **1/16** (a measure). For the night (expose) to the dew and drink for four days.

Beginning of the treatise on the calming of any kind of pain. Remedy for easing the blood vessels: fat **1**, wine sediment **1**,

onion **1**, soot from the wall **1**, bryony fruit **1**, the pea fruit **1**, the wild rue seeds **1**, the Upper Egyptian *sia* (stone) **1**,

incense **1**, myrrh **1**. Cook together and apply on it.

Cooling of the blood vessels (*metu*): jujube leaves **1**, willow leaves **1**, acacia leaves **1**, wild rue **1**, Lower Egyptian salt **1**, garlic **1**. Grind finely, mix together, and apply on it.

Remedy for calming of the blood vessels (*metu*): tomcat oil **1**, petrified wood **1**, resin of the *ikeru* tree **1**. Grind, mix together, and smear with that.

Another: coriander seeds **1**, leather from the sandal maker **1**, the substance (?) *seska* **1**; equally.

Another:

snake oil **1**, wormwood **1**, galenite **1**, honey **1**. Mix together. Smear it with myrrh before.

What to do with a blood vessel (*met*) which quickly protrudes on any limb: the *khesau*

of the *ima* tree **1**, the *tjun* plant **1**, product of the fermentation of honey **1**. Mix together and smear any painful place with that.

Case Hearst 100: 8.4–8.5

Comforting of the blood vessels (*metu*): the *ibu* plant, bryony **1**, Lower
  Egyptian
salt **1**, the sycomore fruits **1**, mash with wheat flour, and place on it.

Case Hearst 101: 8.5–8.6 = Ebers 652: 81.17–81.20

Reviving of the blood vessels (*metu*), refreshing of the blood vessels (*metu*):
  resin, incense, cedar oil, wax, sawdust of the camphor tree,
cedar sawdust, coriander seeds, beef oil. Cook, apply on it, (but) first smear
  with myrrh.

Case Hearst 102: 8.6–8.7

Remedy for calming of the blood vessels (*metu*): sprigs of tamarisk **1**, the
  wam plant **1**. Apply
on it.

Case Hearst 103: 8.7

Another: date **1**, *hemu* of *Ricinus* **1**, juniper berries **1/8** (a measure), honey
  1/16, incense **1/8**. Mix together and apply on it.

Case Hearst 104: 8.7–8.8

Soothing **of the blood vessels (*metu*):** incense,
honey, oil, red clay, wild mint, calamine, myrrh, the *pesedj* fruits; apply on it.

Case Hearst 105: 8.8

Another: sorghum, wheat flour, six-row barley. Grind, cook, and apply on it.

Case Hearst 106: 8.8–8.9

Another: (the stone) great protection, substance (?) *seska*,
cumin, grind, and apply on it.

Case Hearst 107: 8.9–8.10

Another: wax, pine nuts, fresh incense, yellow nutsedge, coriander seeds,
  bryony fruit, the *sar* plant, myrtle,
galenite. Apply on it, first smear it with myrrh.

Case Hearst 108: 8.10

Another: camphor, incense, sorghum, Lower Egyptian salt, honey. Apply on
  it.

Case Hearst 109: 8.10–8.11
Another: beef fat, wax,
sweet myrrh, wild mint, hematite, galenite, incense. Cook into an ointment,
bring to a boil, and apply on it.

Case Hearst 110: 8.11–8.12 = Ebers 694: 85.12
What to do with a blood vessel (*met*), when it is stiff: the *niaia* plant,
Potamogeton;
pound and apply on it, until he gets well.

Case Hearst 111: 8.12–8.13 = Ebers 642: 80.15–80.17
How to make blood vessels (*metu*) accept a remedy: milk (of a woman)
who gave birth to a boy, Lower Egyptian salt, leave overnight in the *hin*
vessel,
until it sours. Smear any painful place with this.

Case Hearst 112: 8.13 = Ebers 643: 80.17–80.18
Another: *pekhekh* of date purée, beer sediment; equally.

Case Hearst 113: 8.13–8.14
Driving away swelling of a blood vessel (*met*): celery, grind with oil;
smear the blood vessel with this.

Case Hearst 114: 8.14
Easing the *shut* disease of blood vessels (*metu*): beef spleen, wheat semolina, hematite, ibex fat, beef innards; apply on it.

Case Hearst 115: 8.14–8.15
Another: incense, Lower Egyptian
salt, the wings and body of the scarab beetle, the substance (?) *seska*, honey; equally.

Case Hearst 116: 8.15–8.16 = Ebers 647: 81.1–81.4
Calming of the blood vessels (*metu*) of the toes: wax, beef fat, acacia leaf,
powder of the plant *tjun*, roots of the *Cynodon*.

Case Hearst 117 a 118: 8.16–8.17 = Ebers 660: 82.18–82.19 = Berlin 50: 4.12
Another: watermelon, Lower Egyptian salt, honey, ibex fat, substance (?)
seska, beef
meat, hematite, carob pod; equally.

Case Hearst 119: 8.17 = Ebers 661: 82.19–82.20
Another: "male" clay, coriander seeds, dates; equally.

Case Hearst 120: 8.17–8.18 = Ebers 662: 82.20–82.22
Mitigating the tremor of a blood vessel (*met*): mussels, date juice, six-row barley,
Lower Egyptian salt, sediment of sweet beer; equally.

Case Hearst 121: 8.18–9.1 = Ebers 693: 85.10–85.12
Cooling of the blood vessels (*metu*): beef fat, donkey fat, both halves of the *pesedj* fruits, peas,
bryony, Lower Egyptian salt; equally.

Case Hearst 122: 9.1–9.2
Revival of the blood vessels (*metu*): myrrh, incense, the *shabet* plant, pine nuts, mix together and
apply on it.

Case Hearst 123: 9.2–9.3 = Ebers 654: 82.1–82.4
Easing the joints of any limb: honey, wax, the highest quality incense, laudanum, milk fat, carob flour, the *sha-*
sha fruits, wild rue seeds. Grind together, cook, and smear with that.

Case Hearst 124: 9.3–9.4 = Ebers 655: 82.4–82.6
Another: juniper berries, tubers (?) of *Astragalus*, bryony,
red clay, celery seeds, incense pellets, juniper seeds (?). Mix together and apply on it.

Case Hearst 131: 9.9–9.10 = Ebers 302: 52.19–52.20
Remedy
for driving away the bitter disease (*dehret*): carob pod, grind with honey, and eat with sweet beer.

Case Hearst 142: 10.1–10.2 = Ebers 695: 85.13–85.14
Setting everything in motion: sculpting clay **1**,
wild mint **1**, the *shasha* fruits **1**, oil **1**, wax **1**. Cook, press, and consume for four days.

Case Hearst 167: 11.9–11.10

Driving away the *meshshut* disease: shed snake skin, sour milk, camphor (?). Grease (the head) with that.

Case Hearst 173a: 11.17–11.18 = Ebers 621: 78.16–78.18
Case Hearst 173b: 11.18–12.1 = Ebers 616: 78.4–78.6

Remedy for treating a finger or a toe: red ocher, a shard of a new *hin* vessel, grind finely with the product
of honey fermentation, bandage the finger or toe with that.
Then you prepare for him a remedy for cooling: acacia leaves **1/4**, jujube leaves **1/4**, ocher **1/32**, green pigment of malachite **1/32**, the insides of a mussel **1/8**. Grind and apply on it.

Case Hearst 174: 12.1–12.3 = Ebers 617: 78.6–78.10

When you find the fingers or toes aching, liquid issues from them, they smell badly, look like worms (*sa*). You say on that: "A disease, which I will treat." **You prepare for him a medicine for extermi-**
nation of the worm (*seped*): the Upper Egyptian *sia* stone **1/32**, the Lower Egyptian *sia* stone **1/32**, cedar oil **1/8**. Grind and apply on it.

Case Hearst 175: 12.3–12.5 = Ebers 620: 78.12–78.16

Treatment of a toe aching:
ocher, natron, (the stone) great protection, red ocher, the *khenenu* stone from the courtyard, flax seed, starch. Mix together and apply on it. **Then you make medicine**
from it: you prepare for him marrow oil, fat, oil, honey. Grind, mix together, and apply on it.

Case Hearst 176: 12.5–12.6

Another remedy: fat,
incense, oil, honey; equally.

Case Hearst 177: 12.6–12.7 = Hearst 188: 12.15–12.16 =
Ebers 618: 78.10–78.11

Remedy for a nail or for a toe: honey **1/64** (a measure), ocher **1/64**, hemp **1/32**, resin
1/32, the *ibu* plant **1/32**. Grind and apply on it.

Case Hearst 178: 12.7 = Ebers 619: 78.11–78.12

Another remedy: honey **1/8**, ocher **1/64**, oil **1/32**; equally.

Case Hearst 179: 12.7–12.8

Remedy for the treatment of the nail

of a toe, which is falling off: treat it with natron, incense, oil, honey, ocher, to
be placed on it preventing its bandage from pressing.

Case Hearst 180: 12.9

What is prepared for a toe: fat, acacia leaves; cook together and spread on it.

Case Hearst 181: 12.9

Remedy, which is prepared for a finger: powder from the *tjun* plant, cook in
oil, and apply on it.

Case Hearst 182: 12.9–12.10

Remedy

for driving away the blood in the toes: grind hulls of acacia finely and apply on it.

Case Hearst 183: 12.10–12.11

Another remedy: a pellet of incense; cook with oil,
make into an ointment and apply on it.

Case Hearst 184: 12.11–12.13

**What is prepared for the nails of the toes, on which it is a wound with an
open mouth:** acacia leaves, carob pod, red ocher,
Lower Egyptian salt, fermented herbal decoction. Cook and apply on it. **Then
you prepare for him:** cedar oil, fat, incense, the seeds
of fennel, carob flour, wax. Mix together and apply on it.

Case Hearst 185: 12.13–12.14

Treatment of a nail on the toes: ibex fat,
hematite, a grain of copper, myrtle, red wood, ocher, wax. Apply on it.

Case Hearst 186: 12.14

Another remedy: fat, incense, ocher, honey; equally.

Case Hearst 187: 12.15

Another remedy: ocher, flax seeds, the *wetyt* of a sycomore, honey, oil; equally.

Case Hearst 188: 12.15–12.16 = Hearst 177: 12.6–12.7 = Ebers 618: 78.10–78.11
Remedy for a nail and a toe: honey
1/8, hemp **1/32**, ocher **1/32**, resin **1/32**, the *ibu* plant **1/32**. Apply it on the nail of the toe.

Case Hearst 189: 12.16–12.17
Another remedy: ocher **1/32**,
oil **1/32**, apply on it.

Case Hearst 190: 12.17
Another remedy: red ocher **1/8**, honey **1/8**; equally.

Case Hearst 191: 12.17–13.1
Another: fresh barley flour, honey **1/16**, ocher **1/32**,
carob pod **1/8**, incense **1/64**, acacia leaves **1/8**, jujube leaves **1/8**, myrrh **1/64**
(a measure). Cook and apply on it.

Case Hearst 192: 13.1–13.2
Another remedy: incense **1/8**, re-
sin **1/32**, ocher **1/32**, the *ibu* plant **1/8**, honey **1/8**.

Case Hearst 193: 13.2–13.3
Treatment of a nail or a toe: red ocher, shards of a new *hin* vessel,
honey, oil. Apply on it.

Case Hearst 194: 13.3–13.4
**Remedy for fingers and toes, for refreshment of the fingers, which is worked
into on the nail:** resin, laudanum, gum, oil,
(the unknown substance) *bedet-hawret*, acacia leaves. Place on it.

Case Hearst 195: 13.4
Treatment of a finger or a toe: fibers of the *qaa* plant; cook in oil. Apply on it.

Case Hearst 196: 13.5
Removing worms (*fenet*) from fingers or toes: red ocher, carob pod, the
henayt stone. Apply it on the fingers or toes.

Case Hearst 197: 13.5–13.6
Remedy for a toe: a salamander,
eviscerate, sprinkle his abdomen (from the inside) with salt. Apply on it.

Case Hearst 198: 13.6
Another remedy: cedar oil, *amem* of a frog; equally.

Case Hearst 199: 13.6–13.7
Remedy for
drying the festering on the nails of the toes: the pea fruit, carob seeds; grind
with honey and apply on it.

Case Hearst 200: 13.7–13.8
Driving away swelling
in the toes: the *tjun* plant fruit; grind with honey and apply on it.

Case Hearst 201: 13.8–13.9
Another remedy: the *Anacyclus* fruit, the pea fruit,
the *tjun* plant fruit, pine nuts. Grind, knead it with honey, and apply on it.

Case Hearst 202: 13.9–13.10
Another remedy: carob pod, the *shasha* fruits, red ocher, honey; equally.

Case Hearst 203: 13.10
Another remedy: *amem* of a *Clarias* catfish, honey. Apply it on the toe.

Case Hearst 204: 13.10–13.11
Driving away the "wheat grain" (*sut*) at a finger: the *seska* substance (?),
the *pesedj* fruits, Lower Egyptian salt, myrtle, honey. Apply on it.

Case Hearst 205: 13.11–13.12
Remedy for driving away trembling in the fingers: rub the fingers
with oil and apply watermelon.

Case Hearst 206: 13.12–13.13 = Ebers 752: 89.20–89.22
Remedy for the *nesyt* disease: the *shenfet* fruits **1/16** (a measure), white six-
row barley **1/8**, green six-row barley **1/8**, juniper berries
1/16, offshoots of bryony **1/16**. Mix together and drink up.

Case Hearst 207: 13.13–13.14 = Ebers 754: 89.23–90.2
Another remedy: figs **1/64** (a measure), *ished* fruits **1/8**, white
oil **1/8**, sweet beer **1/16 1/64** (a measure), honey **1/32**, raisins **1/16**, juniper berries **1/16**. Cook, press, and drink for four days.

Case Hearst 208: 13.14–13.15
Another remedy:
donkey dung, grind finely with wine 1/64 (a measure), drink for four days.

Case Hearst 209: 13.15–13.16
Another remedy: fennel, *Melilotus*, wild rue, garlic, beer.
Pound and drink up.

Case Hearst 210: 13.16 = Ebers 753: 89.22–23
Another: bitter almonds (?) cook with an herbal decoction and drink up.

Case Hearst 211: 13.16–13.17
Driving away the *nesyt* disease from the abdomen: the *ihu* fruits, carob pod,
fennel, sweet beer. Mix together and drink up.

Case Hearst 228: 15.6–15.8
Remedy for calming of the blood vessels (*metu*) in any limb of
a person: wax **1**, fat **1**, pine nuts **1**, yellow nutsedge **1**, incense **1**, coriander
    seeds **1**, bryony (**1**), camphor **1**, the *sar* plant fruit **1**,
myrtle **1**, galenite **1**. Cook together and apply on it, first smear with myrrh.

Case Hearst 229: 15.8–15.10
Another remedy: incense **1**, wax **1**, honey **1**,
goose oil **1**, red clay **1**, wild mint **1**, galenite **1**, calamine **1**, myrrh **1**, fine myrrh
    oil **1**. Cook together and apply on it, until
he recovers.

Case Hearst 230: 15.10
Another remedy for calming of the blood vessels (*metu*) in any limb of a per-
    son: camphor **1**, incense **1**, sorghum **1**, natron **1**, honey **1**. Cook and apply on it.

Case Hearst 231: 15.10–15.11
Another
remedy: wax **1**, fat **1**, myrrh **1**, wild mint **1**, hematite **1**, galenite **1**, incense **1**.
    Cook and apply on it for four days.

Case Hearst 232: 15.11–15.13
Remedy for easing of
the blood vessels (*metu*) in any limb of a man or woman: goose oil **1**,

incen[se 1], [wa]x 1, sweet myrrh 1, dried myrrh 1, yellow nutsedge 1, hematite 1,

galenite 1. Mix together, cook, and apply on it for [fou]r days.

Case Hearst 237: 16.1–16.2

Another remedy for calming of the blood vessels (*metu*): fat 1, wine sediment 1, garlic 1, soot from the wall 1,

bryony fruit 1, the leek fruit 1, the Upper Egyptian *sia* stone 1, fresh incense 1, sweet myrrh 1. Cook together and apply on it.

Case Hearst 238: 16.2–16.4

Another

remedy for cooling of the blood vessels (*metu*) in any limb: jujube leaves 1, willow leaves 1, acacia leaves 1, Lower Egyptian salt 1, the leek fruit 1. Grind finely and apply on it for four days.

Case Hearst 247: 16.11–16.12 = Ebers 612: 77.15–77.17

[. . .]

[aching . . .] the *mesta* drink 1, the *shasha* fruits 1 [. . .] on it for four days.

Case Hearst 249: 16.13–16.14

[Another remedy] for cooling of the blood vessels (*metu*) [. . .]:

[. . .] 1, flour from the *amam* grain 1, acacia leaves 1, flour from [. . .], [app]ly on it.

Case Hearst 250: 16.14–16.17

Another remedy [. . .]

1, coriander seeds 1, pomace 1, sycomore leaves 1, [. . .] 1, date seeds 1, natron 1, [. . .] 1, leaves of the tree *ihy* 1 [. . .]. Apply on it.

Case Hearst 251: 16.17–17.3

Another remedy for coo[ling . . .] [. . .]

the *tjun* plant [. . .], sweet [beer], fat, and [. . .] fat, male [. . .], salt [. . .], sycomore [. . .].

Case Hearst 252: 17.3–17.4

[. . .] kneecap, when it is aching: leaves [. . .] them [. . .].

Papyrus Louvre E4864

Case Louvre E4864, rs 2.4

Remedy for the extermination of a tapeworm in the abdomen: Lower
Egyptian salt, natron, bitter almonds (?) [. . .].

Papyrus London BM 10059

Case London 5: 2.4–3.1

Incantation for the *nesyt* (disease) [. . .]: "tired who comes to the south, tired
who sails to the north [. . .]

you destroy his bones. I do not say, let (them) come to Iunu (= Heliopolis), the
city of Re, the region, where he resides, to Lower Egypt, to [. . .].

What I have found [. . .] drive away [. . .] as he who drives away Nesy and
Nesyt, which are in the body of the N born of N [. . .]

[. . .] life (?) [. . .] and Nesyt [. . .] high [. . .] I give attention [. . .]

[. . .] Bebi before[. . .] amblyopia, which is in [. . .]

[. . .] any [Nesy] and Nesyt, since Nesy [. . .] crosses the primeval ocean [. . .]
find [. . .]

[. . .] in [. . .] **four times** in [. . .] his [. . .] fumigate [. . .]

[. . .] then [. . .]

seal from *shetetut* [. . .] they [. . .] him."

Case London 14: 5.1–6.1

Easing of (what belongs to) the heart (*haty*): limited [. . .] both legs tremble
[. . .]

like women, who come with a male demon of pain and a female demon of pain.
[Destroyed] is the body with beautiful skin, [. . .] Horus, son of Isis [. . .]
Isis [. . .]

the land, when it walks through the land like a jackal. There is not anyone who
would challenge him. I am Wepwawet [. . .] as a child. When they come the
demons of pain [and female demons of pain] to me [. . .]

his [. . .]. Disease, you which were created to cripple, do not approach! Death,
do not reject [. . .] god who sits on his one place, [. . .].

Do not appear against me as the *kaut* blister, as the *serfet* inflammation of the
skin, as the *fenetj* worms, as the *sepy* worms, who come from water. When
they form water [. . .].

When they form the *fenetj* worms, there will not be barley in the whole land,
there will not be offerings to the gods. When the place (around the blisters)
is white [. . .]

[. . .] complete and healthy. The illness thus [. . .]

seven [. . .] in the night barque (*mesketet*) [. . .]

[. . .] withdraws [. . .] (the feast) *denit* [. . .] with the god of the moon, which withdraws [. . .]

[. . .] lean [. . .] they go there, there is not water [. . .]

[. . .] the doors against you [. . .] in this my body and in these [my limbs] [. . .]

[. . .] in these my limbs. They are leav(ing) [. . .] it is not . . .(?) [. . .]

[. . .] red. (It is) their place [. . .] they do not appear in [. . .]

[. . .] fill with water [. . .] divine offerings [. . .]

[. . .] withdraws [. . .] on (the feast of) *denit* [. . .]

[. . .] The Great Ennead, without leaning [. . .]

[. . .] there. Do not fall against [. . .]

[. . .] in this (my) meat, in this my body, in [these my] limbs.

[. . . Recite] this incantation over the base (literally land, which is under foot) [. . .]

[. . .] the pains are enchanted four times. I se[e] [. . .].

Case London 25: 8.8–9.4

Another [. . .] (disease) *nesyt* and (disease) *temyt*: which [Isis] did for her father **in accordance with what was done for** [. . .] the Great Ennead,

which is at the front [of the gods] on the day of the welcoming by the Ennead, which is in the chapel at night, when Osiris opened his mouth to

speak in the *wabet* hall, he says: "My son Horus will fight for me." Thus, his son Horus emerged, who is the Savior of his Father (= Harnedjitef).

In the night, this amulet was found, which came (from heaven) to the great hall of the temple in Gebtu (= Coptos) as the secret of this goddess (= Isis),

by the hand of the lector priest of this sanctuary. When this land was in the darkness, the moon shone over this book on all its journeys.

It was brought as a wonder to His Majesty, King of Upper and Lower Egypt Khufu, the justified. **O these eight** gods, you who came out from

the primeval ocean without clothes and without hair, as for your real names, they are not known: primeval ocean, reed, limitlessness,

darkness, the breath of the demon Khendu, the weapon of the two cobras of the red crown, which destroy non-existence and form the birth, the demon Khendu is for the snake of death, the demon Khepu is for the king. It is he, who will fight for me for the declarations of his father. The joy, which was lacking, is (again) in the cheeks. The cobras (Uraei), which were lacking, are (again) in Dep (= Buto).

. . .(?) Do not descend to N born of N in the night or in the day or in any other time. **This incantation, written down in this book, is to be recited.**

Case London 26: 10.1–10.5

[. . .] The Great Ennead, not to touch with the forehead [. . .]

[. . .] there, they will not fall into [. . .]

[. . .] on this meat on this my body and limbs [. . .].

Case London 37: 13.1–13.3

Incantation for halting blood: "Back, companion of Horus! Back, companion of Seth! The blood is halted, which is coming out from Wenu (=
Hermopolis), the red blood is halted,

which is coming out in (this) hour. You do not know this restraint. Back away
before Thoth!" **This incantation is to be recited over a bead of carnelian
placed into the rectum**

of (a man) or woman. This is the halting of the blood.

Case London 38: 13.3–13.7

This seed, which is of the Weak One (= Osiris Imynehdef), whom Mafdet
accepted into this hall,

where Isis rejoiced and where the testicles of Seth were cut off. Do not hesitate!
Come out, the seed of Horus and the Weak

One (= Osiris), come out against the dead male and the dead female, and others arbitrarily: **The name [of the enemy], the name of his father and the
name of his mother.** O Mafdet, open your mouth (against) this enemy,

[the dead male] and the dead female and the others arbitrarily. Do not let me
see him anytime. **The words recited over the phallus of a donkey from
the *depet* bread, inscribed with the name of the enemy,**

**[the name] of his father, and the name of his mother. To be placed into
meat oil and given to a cat.**

Papyrus Berlin 3038

Case Berlin 1: 1.1

[. . .] drink up. They come out from his rectum immediately.

Case Berlin 2: 1.1 = Ebers 55: 17.9–17.13

Another: date seeds **1/8**, carob flour **1/8**, sweet beer **1/16 1/64** (a measure).
Cook and drink up. It comes out immediately!

Case Berlin 3: 1.2

Another: the *aam* plant, *Anacyclus*. Grind finely with sweet beer. Drunk up by
the (sick) person.

Case Berlin 4: 1.2–1.3 = Ebers 59: 18.7–18.15

Another: the *wam* fruits **1/4**, the *shenfet* fruits **1/4**, the *kher* of the *Avicennia* **1/8**, honey **1/8**, beer **1/64** (a measure).

Pound together, for the night mix with honey. You get up early to [. . .] it. Drink for one day.

Case Berlin 5: 1.3–1.4

Another (remedy) for the extermination of a tapeworm

in the abdomen: the *kher* of the *bekheb* tree, the *djesret* beer **1/16** (a measure). Cook, press, and drink up.

Case Berlin 6: 1.4–1. 5

Another (remedy) for extermination of a tapeworm: the root of the pomegranate tree, the *kher* of *Avicennia*, the *tjehu* of

Moringa. Get up early, pound in a stone mortar with water. To be drunk up by the (sick) person, who (then) spends the night on an empty stomach.

Case Berlin 7: 1.5–1.6

Another: fresh incense, honey, wine.

Merge together. To be drunk by the (sick) person for one day.

Case Berlin 8: 1.6

Another: the *wam* fruits, cumin, [. . .]. Prepare as a morning drink [. . .] swallowed (?) by the (sick) person.

Case Berlin 9: 1.6–1.7

Another, similar to that: the *wam* fruits. Grind finely in a fermented [herbal decoction], strain [. . .].

Case Berlin 10: 1.7–1.9

[. . .] [. . .] dried [root of the pome]granate tree, [. . .]
you [pound] it in a stone mortar [. . .] the root of the pomegranate tree **1/4** [. . .]
[. . .].

Case Berlin 11: 1.9

[. . .] [. . .] **1/4** [. . .] eaten by the (sick) person.

Case Berlin 12: 1.9–1.11

[. . .]

[. . .] **1/4**, honey **1/4**,
[. . .].

Case Berlin 29: 3.5
Remedy for driving away cough: fresh cow sour milk, honey. Eaten by the (sick) person for four days.

Case Berlin 31: 3.6–3.7
Another (remedy) for driving away cough: sour milk, cumin. Soak in honey and give it to (the sick) person to eat for four days.

Case Berlin 32: 3.7
Another: the *shenfet* fruits **1/16**, peas **1/16**, wormwood **1/8**, herbal decoction **1/4**; equally.

Case Berlin 33: 3.7–3.8
Another: gum **1/4**, honey **1/4**; cook. To be eaten by the (sick) person.

Case Berlin 34: 3.8
Another: squeezed dates **1/32** (a measure), honey **1/64** (a measure), sour milk **1/64** (a measure). Mix together and eat for four days.

Case Berlin 36: 3.11–3.12
Another (remedy) for mitigating a fit of coughing: *Melilotus* **1**, sweet beer **1**, oil **1**, myrtle **1**, fermented herbal decoction **1**. Mix [. . .] [. . .] for four days.

Case Berlin 37: 3.12
Another good (remedy) for cough: carob pod **1/16**, milk **1/64** (a measure), white gum **1/32**, honey **1/8**; equally.

Case Berlin 38: 3.12–4.1
Another (remedy) for [. . .]
a fit of coughing: milk, sour milk, milk fat. Drunk by the man or woman for four days.

Case Berlin 39: 4.1–4.2
Another: wine,

Lower Egyptian salt. Grind finely and drink for four days.

Case Berlin 40: 4.2
Another: acacia leaf, honey, sweet beer. Drunk up by the (sick) person.

Case Berlin 41: 4.2
Another: sour milk, cumin. Eat.

Case Berlin 42: 4.3–4.4
Another: pig oil **1/64** (a measure), six-row barley **1/64** (a measure), goose
  oil **1/64** (a measure). Cook, (expose) for the night to the dew and (eat)
  for four days. To be prepared for the man and woman who suffer heat
of the abdomen (?).

Case Berlin 43: 4.4
Another: carob juice, honey; drink up.

Case Berlin 44: 4.4–4.5
Another remedy for driving away cough: the *shenfet* fruits, peas, worm-
  wood, herbal decoction.
Cook and eat for four days.

Case Berlin 45: 4.5
Another: carob pod, *meqret* from the edge of the water, barley flour. Grind
  finely. To be eaten by the (sick) person. Really excellent!

Case Berlin 46: 4.5–4.8
Another: alum,
nehesh (or donkey's tooth?). Grind with wormwood and place on seven
  potter's wheels. You place (it) into a bowl on a bowl (= the fumigation
  vessel), the upper one has been
drilled. You put in it yellow nutsedge, its (other) end is in the mouth of the
  (sick) person, swallowed along with the *peseg* beer by the (sick) person.
Do (this) and you will see (success).

Case Berlin 47: 4.8
Another good (remedy) for cough: sour milk, cumin. Soak in honey.
  Swallowed by the (sick) person for four days.

Case Berlin 48: 4.8–4.11
Remedy

for driving away mucuses in both of his sides: you give him carob pod
to eat for four days, cooked with water, and you prepare (a remedy):
both halves of *pesedj* fruit **1/8**, wormwood (?)
[. . .] fermented [herbal decoction] **1/8**, the *shasha* fruits [. . .] [. . .] **1/8**,
[. . .] **1/8**, cumin **1/64**,
sweet beer **1/16 1/64** (a measure). Cook and drink for four days.

Case Berlin 49: 4.11–4.12 = Ebers 659: 82.16–82.17
Another (remedy) for ea[sing. . .] myrtle [. . .], [. . .], beef spleen, incense, beans.
Cook together and apply on it.

Case Berlin 50: 4.12 = Hearst 117: 8.16 = Ebers 660: 82.18–82.19
Another (remedy): onion [watermelon, Lower Egyptian salt, . . .];
equally.

Case Berlin 51: 4.12–5.1
Another remedy for improvement of calming of blood vessels (*metu*):
myrtle, myrrh, garlic, honey, sweet *Moringa* oil, incense, camphor, flour
from the *bay* fruit, wine. Apply on it for four days.

Case Berlin 56: 5.7–5.8
Another (remedy) for overcoming a *hema* lump
in the lower belly: cracked sycomore fruits **1/8**, carob pod **1/8**, sweet beer
1/32 1/64 (a measure). Drink up.

Case Berlin 58: 5.9–5.11
Another remedy for driving away poisonous substances of a god or
goddess **and poison of a dead male or dead female, driving away**
the tiredness of the heart (*ib*),
[. . .] **of the heart (*haty*) and driving away the forgetfulness of the**
heart (*ib*): beans, fennel, carob pod, *Ricinus* seeds,
[. . .] wild rue seeds. Cook, fumigate (with this the sick) person [. . .].

Case Berlin 59: 5.11–5.12
Another: myrtle, cockroach (or burying beetle?), bryony fruits, wild rue,
the *wam* plant, hemp, the part *mut* of a spinner's mallet (?). Fumigate the
(sick) person with this.

Case Berlin 60: 5,12–6,1

Another: myrtle, lichen from the wall. Place on seven
potter's wheels. Burn with fire, douse with an herbal decoction and girl's
urine. Fumigate the (sick) person with this.

Case Berlin 61: 6.1–6.2

Another: reed,
Anacyclus, pine nuts. Fumigate the (sick) person with this.

Case Berlin 62: 6.2

Another: reed, *Anacyclus*, thyme (?), honey; equally.

Case Berlin 63: 6.3

Another: myrtle, (stone) great protection, scraping stone, fat of a small
cattle. Place (on) fire and fumigate.

Case Berlin 64: 6.3–6.5

Another: honey, fresh moringa oil,
Lower Egyptian salt, girl's urine, donkey dung, tomcat feces, pig's feces,
thyme (?), myrtle. Grind together
and fumigate the (sick) person with this.

Case Berlin 65: 6.5

Another: the *niania* plant; grind finely with fresh moringa oil and (the stone)
great protection. Smear all the doors and all the windows with this.

Case Berlin 74: 7.1–7.2

Fumigation for
driving away the painful substances and all pains: myrtle, lichen, fumigate the person with this.

Case Berlin 77: 7.5

Remedy for treating the heart (of a person) stung (by a scorpion): the
ineb plant, raisins, orpiment, cracked sycamore fruits, hematite, wax,
earth almonds. Fumigate (the stung) person with this.

Case Berlin 109: 9.6–9.7

An ointment for driving away the *nesyt* disease: bryony; cook with pig oil
and girl's urine.

Smear the (sick) person with this.

Case Berlin 110: 9.7
Another: goat's blood, wine. Drink up.

Case Berlin 111: 9.7
Another: watermelon, wine. Drink up.

Case Berlin 112: 9.7–9.8
What is prepared

for a person who is suffering from the *nesyt* disease (demon), which comes from outside: root of the *shas* plant, black powder from the thigh of a draft animal (horse). Smear the (sick) person with this.

Case Berlin 113: 9.9
Another: the best oil of small cattle and fresh *Moringa* oil. Smear with this.

Case Berlin 114: 9.9–9.10
Remedy for driving away the case

of the poisonous substances in the heart (*haty*): figs, grapes, cracked sycomore fruits, honey, cow milk. Cook and press. Drunk up by the (sick) person.

Case Berlin 115: 9.11–9.12
Another: *Anacyclus*, coriander, the *shasha* fruits, wild mint, peas, pine nuts, sorghum. Cook with honey.

Eaten by the (sick) person. (This is) the driving away of all evil substances in the heart (*ib*) of a person.

Case Berlin 116: 9.12–10.2
Another: pine nuts, yellow nutsedge, the *shasha* fruits, (the stone) great protection,

human milk. Drunk up by the (sick) person each morning. This is an effective (remedy for) driving away the painful substances, which tremble (as if) attacked by a dead male or dead female. **What is prepared before**

sleeping: yellow nutsedge, pine nuts, the *shasha* fruits, honey. Eat before sleeping.

Case Berlin 117: 10.2–10.3
Remedy for the effective treatment of the heart: figs **1**,

ocher **1/32**, acacia leaves **1/32**, honey **1/64**, water **1/16 1/64**. Press, leave for the night (exposed) to the dew, and drink for four days.

Case Berlin 119: 10.5–10.7
Remedy for driving away the symp-
toms of painful substances in the tips of all the limbs: figs **1/8**, raisins **1/8**, dates **1/8**, wheat **1/8**, gum **1/16**, water **1/64** (a measure). Leave for the night (exposed) to the dew,
press, and drink for four days.

Case Berlin 120: 10.7–10.9
Another (remedy) for driving away the manifestations of painful substances in both legs: fatty meat half **1/64** (a measure), wine **1/64** (a measure), dates **1/4**, both halves of the *pesedj* fruit **1/4**,
fresh bread **1/8**, juniper berries **1/32**, incense **1/64**, cumin **1/64**, thyme (?) **1/8**, sweet beer **1/16** (a measure). Cook and drink for four days. When he drinks it up, he is to spend his time walking here and there.

Case Berlin 121: 10.9–10.10
Another (remedy) to be prepared after this remedy as an ointment for application: the *afed* part from a goat's leg,
sawdust of the *aru* tree. Grind finely, smear with this many times after drinking up. (This is) destruction of the painful substances in both legs.

Case Berlin 122: 10.10–10.11
Another (remedy) for calming the blood vessels (*metu*) of
the calf and driving away swelling: carob flour, date juice purée, honey. Apply on it.

Case Berlin 123: 10.11–10.12
Another (remedy) for driving away pain in the calf:
bile of a dwarf antelope and bile of a tilapia, apply on it.

Case Berlin 124: 10.12
Another: the plant "donkey phallus"; blend with oil and apply on it.

Case Berlin 125: 11.1
Remedy for driving away swelling in both legs: sorghum, honey, wine. Apply on it.

Case Berlin 126: 11.1–11.2

Another: *aat* vessel of wine from Djahi (= Palestine). Grind with vinegar, apply on it.

Case Berlin 127: 11.2

Another: the *tekhu* plant fruit, honey, wine. Apply on it.

Case Berlin 128: 11.2

Another: the *shebeb* plant, the *tekhu* plant fruit, wine. Apply on it.

Case Berlin 129: 11.2–11.3

Another: the *shasha* plant, natron, honey.
Apply on it.

Case Berlin 130: 11.3

Another: natron, fine (literally sweet) fat, date juice purée. Apply on it.

Case Berlin 131: 11.3

Another: acacia leaf, jujube leaf, ocher, honey. Apply on it.

Case Berlin 132: 11.3–11.4

Another: acacia
leaf, ocher, oil. Apply on it.

Case Berlin 133: 11.4

Another: juniper berries, natron, honey. Apply on it.

Case Berlin 134: 11.4

Another: juniper berries, the pea fruit, honey. Apply on it.

Case Berlin 135: 11.5

Another: ground fennel, the *nesty* of the barley malt. Apply on it.

Case Berlin 136: 11.5–11.6 = Ebers 297: 52.7–52.10

Remedy for driving away mucuses from the abdomen and from any limb:
figs **1/8**, raisins **1/16**, cumin **1/64**,
acacia leaves **1/64**, red ocher **1/64**, the *niaia* plant **1/32**, arugula **1/8**, sweet beer **1/8**. Leave overnight (exposed) to the dew, drink for four days.

Case Berlin 137: 11.6–11.7

Another: barley juice, thickening
to **six 1/64** (a measure).

Case Berlin 138: 11.7–11.11

**Remedy for assuring that all of the mucuses leave, which are wandering in
the meat of a person:** crushed barley **1/64** (a measure), podded carob **half
1/64** (a measure), wormwood **1/32**,

the *aam* plant **1/32**, juniper berries **1/16**, carob pod **1/32**, pine nuts **1/32**, resinous gum **1/32**, water **1/16** *hin*. For the night (expose) to the dew, wash the
crushed barley,

and leave all of that remedy for the night (exposed) to the dew. In the morning, you get up early to put on the pot with water **5** *hin*. Then you make it
thicken **5** *hin*. You place

it on the fire, and you also add to that another **11** *hin* and **13** *hin*. Then cook it,
until the thickening occurs. You remove

it (from the fire) and strain it through a cloth in the very early morning. Drink
for four days.

Case Berlin 139: 11.11–11.12

**Remedy for driving away mucuses when it hurts in the summer or winter
in any limb:** incense, fallow deer's antler. Grate with sweet beer, spread both
his sides with this.

Case Berlin 140: 11.12–12.1

**Remedy for driving away mucuses which hurt
in any limb in the winter:** the *ished* fruits **1/64** (a measure), bread from jujube
1/64 (a measure), oil **1/4**, honey **1/4**. Apply on it.

Case Berlin 141: 12.1–12.2

Another: jujube leaf **1/64** (a measure),
myrtle leaf **1/64** (a measure), mash **1/4**, beef fat **half 1/64** (a measure), sawdust
of the cedar **1/64** (a measure). Apply on it.

Case Berlin 142: 12.2–12.3

**Remedy for driving away mucuses which hurt
in the lower part of the left or right breast:** myrtle, mash. Apply on it for
four days.

Case Berlin 143: 12.3–12.4

**Another (remedy) for driving away mucuses in the urina-
tion:** the *sheny-ta* seeds **1/8**, sweet beer **1/64** (a measure). Drink for one day.

Case Berlin 144: 12.4

Another: the *sheny-ta* seeds **1/8**, honey **1/4**. Drink for one day.

Case Berlin 145: 12.4–12.5

Another: the *sheny-ta* seeds **1/8**, honey **1/4**,
milk **1/64** (a measure). Drink for one day.

Case Berlin 146: 12.5

Another: the *aam* plant **1/32**, carob flour **1/8**, honey **1/8**, the *sheny-ta* seeds **1/8**.
Eat for one day.

Case Berlin 147: 12.5–12.6

Another:
wine **1/64** (a measure), honey **1/8**, the *sheny-ta* seeds **1/8**. Drink for one day.

Case Berlin 148: 12.6–12.8

Remedy for driving away all the bad things which are in the abdomen: herbal
decoction **1/16** (a measure)
the *aamu* plant **1/32**, the *sheny-ta* seeds **1/8**, yellow nutsedge **1/32**, juniper berries
1/16, incense **1/64**, Lower Egyptian salt **1/32**.
Cook, thickening to **half of 1/64** (a measure), and drink for one day.

Case Berlin 149: 12.8–12.9

**Another (remedy) for driving away constipation in the abdomen when it does
not come out:** a male herbal decoction **1**, pomace **1**,
the *sheny-ta* seeds **1**, beer **1**. Drink for one day.

Case Berlin 150: 12.9–12.10

Another (remedy) for driving away blood from the abdomen: the *henen* of
date **1**, beer **1**, the *aam* plant **1**,
oil **1**. Cook. (To be drunk up by the sick) person. Really excellent!

Case Berlin 153: 12.12–13.3

**Examination of the wandering
of excessive painful substances in his limbs.** You prepare for him a medicine for

the extermination of the painful substances and a medicine for the wandering
of the painful substances in his abdomen: fresh fatty

meat **1/64** (a measure), thyme (?) **1/8**, mountain celery **1/16**, incense **1/64**, fresh
bread **1/64**, the *sekhpet* drink **1/16** (a measure), bread from the jujube **1/8**.
Grind finely, cook, and make (from that) the *shat* cake. Eaten by

the person and sweet beer drunk for four days.

Case Berlin 154: 13.3–13.8

Another (remedy for) a deposit (literally a nest) of traveling heat: his abdomen is heavy, his stomach aches, his heart (*ib*) is hot and stings,

his clothing is heavy for him and he does not bear many clothes; his heart (*ib*)
is dark; he feels (literally tastes) his heart (*haty*), which is clouded like (in) a
person who ate

the cracked sycomore fruits; his meat is tired like (with) a person who managed
a distance; when he sits down for excretion, he has a heavy rectum, and it is
not in order

when he passes a stool. You say on him: he has a deposit of the painful substances
in his abdomen, he feels his heart (*haty*). A disease with which I will fight.

When (the deposit) rises in him and a clogging appears, **you prepare for him a
medicine for the treatment of the painful substances and a medicine for
overcoming the painful substances in his abdomen:** earth almonds grind
with water **1/64** (a measure), fresh mash **1/8**, dates

in the white (state) **1/4**, juniper berries **1/16**, *djernet* **1/32**, honey **1/4**, milk **1/8**, the
ished fruits **1/8**, foam (or water for washing) **1/16** (a measure). Grind finely,
(he will get well) quickly.

Case Berlin 155: 13.8–13.10

Another: raw

meat **1/4**, both halves of the *pesedj* fruit **1/8**, thyme (?) **1/8**, the *aam* plant **1/16**,
juniper berries **1/32**, *Potentilla* **1/16**, the *ished* fruits **1/32**, grapes **1/8**, figs **1/8**,
incense **1/64**, the *shenfet* fruits, the *wedja* of dates **1/32**, goose oil **1/8**, sweet beer
1/16 1/64 (a measure). Grind finely, press, and drink for four days.

Case Berlin 156: 13.10–13.11

Another: the *sheny-ta* seeds **1/8**, honey **1/8**,
sweet beer **1/64** (a measure). Drink for four days.

Case Berlin 157: 13.11–14.3

Remedy for mobilizing his repletion, which makes his abdomen heavy.

Prepare for him a medicine for overcoming the painful substances

in the abdomen and turning away the painful substances: figs **1/8**, the *ished* fruits **1/8**, grapes **1/8**, juniper berries **1/16**, *Potentilla* **1/32**, *pesedj* fruit **1/8**, thyme (?) **1/8**, cracked sycomore fruits **1/4**,

incense **1/64**, *Melilotus* **1/8**, mountain celery **1/8**, Lower Egyptian celery **1/32**, fresh bread **1/8**, fatty meat **1/64** (a measure), the *amau* plant **half 1/64** (a measure), goose oil **1/8**, sweet beer **1/16 1/64** (a measure).

Grind, press, and drink for four days.

Case Berlin 158: 14.3–14.4

Examination of a person whose abdomen is distended and mobilizing his repletion. Prepare for him a medicine for removing the painful substances

from the abdomen: the *aam* plant **1/8**, the *ished* fruits **1/8**, goose oil **1/8**, sweet beer **1/16 1/64** (a measure). Grind finely, press, and drink for four days.

Case Berlin 159: 14.4–14.5

Another: *Moringa* oil **1/8**, honey **1/8**, jujube leaves

1/8, acacia leaves **1/8**, myrtle leaves **1/8**. Leave for the night (exposed) to the dew, mash with water, and pour into the rectum for one day.

Case Berlin 160: 14.5–14.6

Another: the *ished* fruits **1/8**, figs **1/8**, *Potentilla* **1/8**,

sweet beer **1/16 1/64** (a measure); cook. Drunk up by the person with this disease.

Case Berlin 161: 14.6–14.9

When you examine a person who has symptoms of the painful substances on the tips of both his hands so that the painful substances travel

here and there. When you examine a person with symptoms of the painful substances on the tips of both his hands, he has agony in his face and moreover his meat looks like worms,

Moringa oil of his blood is in his meat, acting against him. You say on that: he has the symptoms of the painful substances on the tips of his hands. A disease which I will treat. **You prepare for him**

a mash from barley, he will eat (it) every day, but do not give him anything hot to eat.

Case Berlin 162: 14.9–14.11

Another: thyme (?) **1/8**, fatty meat **1/64** (a measure), both halves of the *pesedj* fruit **1/16**,

Melilotus **1/8**, the *temem* of dates **1/8**, the *shenfet* fruits (?) **1/8**, incense **1/32**, cumin **1/32**, juniper berries **1/16**, sweet beer **1/16** (a measure), the *djesret* beer **1/16** (a measure), *sau* of dates

1/8. Leave for the night (exposed) to the dew, press. To be drunk by the person for four days.

Case Berlin 163a: 15.1–15.5

Beginning of the collection for understanding the painful substances, which was found among the ancient books in the chest for documents under the feet of Anubis

in Sekhemu (Letopolis) at the time of His Majesty, King of Upper and Lower Egypt Den, the justified, when he aged. It was brought to His Majesty, King of Upper and Lower Egypt Senedj, the justified

because of its exceptional nature. This book set loose immobile legs, through the scribe of the divine words, the great of the excellent physicians, who pleased god.

What was performed (because of this) book, was a procession at sunrise and offerings of bread, beer, and incense on the fire in the name of Isis the Great, Horus Khentykherty,

Khonsu, Thoth, and the god(-child), who is in the abdomen (of his mother).

Case Berlin 163b: 15.5–15.6

Instructions for a person (against) all diseases which appear in him. His head has inside twenty-two arteries (*metu*), which lead

the air (winds) to his heart (*haty*), and they are the ones who provide air to all of his limbs.

Case Berlin 163c: 15.6–15.8

Two arteries (*metwy*) are in his (two) breasts. They are the ones who provide heat to the rectum.

What is prepared for them as a medicine: fresh dates, *hemu* of *Ricinus*, seeds (?) of the sycomore, water; pound

together and (give) to the person to drink up. He gets well in four days.

Case Berlin 163d: 15.8–15.9

Two arteries (*metwy*) are in his two thighs. When both of his thighs hurt and both of his arms are flaccid, it is

an arterial braid of his thighs which is causing the disease.

What is prepared for him as a medicine: myrtle, water for
washing, dill seeds, blend with honey, apply to the neck. (He will) get well
in four days.

Two blood vessels (*metwy*) are in his
upper arm. When his shoulder hurts and he has mucuses in his fingers, **you
say on it**: this is mucuses. **What is prepared for that as a medicine:**
this is for (inducing) vomiting: fish and wild rue or meat. When you do it, you
say: **(this is) a medicine, prepared for him**. You apply
on his fingers: watermelon and strong beer. The relief in his arms (comes) in
four days.

**Two blood vessels (*metwy*) are of his neck, two blood vessels (*metwy*) are
of his forehead,**
**two blood vessels (*metwy*) are in his eyes, two blood vessels (*metwy*) are in
his eyebrows, two blood vessels (*metwy*) are in his nostrils, two blood
vessels (*metwy*) are in his right**
ear, the breath of life comes into them, **two blood vessels (*metwy*) are in his
left ear**, the breath (of death) comes into them.

They go jointly to
his heart (*haty*), they divide at his nose and join in his rectum. The disease
of his rectum appears in them, with excretion they cause its arrival, death
begins with the blood vessels (*metu*) of his two legs.

What is prepared as a remedy, it is a remedy acquired from an outstanding
physician, who satisfies god:
First prepare cow milk **eight times 1/64 (a measure)**, place into a pot. When
it first rises up, then it is hot.
Add vinegar, strain through a cloth, add to that honey **1/4**. Drink for four
days.

What is prepared afterwards: milk of a small cattle,

which is boiled **four times 1/64** (a measure), honey **1/4 equally**. You add "milk fat" of oil **half 1/64** (a measure) or human milk **half 1/64** (a measure). Pour

into his rectum, he remains lying until daybreak.

Case Berlin 163h: 16.9–16.10

What is prepared afterwards: fresh *Moringa* oil **1/4**, honey **1/4**, fermented herbal decoction

three times 1/64 (a measure), Lower Egyptian salt **1/16**. Pour into the rectum for four days.

Case Berlin 163h: 16.10–16.11

What is prepared afterwards: honey **half 1/64** (a measure), fresh *Moringa* oil **half 1/64** (a measure),

fermented herbal decoction **1/16** (a measure), sweet beer **1/64** (a measure), Lower Egyptian salt **1/8**. Pour into the rectum for four days.

Case Berlin 163h: 16.11–16.12

What is prepared afterwards:

fresh *Moringa* oil **half 1/64** (a measure), sweet beer **1/16 1/64** (a measure), Lower Egyptian salt **1/8**. Pour into the rectum for four days.

Case Berlin 163h: 16.12–17.1

What is prepared afterwards:

honey **half 1/64** (a measure), *Moringa* oil **1/4**, sweet beer **1/64 1/64** (a measure). Pour into the rectum for four days.

Case Berlin 164: 17.1–17.6

Remedy for driving away

the painful substances in the abdomen, retention of the painful substances and constipation of the rectum: honey **1/4**, *Moringa* oil **1/8**,

sweet beer **1/64 1/64** (a measure). Pour into the rectum for four days. **The art of the physicians:** honey **1/64** (a measure), *Moringa* oil **1/64** (a measure), herbal decoction **1/16** (a measure),

Lower Egyptian salt 1/16. Pour into the rectum for four days. **What is prepared against that as a remedy afterwards, when he has constipation,**

to cause it to leave: flour from beans strained through a cloth **half 1/64** (a measure), boiled water **1/16** (a measure). Pour

into the rectum, so that it leaves quickly. Really excellent!

Case Berlin 165: 17.6–17.7

Remedy for a person, who excretes large amounts of blood:

honey **half 1/64** (a measure), fresh *Moringa* oil **1/4**, sweet beer **1/64 1/64** (a measure). Pour into the rectum for four days.

Case Berlin 166: 17.7–17.8

What is prepared for a person

having pain during urination: fresh *Moringa* oil **1/4**, Lower Egyptian salt **1/16**, herbal decoction **1/16 1/64** (a measure). Pour (into the rectum) for four days.

Case Berlin 167: 17.9–17.10

Remedy for a person with the evil *qesnet* disease: human milk **1/64** (a measure), *Moringa* oil **1/64** (a measure), oil **1/16 1/64** (a measure), Lower Egyptian salt **1/16**, herbal decoction **1/16** (a measure). Pour into the rectum for four days.

Case Berlin 168: 17.10–18.1

Remedy for driving away the painful substances:

fresh *Moringa* oil **1/8**, honey **1/8**, acacia leaves **8 *ro***, jujube leaves **1/8**, myrtle **1/8**, sweet beer **1/16 1/64** (a measure). Pour into the rectum for four days.

Case Berlin 169: 18.1–18.2

Remedy for the *henhenet* lump on both legs: honey **1/4**, fresh *Moringa* oil half **1/64** (a measure),

Lower Egyptian salt **1/32**, sweet beer **1/16 1/64**. Pour into the rectum for four days.

Case Berlin 170: 18.2–18.3

Remedy for overcoming the painful substances in the abdomen: *Moringa* oil **1/4**, herbal decoction

1/64 and half 1/64 (a measure). Pour into the rectum for four days.

Case Berlin 171: 18.3–18.4

What is prepared (for) urination, when it aches: honey **1/8**, fresh *Moringa* oil **1/4**, "milk fat" of oil **1/8**,

Lower Egyptian salt **1/16**, herbal decoction **1/16** (a measure). Pour into the rectum for four days.

Case Berlin 172: 18.4–18.6

Good remedy for the *khayt* disease: fresh *Moringa* oil **1/8**, honey **1/8**, oil **1/64** (a measure), "milk fat" of oil **1/64 1/64** (a measure), human milk **1/64** (a measure), sweet beer **1/64** (a measure), Lower Egyptian salt **1/16**.

Pour into the rectum for four days.

Case Berlin 173: 18.6–18.7

Another (remedy) for any kind of evil *qesnet* disease: "milk fat" of oil **1/64** (a measure), Lower Egyptian salt **1/8**,

carob juice **1/64 1/64** (a measure), sweet beer **1/64** (a measure). Pour into the rectum for four days.

Case Berlin 174: 18.7–18.9

Another remedy for a blood vessel (*met*) which itself quivers and hurts when walking,

and for breaking the painful substances: *Moringa* oil **1/64** (a measure), honey **1/4** (a measure), oil **1/64** (a measure), Lower Egyptian salt **1/16**, sweet beer **1/64** (a measure). Pour

into the rectum for four days. **Another (remedy) afterwards:** *Moringa* oil **1/4** (a measure), honey **1/4** (a measure), sweet beer **1/64** (a measure). Pour into the rectum for four days.

Case Berlin 175: 18.10–18.11

Another: fennel grind with water and strain **1/64 and 1/64** (a measure), honey **half 1/64** (a measure), *Moringa* oil **half 1/64** (a measure), sweet beer **1/64** (a measure). Grind finely and pour

into the rectum for four days.

Case Berlin 176: 18.11–18.12

Another: carob juice **1/64 and 1/64** (a measure), honey **half 1/64** (a measure), sweet beer **1/64 and 1/64** (a measure).

Pour into the rectum for four days.

Case Berlin 177: 18.12–19.1

Another: honey **1/4**, *Moringa* oil **1/8**, Lower Egyptian salt **1/4**, the *debyt* drink from sweet date

mash **three 1/64** (a measure). Pour into the rectum for four days.

Case Berlin 178: 19.1–19.2

Another: honey **1/4**, Lower Egyptian salt **half 1/64** (a measure), the *debyt*

drink from sweet date mash **three 1/64** (a measure).
Pour into the rectum for four days.

Remedy for

driving away the *shepen* disease in the urine: wine **1/64** (a measure), a grain of copper **1/32**, Lower Egyptian salt **1/32**. Pour into the rectum for four days.

Remedy for drinking which is prepared when the remedy is in preparation: wheat semolina **1/64** (a measure), water **1/4 1/8 1/16 1/64** (a measure), oil **1/8**,

honey **1/8**. You add its (the relevant) water to the pot. Once it first starts to boil after warming up,

(you add) wheat semolina. Once it again begins to boil after warming up, you add its oil, so that it

cooks with this. You add honey the moment it is thickened to **six times 1/64** (a measure). Leave for the night (exposed) to the dew. Drunk

by the (sick) person.

Red oil. What is prepared as a remedy for the heart after its heat (occurs). The *desher* plant **1/8**,

wheat semolina **1/64** (a measure), pulp of carob pod **1/32**, honey **1/8**, oil **1/8**, water **1/4 1/8 1/16 1/64** (a measure). You add

its (the relevant) water and its semolina into the pot. Once it first begins to cook after warming up, you add the *desher* plant.

As soon as it again begins to boil, you add the pulp of carob pod. As soon as it again begins to boil, you add

its oil, so that it cooks gently. You add honey the moment it is thickened to

six times 1/64 (a measure). Leave for the night (exposed) to the dew, strain through a cloth. To be drunk by the (sick) person for four days.

Another oil: yellow nutsedge **1/64** (a measure), fresh

dates **1/64** (a measure), the *ihu* fruits **1/8**, sorghum **1/64** (a measure), water **1/16** (a measure). Leave overnight (exposed) to the dew. Blend with your hand, strain through a cloth, leave overnight (again exposed) to the dew. To be drunk by the person for four days.

Case Berlin 187: 20.6-20.7
Remedy which is prepared for driving away the painful substances
[. . . excre]tion of blood: goose oil **1/64** (a measure),
the *henen* of date **1/64** (a measure), sweet beer **1/64 1/64** (a measure). For the
night (expose) to the dew, drink for four days.

Case Berlin 188: 20.7-20.9
Another: wormwood (or chaste tree) **half 1/64** (a measure), the
aru tree fruit **1/16**, coriander **1/32**, honey **1/32**, sweet beer **three 1/64** (a measure). For the night (expose) to the dew, pulp with your hand with
that beer, strain through a cloth, and drink for four days.

Case Berlin 189: 20.9-21.3
Spell for the remedy for drinking up: you can wake up well, you who remain
forever!
Driven away is any kind of disease which is before you. Your mouth is opened
by Ptah and your mouth is opened wide by Sokar with the aid of his metal
stylus.
This remedy, be set loose of the burden, away with weakness, he who is on his
stomach will be set loose, as done by Isis, the goddess. The seed of the dead
will be driven away, the dead who is in the limbs of N born of N. **Words
recited by**
Nephthys, they are useful for him (= the sick person), like when the Falcon
eats, like when a bird is struck, like when the sea
listens to Seth's voice.

Case Berlin 190: 21.3-21.9
Spell against an enemy [. . .]: protection is given to me such as the enclosed
earthwork, which Isis (encircled) with the ends of her hair. A fever will not
come down to me, will not divide
(my) body. He will be found, who divides the body, raised the lake, opened the
coffins in Abdju (= Abydos), broke the planks of the divine barque, beat the
waves of the lake. When he is found, he will be destroyed!
I am Horus, who spent the night [. . .]
and who spent the day in Abdju. My staff assures (my) protection. Be greeted,
willow staff, which assures the protection (of my) body, tip (of the rod)
from sacred acacia.

Seven Hathors assure the protection of bodies, so that (my) body [. . .] was
untouched [. . .] like the rise of Re for the land (= Egypt).

(My) protection is my hand, it is Isis the Great, who used the art of Re through
a physician, who pleases the god.

Case Berlin 191: 21.9–21.11

What is prepared for the abdomen when it aches:

I am Horus, son (of Osiris) inside his temple, who comes to see what has happened [. . .] **Recite** over the (abdomen), grind pomace

in water. Drunk up by the (sick) person, and he recovers quickly.

Case Berlin 204: verso 3.1–3.12

[. . .]

Anacyclus fruit **1/64**,

cumin **1/64**,

pine nuts **1/64**,

juniper berries **1/8**,

the *ankh-imy* plant **1/4**,

melilotus **1/32**,

acacia leaves **1/32**,

[. . .] wild rue (?) **1/64**,

honey **1/8**,

sweet beer **two 1/64** (a measure).

Cook on the heat of the ashes.

Drunk up (by the sick) person.

Chester Beatty Papyri
Case Chester Beatty V: verso 4.1–4.9

The book of the incantation of half the head. O Re, Atum, Shu, Tefnut,
Geb,

Nut, Anubis, the foremost of the divine hall, Horus, Seth, [Isis], Nephthys,

The Great Ennead, The Small Ennead! Come and look at your father, who
appears

surrounded by luster [to see] the horn of Sakhmet. Come remo[ve] this enemy,
dead male

and dead female, enemy male and female, [who] are in the face of N born by
N. To be recited over a [croco]dile

from clay with a seed of grain [. . .] in his mouth and with eyes from faïence
in[set] in his head.

[To be bound] together and to have drawn the figures of the gods on a scarf of fine cloth, which is put on his head. Recite (over) a statuette of Re, Atum, Shu, Mehit, Geb, Nut, Anubis, Horus, Seth, Isis, Nephthys,

the oryx with the figure of Horus standing on its back, having a spear.

Case Chester Beatty V: verso 4.10–6.4

Another book for driving away migraine. The head of N born of N is the head of Osiris

Wennefer, on whose head was placed those 377 divine uraei and they spit flames [. . .],

to make you leave the head of N born of N, like (from that) of Osiris. If [you do not leave] the temple of N born of N,

I will burn your [soul] and I will ignite your corpse, I will be deaf to your [. . .] wish toward you, I will have you be seized [. . .] If you are a god, I will demolish [your] sanctuary, I will [. . .]

your tomb, so you could not receive incense [. . .], so you could not receive

water and excell[ent. . .], so you could not meet with the followers [of Horus]. If you do [not heed]

(my) words, [I will have] the heavens overturned, I will set a fire among the Lords of Iunu (= Heliopolis), I will cut off the head of the co[w from] the entrance hall of Hathor, I will cut off the head

of the hippopotamus from the entrance hall of Seth, I will have Sobek seated wrapped

in the skin of a crocodile, I will have Anu[bis] seated [wra]pped [in] the skin of

a dog. I will have the heavens divided in their middle, I will have

the seven [Hathors] fly in smoke to the heavens, I will cut off [. . . , I will have]

the eye of Seth blinded. Well then, leave the temple of N born of [N]. I will prepare [. . .]

an amulet, mentioning their names **on this day. To be recited** over the[se go]ds drawn [on fine] cloth to be placed on the [temple] of a person. **(the symbols follow, depicting a jackal, [. . .] seated god (3×), divine eye (4×) and uraei (4×))**

Case Chester Beatty V: verso 6.5–6.7

Beginning of the incantation of the *hek* disease. Flow out! Leave from the left temple [. . .] you came

. . . [. . .] give your [. . .] far [. . .]. **To be recited seven times,**

and you take your left hand into your right hand, **seven incantations**.

Case Chester Beatty VI.1: recto 1.1–1.7
[. . .]
[re]ctum aching:
milk fat [. . .],
herbs. Grate in a mortar, strain
through a [cl]oth, blend
with honey; form a pellet for
the rectum, until (the sick person) quickly recovers.

Case Chester Beatty VI.2: recto 1.8–2.9
[. . .] the discharge [. . .]
[. . .] the swelling of the ulcers
crushing of the ulcers in
the rectum, soothing the blood vessels
of the rectum, driving away the scratching
[. . .] of a woman:
[. . .] salt,
myrrh [. . .],
salt [. . .],
human milk [. . .],
honey [. . .],
incense [. . .],
goose oil [. . .].
Mix toge[ther] [. . .]
for 2[+ x] days.

Case Chester Beatty VI.3: recto 2.10–3.9
What is prepared against that [. . .]
afterwards: flour from [. . .]
goose oil [. . .]
powder from fri[t. . .]
honey [. . .],
[. . .] 1/12
[. . .] 1/16
[. . .] 1/64
[. . .] 2   4
[. . .] 1   12
[. . .] 1/16
[. . .] 1

[. . .] rectum
[. . .].

Case Chester Beatty VI.4: recto 3.10–3.13
[. . .] rectum
[. . .] **1**
[. . .]
[. . .].

Case Chester Beatty VI.5: recto 4.1–4.10
**Another medicine that is prepared for crush-
ing ulcers:**
scales of sea fish,
yellow nutsedge from oases,
flax leaves,
the *mesta* drink.
Blend together
with this, you make twelve
pellets and place four
pellets into his rectum, until he recovers.

Case Chester Beatty VI.6: recto 4.11–5.5
Another (remedy), which is prepared afterwards: the remnant
fennel 1,
goose oil 1,
honey 1.
Make a sachet from cloth, you make four pellets and one of them is placed in
the rectum every day. If you find
blood behind him, which flows out (like) water, you prepare for him: juniper
berries crush, expose to the dew, apply it on every
(affected) limb, until he recovers. If you find blood behind him, which flows
out for seven days, you make for him a remedy:
galenite, ibex fat, sorghum. Grind finely together, form into four pellets, and
for the night (expose) to the dew. Place
into the rectum, until he recovers.

Case Chester Beatty VI.7: recto 5.5–5.6
Remedy for any kind of thing in the rectum: carob flour **1**, Lower Egyptian
salt **1**, natron **1**,

salt from the east **1**.

Case Chester Beatty VI.8: recto 5.6–5.7
Another (remedy) similar to that: the *khes* of the *ima* tree **1**, carob pod **1**, honey **1**,
natron **1**. Mix together and apply on it for four days.

Case Chester Beatty VI.9: recto 5.7–5.8
Remedy for driving away turning in the rectum: flour from beans,
Lower Egyptian salt, goose oil, decoction from barley, honey. Mix together and apply on the rectum for four days.

Case Chester Beatty VI.10: recto 5.8–5.12
Another remedy
for crushing ulcers, driving away heat in his rectum, in the urinary bladder, on (the body part) *sak-mesha*
of a man or woman: natron **1**, red ocher **1**, incense **1**, cedar oil **1**, honey **1**, dried myrrh **1**, aromatic
myrrh **1**, almond tree nuts **1**, the *tjun* plant fruit **1**, pine nuts **1**, reed **1**, fine fat **1**, sweetgum **1**, the *qeneny* plant **1**,
(tree) [. . .] **1**. Grind finely, apply on it, until he recovers.

Case Chester Beatty VI.11: recto 5.12–6.1
Another remedy for the entry of the urinary bladder, driving away *shen-fet* and driving away
any kind of [disease] in the rectum of a man or woman: sesame oil **1**, oil **1**, honey **1**, Lower Egyptian salt **1**, human
milk **1**. Pour into the rectum for four days.

Case Chester Beatty VI.12: recto 6.1–6.2
What is prepared for application afterwards: myrrh **1**, goose oil **1**, cumin **1**, incense **1**, honey **1**. Mix together, apply on it, until he recovers.

Case Chester Beatty VI.13a: recto 6.2–6.6
When it spews like a scheme (of demons),
ulcers on the urinary bladder, phlegm on his joints, he excretes water between his buttocks, his limbs are
hot and having pain, his urination is agonizing, when it proceeds, his rectum strains and its proceeding

does not end. You say on that: it is the strain of his rectum. A disease which I will fight.

You make a remedy for his recovering:

goose oil **1/64** (a measure), honey **1/64** (a measure), human milk **three 1/64** (a measure). Pour into the rectum for four days.

Case Chester Beatty VI.13b: recto 6.6–6.8

Another remedy to be prepared

afterwards: juice from sorghum **1**, juice from hemp **1**, juice from the *kebu* plant **1**, fresh mash **1**, goose oil **1**, offshoots of

a lotus **1**, acacia leaves **1**. Mix (into) one and pour into the rectum for four days.

Case Chester Beatty VI.14: recto 6.8–6.10

Comprehensive handbook of medicines of a physician. Remedy

for driving away the *ahhu* disease in the chest, tending of his side and cooling of the rectum: earth almonds **1/64** (a measure), fresh dates **1/64** (a measure), gum **1/32**,

juniper berries **1/32**, anise **1/16**, ocher **1/32**, honey **1/32**, water **1/16 1/64**. Press (and drink) for four days.

Case Chester Beatty VI.15: recto 6.10–6.11

What is prepared as an enema (= clyster)

afterwards: old honey **1/64** (a measure), fresh *Moringa* oil **half 1/64** (a measure), Lower Egyptian salt **1/8**, [. . .].

Case Chester Beatty VI.16: recto 6.13A+12

Another remedy for the tending of the chest, cooling of the heart (*haty*), cooling of the rectum and for driving away any kind of her heat: fresh dates **1/64** (a measure), the cracked sycomore fruits **half 1/64** (a measure), grapes **half 1/64** (a measure), sorghum **1/4**, earth almond **1/64** (a measure),

honey **1/4**, water. For the night (expose) to the dew, press, (and drink) for four days.

Case Chester Beatty VI.17: recto 6.12–6.13

What is prepared as an enema afterwards: milk of a small cattle, honey. Pour into the rectum for four days.

Another remedy for cooling of the heart (*haty*), cooling of the rectum, and revival of the arteries (*metu*), which is prepared

in the summer: earth almonds milled **1/64** (a measure), fresh dates **1/64** (a measure), pine nuts **1/16**, a *hemu* of *Ricinus* **half 1/64** (a measure),

honey **1/4**, water **1/16 1/64** (a measure). Drink for four days.

Case Chester Beatty VI.19: recto 7.2–7.3

Another remedy to be prepared afterwards as an enema: honey **half 1/64** (a measure), fresh *Moringa* oil **1/4**,

sweet beer **1/32** (a measure). Pour into the rectum for four days.

Case Chester Beatty VI.20: recto 7.3–7.4

Another remedy for driving away heat in the heart (*haty*): fresh dates **1/64** (a measure), honey **1/4**,

sweet beer **1/32** (a measure). Pour into the rectum for four days.

Case Chester Beatty VI.21: recto 7,4–7.5

Another remedy to be prepared later as an enema: Lower Egyptian salt **1/4**, milk fat **half 1/64** (a measure),

carob juice **1/32** (a measure), sweet beer **1/32 1/64** (a measure). Pour into the rectum for four days.

Case Chester Beatty VI.22: recto 7.5–7.6

Another remedy for cooling of the heart (*haty*), a driving away heat in the rectum: grapes **1/64** (a measure), earth almonds **1/64** (a measure), anise **1/16**, honey **1/8**, water **1/16 1/64** (a measure). Press and drink for four days.

Case Chester Beatty VI.23: recto 7.6–7.8

Another remedy for driving away heat

in the rectum: grape seeds **1/16**, muskmelon leaves **1/16**, fresh dates **1/8**, mash **1/32**, water **1/32** (a measure). For the night (expose) to

the dew and drink for four days.

Case Chester Beatty VI.24: recto 7.8–7.9

Another remedy to be prepared later as an enema (for) driving away heat in the rectum and its cooling: hemp

1/4, carob pod **1/32**, the *mesta* drink **1/16 1/64** (a measure). Pour into the rectum for four days.

Case Chester Beatty VI.25: recto 7.9–7.10

Another remedy, which is prepared for driving away heat in the heart
   (*ḥaty*)

and cooling of the rectum: grapes **1/64** (a measure), bryony fruit **1/64** (a measure), carob pod **1/32**, honey **1/32**, water **1/16**. Press (and drink) for four days.

Case Chester Beatty VI.26: recto 7.10–7.12

Another (remedy),

to be prepared later as an enema: beef brain **1/64** (a measure), cooked milk
   1/64 (a measure), fresh *Moringa* oil **1/32** (a measure), honey **1/64** (a measure). Pour into the rectum
for four days.

Case Chester Beatty VI.27: recto 7.12–7.13

Another remedy for driving away heat: figs **1/8**, the *ished* fruits **1/8**, the
   qesenty stone **1/32**, wheat semolina **1/8**, water **1/64** (a measure). Press
and drink for four days.

Case Chester Beatty VI.28: recto 7.13–7.14

Another remedy to be prepared as an enema: flour from beans **1/3[2]**, salt
   1/32, oil **half 1/64** (a measure), honey **1/4**,
sweet beer **1/16 1/64** (a measure). Pour into the rectum for four days.

Case Chester Beatty VI.29: recto 7.14–8.1

Another (remedy) to be prepared on this day: the *ished* fruits **1/8**, the *qesenty*
   stone **1/32**, wheat semolina **1/8**,
honey **1/32**, water **1/32** (a measure). Press and drink for four days.

Case Chester Beatty VI.30: recto 8.1–8.3

Another remedy to be prepared as an enema [. . .] [. . .]
pine nuts **1/16**, the *shasha* fruits **1/16**, wild mint **1/12**, carob pod **1/12**, the
   cracked sycomore fruits [. . .] into the rectum for
four days.

Case Chester Beatty VI.31: recto 8.3–8.4

Another (remedy) to be prepared as a drink for driving away the burning
   in the painful substances: earth almonds [. . .]
1/4, honey **1/4**, water **1/16 1/64** (a measure). Press and drink for four days.

Case Chester Beatty VI.32: recto 8.4–8.5
Another (remedy) to be prepared afterwards as an enema [. . .]
cooling the sides: figs **1/8**, the *ished* fruits **1/8**, anise **1/8**, grapes [. . .].

Case Chester Beatty VI.33: recto 8.5–8.6
[. . .][. . .]
1/8, barley semolina **1/8**, earth almonds **1/8**, honey **1/8**, ocher **1/32**, water **1/16 1/64** (a measure). Press and drink for four days.

Case Chester Beatty VI.34: recto 8.6–8.7
[. . .]
barley semolina **1/8**, pine nuts, honey **1/8**, water **1/16 1/64** (a measure). Press and drink for four days.

Case Chester Beatty VI.35: recto 8.7–8.8
Another [. . .]
1/8, grapes **half 1/64** (a measure), honey **1/8**, water **1/16 1/64** (a measure). Press and drink for four days.

Case Chester Beatty VI.36: recto 8.8–8.9
Another: figs [. . .],
1/64 (a measure), carob pod **1/32**, grapes **1/8**, garden cress **1/64**, incense **1/64**, water **1/16 1/64** (a measure). Press [. . .].

Case Chester Beatty VI.37: recto 8.9–8.11
[. . .]
in the side: the cracked sycomore fruits **1/8**, grapes **1/8**, garden cress **1/64**, incense **1/64**, cumin [. . .]
sycomore leaves **1/8**, carob pod **1/32**, sweet beer **1/16 1/64** (a measure). For the night (expose) to the dew, press, and drink for four days.

Case Chester Beatty VI.38: recto 8.11–8.13
Another: bile [. . .], Lower Egyptian
salt **1**. Grind finely, form a pellet to be swallowed by the (sick) person. Herbal decoction **1/64** (a measure) [. . .]
sweet [beer] **1/16 1/64** (a measure). Pour into the rectum for four days.

Case Chester Beatty VI.39+40: recto 8.13–8.14
What is prepared after (that as an) enema: the cracked sycomore fruits **1/8**,

the seeds [. . .],
the *ished* fruits **1/8**, water **1/16** (a measure). Press and drink for four days.

Case Chester Beatty VI.41: recto 8.14
What is prepared later as an enema: acacia leaves [. . .].

Case Chester Beatty VI: verso 2.2–2.5
Book for driving away the demon Nesy and female demon Nesyt:
Back! Fall (on) your face! You will not be in the heavens, you will not be on the
earth! You are not in the underworld, and you are not in the primeval ocean,
you are not in the created beings,
you are not in a god or in a goddess! Do not come to N born of N, and do not
enter him! Do not do
to him what your usual scheme is! Beware of his right side(?) and N born of N.

Case Chester Beatty VI: verso 2.5–2.9
Another spell: These four
shining spirits (*akhu*), you are those who patrol over Osiris. The patrol,
which you conduct over Osiris, you will conduct the same way over N born of
N, not to make him killed
by any dead male or any dead female, any male adversary or any female adversary which is in any limb of N born of N. The four gods
is the name of these seven.

Case Chester Beatty VIII: recto 5.1–5.3
[. . .] afterwards: Prepare the offerings for the gods and make a remedy for getting out of the seed of a god from the abdomen of a man or woman
and getting out of a god from the abdomen [. . .] any [dead male] and dead
female, any diseases, against which is prepared: honey **half 1/64** (a measure),
incense **half 1/64** (a measure), fresh *Moringa* oil **half 1/64** (a measure), wine
half 1/64 (a measure).
Drink up by a man or woman.

Papyrus Leiden I 343 + I 345
Case Leiden recto XXVI 12–XXVIII 5
**Another incantation for an inflammation, which appears on the *sedja* part
of the leg:**
[This your blood] is Re's, this your injury is Atu[m's on] the day when your
heads were

cut off in the fields of Iaru. The heavens are broken, the earth rages,

the heavens are in confusion, the earth is suffocating. If you do not heed what
I say, I will not give

him the eye of Horus, I will not give him the testicles of Seth in this land forever. Turning away of the inflammation

is this to drive away the activity, so the gods were reconciled in their sanctuaries.
Driven away was the activity of a god, the activity of a god-

dess, the activity of a dead person was driven away [. . .] **Recite this incantation four times**.

Case Leiden verso IX–X.2

[. . .] from the arm of N born of N. O evil effect, disease, dead,

[. . .], male enemy, female enemy, who is in him. Behold, Re awaits you so he
rises, and Atum so he sets, to remove yourself from the arm,

[. . .] N born of N. O evil effect, disease, beware, Khontamenty awaits you, so
the justified comes out [. . .]

[. . .] to remove yourself from the arm of N born of N. O evil effect, disease,
behold, Horus awaits you [. . .]

[. . .] Apophis, to remove yourself from the arm [. . .]

[. . .], to illuminate the land with his eye, to remove yourself from [. . .]

[. . .]

[. . .]

[. . .]

[. . .] in the Great Place. You came, so [. . .]

Heh, to seize the voyage of the sacred barque. You came to scare off the sun
(Aton) [. . .].

Come out, come out, to remove yourself from the arm of N born of N. Your
poison will not arise in him. **Recite the words over myrrh, [. . .] of an
ibex,**

**the *nui* plant, the blood of a billy goat, the *mesta* drink. Grind together and
apply on it [. . .].**

Case Leiden verso XXIII

Spell for the legs when they ache: painful substances fall on their faces, painful substances descend into their blood as the gods descend to their Djatu
(?) under the power of the staff of Khentyirty,

who is the foremost of Khemu (= Letopolis). I was released by Horus, [. . .]
defeated by Seth. Fall, pains of his legs, by which acts [. . .] Thoth [. . .]

[. . .] every pain, which [. . .]

[. . .] me [. . .]
[. . .]
[. . .]
[. . .]
[. . .]
[. . .] They enter into his eye to [. . .].

Case Leiden verso XXVI.7–9
[Reme]dy for driving away swelling in both legs or in any limb [. . .]
[. . .] in(k) **1**, carob flour **1**, dates **1**, [. . .]
[. . .] together with honey. Apply on it for four days.

Case Leiden verso XXVI.9–10
Another remedy: human
feces **1**, red ocher **1**, pomace **1**, fermented herbal decoction. Apply on it.

Case Leiden verso XXVI.11
Another remedy: date seeds **1**, pomace, natron **1**. Grind finely and apply on it.

Case Leiden verso XXVI.11–12
Another:
the *shenfet* fruits, Lower Egyptian salt, herbal decoction. Apply on it.

Cairo Ostraca from Deir el-Medina
Case O.DeM 1091 verso 1
Remedy for the heart (*haty*) [. . .].

Case O.DeM 1216
[. . .] of the abdomen, when it aches: Abdomen, abdomen! O Isis [. . .]
abdju from gold twice on the coast of the sea from [. . .]
[. . .] this *akh* creature, continues the pain of his abdomen [. . .]
adversary. When he does [. . .] pain of his abdomen [. . .]
[. . .] stands in his harm [. . .].

4

INTERNAL DISEASES
AND THEIR TREATMENT

The basic question in writing a medical commentary of ancient Egyptian cases for this volume was whether we should interpret material for internal medicine according to the arrangement of the cases in the individual medical papyri or divide them into groups according to their content. After careful consideration, we selected the second approach, better suited to a medical evaluation of the cases, which moreover allows a comparison of the treatment methods and their assessment within the thematic units. In contrast to that, the original form of the ancient Egyptian texts and order of the cases and prescriptions in them are indicated in the translations in Chapter 3. It can be noticed here that the arrangement of the cases in the text does not always reflect their thematic focus. On the contrary, the texts were usually written down and copied from various older sources so that the cases were sometimes in groups and other times individually listed, placed in diverse parts of the papyri, and separated from each other by cases of entirely different medical focus.

For the better orientation of the reader, we have arranged the cases relevant to the topic of internal medicine discussed in this volume according to anatomical or physiological categories. At the same time, thematically similar cases were grouped for each of them from various papyri. A coherent "cocktail" thus emerged, in which the contributions of the individual ancient Egyptian texts combine or complement, usually without contradicting one another.

Neither the Ebers Papyrus nor any other texts discussed in this volume was arranged entirely thematically. Moreover, some cases repeated or were not recorded correctly. These omissions and diagnostic errors make the commentary of the cases and prescriptions very difficult.

The structure of the commentary typically reflects the categories which arise from the cases and prescriptions of the Ebers Papyrus and whose predominant number create a solid base. Analogical internal cases or prescriptions from the other nine preserved texts were added to it.

Whereas some cases are described separately in the commentary, other times they are thematically related groups of cases and prescriptions, furnished with a joint heading in the original, conceived as partial units of these symptoms of internal diseases. In such groups, we present at the end of each case its number with a shortening of the headings of the individual papyri, so that the interested reader can look for and check the translated version of the case (see Chapter 3). At the beginning of the cases, we present their original names, if they exist, or their focus. At the same time, we try to interpret the terminology of contemporary anatomy and subfields of internal medicine to bring it closer to today's reader.

From the perspective of modern medicine, it is necessary to emphasize that our categories of illnesses (nosological units), established for the first time during the second half of the nineteenth century and complemented to this day, were not known even in embryonic form in the medicine of the ancient Egyptians. The medical texts most often contain names of symptoms, which were among the commonly known terms of the general language, comprehensible at that time for the majority of the people. Rarely, it is possible, for example with the symptoms of angina pectoris (Eb 37) or with other cases (Eb 36, and 38–43), to consider the connection of more symptoms into syndromes.

We have divided the commentaries on the internal cases or prescriptions into fifteen sections, the first two of which introduce the reader to the issue of the then differentiated symptoms of internal diseases and their treatment (pages 168–70). The following section provides a look into the sphere of magical treatment, which was an indelible component of rational treatment for the entire pharaonic civilization (pages 170–77).

Other special sections follow one another, not according to the contemporary anatomical approach of "from head to toe," but according to their importance and connection in the ancient Egyptian embryonic concept of anatomy, physiology, and pathology (in detail in the forthcoming third volume of this series). In order to introduce them to today's reader, mainly from the ranks of physicians and other healthcare workers, we include with their titles, selected according to the division of the material, the currently used Greco-Latin terminology of the clinical fields in parentheses, to which we dare to more or less compare the ancient Egyptian category *(cum maximo grano salis)*. In that, we have divided contemporary gastroenterology into its subfields (pages 211–63), we have named today's non-existent fields of phlegmology (pages 272–87) and melalgia (pages 292–307) ourselves for completeness. The following sections thus emerged:

1 Ingredients of the Medical Preparations for Internal Problems
2 Medical Examination
3 General Magical Enchantments
4 Heart and Arteries (cardiology and angiology)
5 Lungs and Chest (pulmonology)
6 Stomach and Liver (gastrology and hepatology)
7 Abdomen and Intestines (enterology)
8 Rectum (proctology)
9 Urinary Tract (urology)
10 Mucuses and Worms (phlegmology and helminthology)
11 Head (as a whole, neurology)
12 Limbs (melalgia)
13 Stiffness and Contortion (orthopedics)
14 Non-Arterial Blood Vessels (i.e., Veins) (angiology)
15 Pain (Unlocalized) and an Illness (Unspecified)

In the section devoted to the head (pages 287–92), other specialized fields were left out, for example, *dermatology*; oral, tooth, jaw, and facial medicine (stomatology); eye medicine (ophthalmology); and aural, nasal, and laryngeal medicine (otorhinolaryngology), and others which today do not belong to the sphere of internal medicine, so they will be included in the forthcoming third volume of this series.

It was not possible to put all of the cases cited in the papyri clearly into the individual categories. Some include two or more categories and it was necessary to decide what the main diagnosis was, according to which it was placed in our commentary. Sometimes, such cases follow those described in more detail and could represent their alternative. Elsewhere, the thematic evaluation was extremely difficult. It is necessary to remind the reader that the Egyptian authors of the preserved medical texts made mistakes themselves, which makes the interpretations of individual cases even more complicated. A large group comprises diseases or symptoms whose ancient Egyptian names are not yet translatable, nor is the method of treatment. Although they often repeat, they do not provide a key to their identification. It is difficult to deal with the preserved fragments of the prescriptions, where the name of the case, symptoms of the disease, prescribed treatment, or all except the ingredients of the recommended prescriptions are lacking.

In the quoted prescriptions for treating the symptoms of the diseases, we have adjusted the order of the treatment ingredients so that most often, the plant-based are listed as the first-named preparations translated into English, less often the animal or mineral medicines, which are mostly comprehensible for the reader. After them come the medicines with exclusively ancient Egyptian names, which have remained untranslatable and are incomprehensible. Further then come mainly disgusting or ineffective substances added apparently for magical reasons, and ultimately substances to improve the medicine's taste (mostly honey) and solvents such as beer, wine, oils, juices, or water. In those prescriptions where precise amounts of additives are determined, they are additionally arranged according to the recommended amount. Thus, the reader has the opportunity to imagine very precisely the composition and consistency of the individual medicinal mixtures.

Ingredients of the Medical Preparations for Internal Problems

Some ingredients used for the preparation of medicinal remedies were presented already in the first volume of this series in the sections devoted to surgery and the treatment of women and children (Strouhal et al. 2014, 25–27 and 102–106). However, a much greater variety of ingredients can be found in the prescriptions for the treatment of internal diseases that we deal with in this volume. These were medicines prepared from a wide range of ingredients of plant, mineral, and animal origin, diverse liquids, and other substances.

In some cases, it is possible to judge the efficacy of the prepared mixtures and it is clear that ancient Egyptian physicians—just as healers in many ancient cultures—utilized the favorable features of many herbs, fruits, and spices, which we are able to investigate, describe, and only now verify scientifically in modern, well-equipped laboratories. We could find similarly broad empirical knowledge in later European rootstocks or today's traditional herbalists; the continuous development of similar experiences can be attributed to thousands of years of experience of traditional Chinese doctors.

However, our understanding of the prescriptions from the preserved papyri is, unfortunately, rather limited, as we cannot translate satisfactorily about half of the Egyptian ingredient names. Some names of plants or minerals are not clearly identified, as these names are not attested elsewhere than in the medical prescriptions. Experts argue about the exact meaning of many of these ingredients, especially those of plants, which are often judged only by their medical use (see for instance Manniche 1989, Germer 2008).

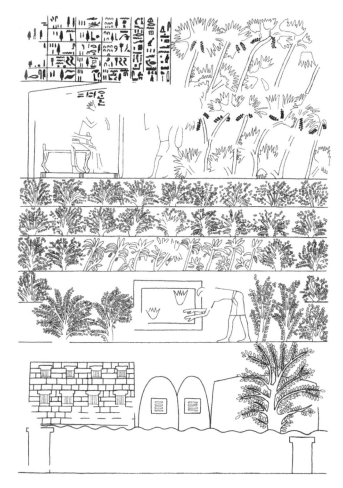

Fig. 6. A large garden with herbs, bushes, trees, and palms surrounds the house of the builder Ineni (Eighteenth Dynasty, tomb of Ineni (TT 81), after Manniche 1989, 11)

The meanings of the names marking some parts of the plants are similarly unclear. For instance, the Egyptian term *peret* could label both the seed and the fruit, so that we can deduce its suitable English equivalent only from the context of the individual plants in the prescriptions. With some ingredients, the determination is obvious, such as the seeds of dill or fennel or the fruits (berries) of juniper or bryony. Yet it is not possible to decide with certainty elsewhere, whether the seed or fruits was used, such as with bindweed, castor oil plant, or willow.

As with plant ingredients, a number of names of mineral ingredients and stones, and even some animals or parts of their bodies, cannot be translated satisfactorily. For unspecified ingredients in the translations and commentaries, we have therefore left their Egyptian names in italics.

The ingredients are listed one after another in individual cases and prescriptions, often with precise quantities, similar to today's cookbooks. Sometimes the text also contains a description of the preparation process with information on whether it is necessary to crush or grind the ingredients, mix together or add gradually, whether the mixture should be boiled, strained, or reduced, left standing overnight, or other instructions. However, a number of prescriptions are limited to a very brief list of ingredients without further instructions.

Units Used in Prescriptions

A large part of the prescriptions for the treatment of internal problems contains precisely set amounts of the individual ingredients. The usage of larger and smaller units shows an immense precision, and the ingredients were often carefully measured, even in very small amounts. Such precise dosage makes sense especially with ingredients that could be dangerous for people, for example with the castor oil plant *(Ricinus)* or psychotropic wild rue *(Peganum harmala)*. Yet, even with the safe mixtures, the ingredients were often measured precisely, which indicates that Egyptian physicians built on a very long empirical tradition of the effects of various species of plant and mineral substances, oils, honey, and many other ingredients and their combinations.

We can interpret a number of mixtures rather as dishes than as medicines, which shows that Egyptians sometimes put stress on the proper or balanced nutrition, which could benefit or relieve the patient. It is particularly clear with intestinal or stomach problems, but also in other cases when a special diet was recommended.

Despite the undoubted experience of many, many generations of Egyptian physicians, which are reflected in the preserved medical texts, it is, nevertheless, natural that the healing potential of Egyptian medicine was relatively limited in comparison with today's Western medicine.

The units that we find used in the preserved prescriptions in this volume also appeared in the prescriptions in the first volume of this series, where they were briefly presented (Strouhal et al. 2014, 102–103, for a detailed summary of the units, see also Westendorf 1999, 521–24). However, for the sake of clarity, we now provide more precise information on the amount of the ingredients in the commentaries so that the reader can create a good idea of the relative proportions of the ingredients used.

The basic unit of volume in Egypt comprised the Egyptian *heqat*, whose fractions from 1/2 to 1/64 we can find in the prescriptions, especially in connection with the measurement of liquid binding agents (water, wine, beer) or loose materials (grains, semolina, and others). A tenth of the measure, hence 1 *hin*, was not only a hollow measure, but also the name of a container in which

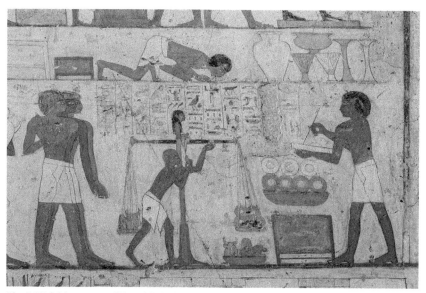

Fig. 7. Weighing commodities with the help of various weights in the shape of animals (Eighteenth Dynasty, tomb of Rekhmire (TT 100) in Sheikh Abd el-Qurna, photo © Archive of the Czech Institute of Egyptology, Faculty of Arts, Charles University, Martin Frouz)

a particular medicine was sometimes mixed or given to the patient. Thus, we can assume that some types of containers were produced at a set size and used as measuring cups.

In terms of the prescriptions, the most frequently used measurement is 75 ml, which is 1/64 of a *heqat*. For simplicity, we can compare it to the popular measurement from our 1 cup kitchen recipes, which corresponds to 250 ml. Our popular cup thus corresponds to 3.33 times the ancient Egyptian volume of 1/64 of a measure. For the reader's easier orientation, we provide similar modern equivalents:

1 *hin* = 480 ml	1.92 cups
1 measure = 10 *hin* = 4.8 l	19.2 cups
1/2 measure = 2.4 l	9.6 cups
1/4 measure = 1.2 l	4.8 cups
1/8 measure = 600 ml	2.4 cups
1/16 measure = 300 ml	1.2 cups
1/32 measure = 150 ml	0.6 cups
1/64 measure = 75 ml = 5 ro	0.3 cups

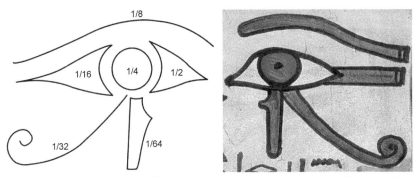

Fig. 8. The eye of Horus, whose individual parts served as symbols for the fractions of the grain unit (Eighteenth Dynasty, tomb of Sennefer (TT 96), photo © Sandro Vannini, drawing Hana Vymazalová)

Besides the *hin* and *heqat* units, the ancient Egyptian medical texts also feature ingredients for which their amounts are given with no specific units mentioned. This makes it difficult for us to interpret the quantities of these substances. On the one hand, we can understand the numbers in these prescriptions simply as the ratio of the individual ingredients used. It is, however, also possible to interpret them as quantities given in yet another unit, namely, the unit *ro* (see also Westendorf 1999, 521–24).

The unit of 1 *ro* was used for small amounts of ingredients, and it corresponds to 15 ml or our tablespoon. In today's kitchens we can find a cup and its smaller parts in the form of small plastic or metal measuring cups used in baking and cooking. In the same way, measuring spoons for a tablespoon and a teaspoon, corresponding to 5 ml, and its smaller parts are available as well. Similar measuring cups existed in ancient Egypt. We find measuring cups of various types not only in ancient Egyptian depictions but even in archaeological excavations where several examples have been found (see for instance Pommerening 2005). The prescriptions (recipes) in medical texts count on not only tablespoons, but also smaller parts, namely 1/2 to 1/64 of this unit, which is a very small amount of liquid or loose ingredients. For comparison, today's commonly used 1/4 teaspoon corresponds to 1.25 ml—and Egyptian recipes use even 1/5 of this amount, which we can imagine perhaps as a pinch. For simplicity in the following list, and also in the commentaries, we round the small fractions of the unit *ro* so that the reader can more easily conceive the mentioned amount:

1 *ro* = 15 ml
1/2 *ro* = 7.5 ml (= 1/64 *hin*)
1/4 *ro* = 3.75 ml ≈ 4 ml

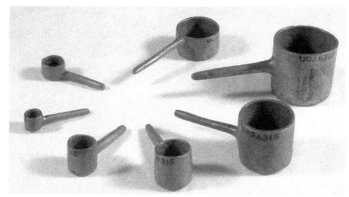

Fig. 9. Measuring cups for small amounts of loose and liquid ingredients (Eighteenth Dynasty, Naqada, Petrie Museum of Egyptian Archaeology UC 26315, photo © Petrie Museum of Archaeology, University of London)

1/8 *ro* = 1.875 ml ≈ 2 ml
1/16 *ro* = 0.937 ml ≈ 1 ml
1/32 *ro* = 0.469 ml ≈ 0.5 ml
1/64 *ro* = 0.234 ml ≈ 0.25 ml

It is worth noting that these small units of volume appear in recipes with ingredients such as peas, incense, dates, or onions. This seems to indicate that the ingredients may have been prepared in a milled or finely ground condition to allow the smallest amount to be measured.

The Egyptian originals express the difference between these two types of units, the *heqat* and the lesser unit *ro*, with the aid of two types of fractions. Fractions of a *heqat* measure were recorded with special signs, the so-called fragments of Horus's eye (see also Vymazalová and Coppens 2010, 61), whereas ordinary fractions were used for parts of the unit *ro*.

In a careful reading of some prescriptions, we can notice that the presented amount of the ingredients is sometimes somewhat strange; it is thus possible that the authors of the texts sometimes accidentally recorded one type of fraction instead of another, or by mistake left out some ingredient. For instance, in the Ebers Papyrus in the prescription Ebers 23, a curative drink is to be prepared, which was subsequently left to be reduced to 225 ml, but the recipe itself states only 7.5 ml of herbal decoction, but no liquid binder in a greater amount. It is possible that the scribe forgot to include a larger amount of water in the prescription, or he made other mistakes when he copied the text from earlier models. From today's perspective, such typographical errors have little impact on the assessment of the potency of the mixture concerned. However, other recipes are quite easy to understand.

Ingredients of Plant Origin

Plant ingredients used for the preparation of remedies against internal diseases include various types of green herbs and their fruits and seeds, which are used to this day as spices, salads, grains, legumes, nuts, and seeds, many species of fruits and vegetables, parts and various products of woody plants, and more. These ingredients are numerous and diverse, and therefore it is not possible to name them all. We therefore present in this passage mainly those more important and known substances, whose effects on the human body can be judged from the perspective of modern science (for the medicinal effects of herbs, see for instance Korbelář 1990). The reader might have encountered some of them already in Strouhal et al. 2014. Other ingredients and unknown species of plants are listed in full in the translations and commentaries.

Identification of the ancient Egyptian names of plants is not simple. From the depictions in the Egyptian temples and tombs and also from archaeological research, various types of flowers, fruits, and woody plants are attested, but we often do not know their Egyptian names (see Germer 1985 and Germer 2008, 173–368).

For example, Tutankhamun's tomb contained items and grave goods produced from more than sixty types of plants, which grew in Egypt in his time or were imported (Germer 1989). The burial equipment of the young king included a number of floral decorations, linen garments, food offerings in baskets and ceramic vessels, precious oils in beautiful containers, and also small statues and furniture produced from various types of wood (Germer 1989, 1–3). We know the appropriate Egyptian name only for some of them (Germer 1989, passim).

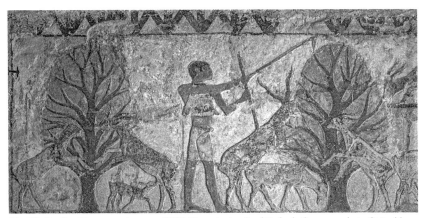

Fig. 10. Goatherd in an acacia grove (Fifth Dynasty, tomb of Nefer in Saqqara, photo © Archive of the Czech Institute of Egyptology, Faculty of Arts, Charles University, Martin Frouz)

Attributing their meanings to their Egyptian names is just as difficult as it is to determine the names of the attested plants. The prescriptions from the medical texts do not contain any signs or context which would hint at the identification of the names, besides their medical usage. In the identification of the individual ingredients, it is possible to start from an earlier dictionary of names of the ingredients in the series *Grundriss der Medizin der Alten Ägypter* (Deines and Grapow 1959) or from the general dictionaries of Egyptian (Erman and Grapow 1926–61; Hannig 1995). The latest and much more detailed study by Renate Germer focuses directly on the plant ingredients (1979, 2002, 2008). We can also introduce the English reader to the work with a similar focus by Lisa Manniche (1989).

With many herbs, the identification of the Egyptian names is difficult and unclear and is still a subject of debate by experts (see especially the detailed discussion in Germer 2008). Sometimes the proposed meaning of these ingredients does not quite correspond from the healer's perspective to their usage in the preserved prescriptions. Other times, the usages correspond to certain well-known herbs, but their appearance in Egypt in antiquity is not always attested. Despite the effort to translate the ancient Egyptian plant names, the meaning of a large part of them remains disputable.

With the prescriptions devoted to the treatment of internal problems, there are many digestion-improving herbs, for instance *Melilotus (afa)*, which works against flatulence, or *Anacyclus* or *Achillea ptarmica (shames)*, from which all parts of the plant were used, not just the fruit, roots, and leaves. Good digestion is also supported from tubers of yellow nutsedge *(giu)*, today called earth almonds, chufa nuts or tiger nuts *(wah)*, due to the high content of fiber. It is moreover beneficial to the blood vessels thanks to its containing rutin. Besides yellow nutsedge, sedges *(iaru)*, *Juncus (sut)* and various species of *Phragmites (isy, nebit, tewer)* also appear in the prescriptions. The use to this day of garden cress *(semty)* and arugula *(gengenet)*, which inter alia have diuretic effects, is generally beneficial, but the determination of these ingredients is not entirely clear (see Germer 2008, 115 and 148). *Astragalus*, or milkvetch, *(rekrek)* also has diuretic and calming effects, and *Cynodon*, or scutch grass, *(kadet)* is also beneficial for urinary tracts and digestion.

The determination of mallow (whose Egyptian name meant "mouse tail": *sedj-penu*) is not entirely certain. It has anti-inflammatory and astringent effects and helps dissolve mucus. *Potamogeton (nesha)* also acts as an astringent and, moreover, is refreshing. The identification of *Potentilla*, or cinquefoil (Germer 2008, 129) is just as uncertain. Its supposed name in Egyptian means "feather of the god Nemty" *(shut Nemty)*, and it helps against cramps and is often used during diarrhea or menstruation. For female problems, chaste tree or vitex *(saamu)* is recommended to this day; however, some experts exchange it for ragweed, which seems in certain Egyptian recipes as a more suitable herb for its antibacterial and antiviral effects. Also uncertain is the determination of fenugreek *(hemat)*, which facilitates healing, or hemp *(shemshemet)*, whose Egyptian name, due to its similarity to the Arabic *simsim*, is sometimes translated as sesame (for the various meanings of these Egyptian names, see Manniche 1989; Germer 2008). Psychotropic effects can also be had by *Peganum harmala*, or wild rue, *(djais)*, which is also a bactericide and insecticide and is recommended for stomach problems and against parasites.

We also find poisonous herbs in Egyptian recipes. Bryony *(khasyet)*, whose fruits, roots, rhizomes, and offshoots were used in the prescriptions, was used in small dosages as a diuretic or to cause vomiting. Ricin *(kaka, degem)* was used in the form of leaves, roots, and mainly the seeds, the oil of which was detoxified by boiling in water. The usage of some parts of the lotus *(seshen)* must have also been dangerous. To this day, its rhizomes are used to help dissolve mucus and are recommended for a cold.

The taste and other medicinal effects were assured according to the recipes in the texts by various types of spices such as wild mint *(ibsa)* or dill *(imset)*. Anise *(inset)* has calming effects, helps dissolve mucus, and favorably influences digestion. In the same way, cumin *(tepnen)*, coriander *(shau)*, or juniper *(wan)*, which moreover acts as a diuretic and tonic, are recommended against gas and to strengthen the appetite for food. These spices help against a cold as well. Similarly, fennel, and especially its seeds, also acts against bloating, improves digestion, and facilitates and promotes expectoration (coughing up mucus). Thyme *(inek* or *innek)*, usable with similar problems, has a strong antiseptic effect, but the determination of this herb is not entirely convincing and other times is considered to be conyza (see Germer 2008, 29), which is recommended during urological problems for its diuretic effect and is also beneficial for stopping light bleeding. The determination of wormwood *(sam)* (see Germer 2008, 111 and 132) is also not entirely certain. It has anti-inflammatory and stimulant effects, especially in the case of the digestive and urinary tracts, and against parasites. The same for poppy seed *(shepen)*. Besides the poppy seed itself, its tincture (infusion) from dried juice from immature poppies or laudanum *(iber)* was used, which was recommended not only against pain but also for cough or diarrhea. The use of laurel fruits *(paaret)* is also attested, whereas the laurel (or bay) leaf does not appear in medicinal recipes.

Very beneficial especially (but not only) for digestion is flaxseed *(inyt n mehy)* and just as valuable are pine nuts *(peret-sheny)*. Of the dried fruits, bitter

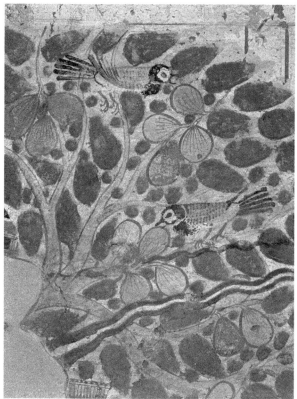

almonds *(hemayt)* might also have been used, but their determination is not entirely certain (Germer 2008, 94).

Other components of the medicinal recipes were legumes such as peas *(tehu)*, beans, or green beans *(iuryt)*, which are a source of proteins and fiber. Of the cereals, we often encounter barley and wheat in the recipes in the form of grains, flours, or mashes. The use of gluten-free sorghum is also common. The meaning of the name for the cereal grain *amaa* or the name *besha*, which could indicate a type of cereal or malt, is not entirely clear.

Vitamins and fiber were provided by medicinal mixtures of various types of vegetables, such as wild carrot *(kheper-wer)*, whose determination is not entire clear (Germer 2008, 101), or celery *(matet)*, which not only supports digestion, but moreover acts as a diuretic and anti-inflammatory ingredient. Its seeds were used as well and even mountain celery appears in the recipes *(matet khasut)*, which is sometimes considered to be parsley (Bardinet 1995,

429). Onion acts as a natural antibiotic and moreover has a diuretic effect and supports expectoration.

In the recipes we also find many types of fruits, which gave the medicinal mixtures not only vitamins and minerals but also the necessary sweetness. Frequent ingredients are especially raisins *(wenesh)* or grapes *(iareret)* but also various types of melon, such as muskmelon *(shespet)*, watermelon *(bededuka)*, or the unidentified melon *shebet*. Digestion was benefited by the use of figs *(dab)* and the sycomore fruits *(nehet)*, which appeared in the recipes in various stages of ripeness and preparation. Dates *(bener)*, their juice *(beniu)*, or their purée *(sermet)* often occur in the recipes; even date seeds ground into a powder were used.

Ceratonia, or carob tree *(nedjem)* was widely used in the recipes. Its fruits *(peret nedjem)*, thus the carob pods *(djaret)*, are known as St. John's bread. By drying and milling, carob is acquired from them, which is beneficial to digestion and inter alia lowers cholesterol.

The recipes for the preparation of medicinal remedies also include various parts and products of woody plants, such as leaves, bark, sawdust, gum, and other parts of the common fig tree *(dab)*, sycomore *(nehet)*, acacia *(shenyt)*, *Ziziphus jujuba (nebes)*, or willow *(tjeret)*. The determination of camphor *(tishepes)* is uncertain. It has antiseptic and anesthetic effects and helps with blood supply. Some experts, however, prefer to translate this Egyptian name as cinnamon (Manniche 1989, 104). Doubts also dominate with the determination of myrtle *(khet-des)*, which is often confused with *Sesbania* (Germer 2008, 104). We also find among the ingredients of the recipes the pomegranate *(inhemen)*. A much valued ingredient was cedar *(ash)*, the oil of which *(sefetj)* is antiseptic and also works against gas and to support excretion. The oil from the seed of the *Moringa* tree *(bak)* has an anti-inflammatory effect.

Resins also had great usage, whether it was incense *(sentjer)*, myrrh *(antyu)*, or the resins of various other trees, natural gum, starch, and balsam.

Other than these identifiable (although often not entirely) plant ingredients, we find in the recipes dozens of names of plants, fruits, and seeds whose meaning we do not know today, and therefore it is not possible to consider their effect. It may be worth mentioning the *pesedj* fruit, which is sometimes considered to be henbane (nightshade), but it was perhaps rather the hull of some legume (see the discussion in Germer 2008, 73). The *shasha* fruit is sometimes translated as valerian (Bardinet 1995, 401), but this determination is very uncertain. The meaning of the expression *khet-awa* is also discussed, which is sometimes translated as petrified wood (Hannig 1995, 623), but at other times is interpreted as aloe (Germer 2008, 102).

Ingredients of Animal Origin

Honey (*bit*, see Vachala 2014, 234–37) had an irreplaceable significance in Egyptian medicine because of its antibacterial and fungicidal effects, and it provided sweetness and flavor to the mixtures. Wax was also used.

Milk (*irtet*) had wide usage, and could be from a cow, donkey, or small livestock (that is, a goat or sheep), or sometimes even from a human. Mainly, the milk of a mother who had given birth to a boy was recommended, which refers to the protective power of the goddess Isis, mother of the god Horus. Sour milk (*semi*) and milk fat (*mehwy* or *mehut*) appear among the additives.

Oil or fat (*merhet*) appears not only as a binder in many recipes; it sometimes is more closely identified as white (*hedj*) or fresh (*maat*). Often, the type of animal oil (*merhet*) or fat (*adj*) is more specified, such as oil or fat of a cow, donkey, ram, pig, goose, or duck, but also ostrich, antelope, ibex, tomcat, mouse, and lizard occur in the texts. To acquire fat from a snake, lion, crocodile, or hippopotamus was certainly dangerous and expensive.

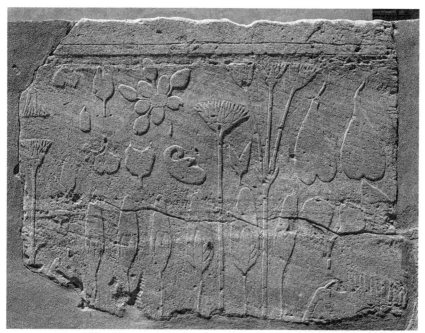

Fig. 12. The so-called botanical garden in Karnak captures diverse types of plants and fruits that the Egyptians encountered during military campaigns abroad in the reign of Thutmose III (Eighteenth Dynasty, Karnak, photo © Archive of the Czech Institute of Egyptology, Faculty of Arts, Charles University, Martin Frouz)

The most commonly prepared meat in the preserved recipes was beef, which was available to the noblemen but was not, however, part of the ordinary diet of the common people, who might have perhaps eaten it during important festivals. Besides meats in the recipes, we also find beef marrow, spinal marrow, brain (or offal), spleen, and tongue.

Animal blood *(senef)*, namely cow's, pig's, or goat's, was added to some medicines, as was also bile *(weded)*, namely cow's, antelope's, or Nile tilapia's. We also find among the ingredients the testicles of a donkey, which were apparently to have the fair color of the coat. A component of some recipes was skin of either a cow or a hippopotamus.

Not very often we find eggs and their parts in the recipes, specifically ostrich eggs, goose yolk, or the yolk from the eggs of the pintail. Much more often, there are ingredients from fish, including bones, for instance of the Nile perch or tilapia, the skulls of a catfish or *Synodontis*, the bile and fat of a red mullet *(adju)* and other, unknown, fish *(abdju)*. Rarely, a salamander, tadpole, frog, or a tortoise shell was also added to medicines. We also find cuttlefish bone or freshwater mussels among the ingredients.

Many recipes also included disgusting substances, especially dung or droppings *(hes)* of various animals including tomcats, dogs, donkeys, pigs,

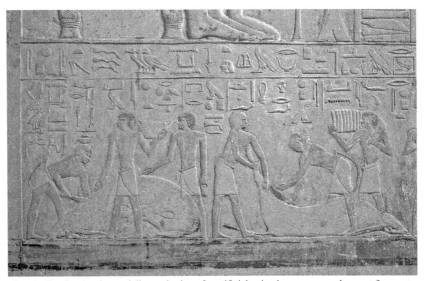

Fig. 13. The slaughtering and dismembering of sacrificial animals was among the most frequent scenes depicted in the tombs of the Old Kingdom, expressing the desire of the dignitaries to enjoy plentiful offerings in the next world (Sixth Dynasty, mastaba of Neferseshemptah in Saqqara, photo © Hana Vymazalová)

crocodiles, or birds, and even human feces. Repugnant ingredients can also include a girl's urine.

Ingredients of Mineral Origin
Mixtures for the treatment of internal diseases contained a wide range of ingredients of mineral origin. A large number of them are, however, difficult to identify. Salt *(hemat)* was often added to the concoctions, which acts osmotically and adds flavor to the mixture. Serving a warm solution of salt has a slightly emetic effect. The salt is sometimes specified as Lower Egyptian (from the Delta), which is sea salt obtained through evaporation. Less often mountain salt is specified. Natron *(hesmen)* or cleansing natron *(hesmen wab)* appears less often in the recipes, used sometimes in the form of a powder or a solution.

The ingredients also included malachite *(wadju)* in the form of a powder or pellets, and galenite *(mesdemet)*, both minerals used for the production of green and black eye makeup. Black flint *(des kem)*, pumice *(weshbet)*, and hematite (*didi* or *bia*), which thanks to its coloring is usually connected with treatment of blood diseases, are also used.

Calamine *(hestem)* could be beneficial as it contained zinc; copper *(hemty)* was also used in the form of cinders, chips, or grains. Orpiment *(kenit)* is dangerously toxic, and was therefore used only in concoctions intended for fumigation.

Ingredients such as mud *(shefshefet)*, Nile mud *(kah)*, and clay *(ta)*, as well as gypsum *(besen)*, were commonly accessible. The popular ingredients of remedies included ocher *(sety)* and red ocher *(menshet)*, red clay *(peresh)*, and chalk *(meni)*. On the other hand, the rare ingredients were amber *(sehret)* and asphalt, in Egyptian called "mountain oil" or "oil from a foreign land" *(merhet khaset)*. Also, red, seemingly orpiment glass, appears sporadically.

As with plant additives, a number of names of mineral substances are not reliably determined, and with some not even their origin can be specified. Of particular note is the often-occurring stone *sa-wer*, whose name means "great protection" but according to some experts it is a substance of plant origin (see Germer 2008, 106–107). In the recipes we frequently encounter the stone *qesenty*, whose determination is not certain but which is found in wide usage in a number of areas of ancient Egyptian healing.

Other and Unknown Types of Ingredients
An entire range of other ingredients in the recipes for medicinal concoctions in the preserved texts rank among the common foodstuffs. These include particularly liquids such as wine *(irep)*, or the more commonly accessible beer *(henqet)*, sometimes sweet beer *(nedjmet)*, other times strong *(djesret)*, beer

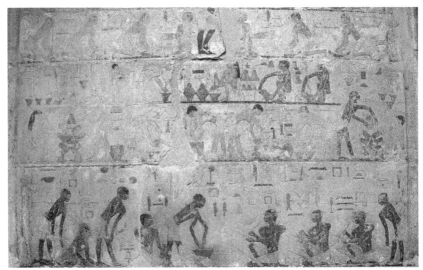

Fig. 14. Preparation of beer in an ancient Egyptian brewery (Fifth Dynasty, the tomb of Ty in Saqqara, photo © Sandro Vannini)

sediment or dregs *(tahet)*, or foam *(iayt)*. Water *(mw)* was also used for the preparation of drinks and medicinal remedies, and sometimes a juice was pre-pared as a watery solution with additives from barley, sorghum, cannabis, or carob, and others. Dew *(iadet)* was used, particularly during the preparation: various mixtures were left to stand overnight "exposed to dew," which could help the binding of the individual ingredients.

A significant role in the preparation of medicines was played by decoctions from herbs *(hesa)*, sometimes fermented *(hesa awayt)*, and also mash *(ah)*, which might have been prepared from dates (?). The meanings of other liquids or drinks are unknown, including *ibkhi, mesta, pa-ib, sekhpet,* and *sedjer*. The recipes also contained various types of baked goods including fresh or roasted bread, jujube bread, baker's yeast, or dough. Some names of ingredients are still entirely incomprehensible to us, so it is not possible to even determine what type of substance it was. The meaning of the phrase *khemtu* from *djesfu* or the names of the substances *meqret, nehesh,* or *djat* are not known for instance.

Medical Examination

Whereas in the case of the examination of injuries and fractures, the cause of the problem was usually known (Strouhal et al. 2014), with internal diseases the ancient Egyptian physician examining the patient had only a relatively lim-ited variety of physical methods available, which supplemented the skimpy anamnestic data and specific complaints of the patient. What was important was the physician's observation of the appearance and behavior (aspection) of the ill and obvious manifestations of his diseases, for instance a cough, painful places, breathing or digestive problems (symptomatology). If necessary, the physician used his touch (palpation), for instance in palpating the intestines or monitoring the pulse of the artery to assess the rate of heart rhythm over his own (see also Strouhal et al. 2014). Tapping (percussion) combined with listening (auscultation) is not attested in the papyri. Rarely, there are body temperature estimates based on manifestations (symptoms) such as feeling of heat, sweating, chills, or tremors. The determination of the heat of some organ and the effort of the physician to cool it is often repeated. The attention of the physician was also aroused by changes in the color of the skin—especially the face, lips, mouth, and tongue—and the patient's information on bad tastes in the mouth, heartburn, or perception of bitterness of bile origin. These included the manifestations of bleeding, for instance vomiting blood, an admixture of blood in the stool in hemorrhoids or in the urine, which are frequent with schistosomiasis, one of the most widespread parasitic diseases, which affects especially the villagers of those times living in unhygenic conditions. The names of the groups of cases in the papyri are not always clear. They speak of strengthening, comforting, or correcting the organ, curing or relieving the disease, and other examples.

The ancient Egyptian conception of health and illness shows that the basic manifestation of a number of diseases was an obstruction in one of the tubes, called *metu* in Egyptian, which spread through all parts of the body (see Vymazalová and Coppens 2011, 195–96; Nunn 1996, 44–49). Those included mainly the digestive tract, especially the stomach and the intestines, in which the symptoms of obstruction appeared, in the translations of the texts often referred to as "constipation of the stomach," through the complete stoppage of the passage of the contents (ileus). Problems in digestion could form blockages as a consequence of the usage of spoiled or inappropriate foodstuffs or creating clumps (convolutes) of coagulated or baked blood (e.g., Eb 198), or parasitic worms. Egyptian physicians therefore devoted great attention to precisely these symptoms and were the first in the world then to begin to notice the stools of the ill. On the contrary, we do not find mentions of an interest in examining the urine or even explicit mentions of its appearance.

Anamnestic data, which the patients shared about themselves with physicians, or physician's questions to the ill to be able to discover his problem and begin treatment, are relatively rare in the texts. The authors of the medical texts wrote them not for patients, the majority of whom did not know how to read and write, but for physicians, who judged the case and then interpreted the treatment instructions to the ill. The texts also recommended the preparation of the prescribed medicines in the form of mixtures, mashes, drinks, suppositories, ointments, or substance for inhalation. The job of a pharmacist is not attested in ancient Egypt, and it seems from the medical texts that the healing mixtures were prepared by the physician himself (Westendorf 1999, 489–90). In some cases, the additives were so common that the mixture might even have been prepared by the relatives of the ill under domestic conditions according to the physician's instructions (Vymazalová and Coppens 2010, 230). We could label the producers of linen bandages and orthopedic aids as assistants of physicians (more in the forthcoming third volume of this series).

The use of medicines by the ill was usually ordered standardly "for four days," which apparently was the popular number of Egyptian medical numerology at the expense of the elsewhere common 3, 7, 9, and 13 (for their symbolism, see Goedicke 1986; Wilkinson 1999, 126–47; and Rochholz 2002). In the ancient Egyptian conception, the number 4 expressed unity and completeness. Its symbolism was apparently influenced by four cardinal directions, which, however, did not always have to be directly manifested in the symbolic use (Wilkinson 1999, 133–35; and Goedicke 1986, 128). At other times, the medicine was used only once or for one day, but sometimes the texts do not specify the duration of use. Exceptionally, the medicinal compounds were to be used repeatedly for a prolonged period of time. We include this information in our commentary where the recommended duration of the medicine's use varies or is specific in some way.

In the commentaries of the medical papyri, we considered it appropriate to include not only the medical terms understandable to the general readership but also the terms of the Greek-Latin terminology internationally recognized by healthcare professionals.

General Magical Enchantments

Whereas injuries and problems treated with a knife (discussed in Strouhal et al. 2014) had a clear cause, the illnesses hidden inside the body were difficult for ancient Egyptian physicians to understand, and in the conception of Egyptian medicine and religion they were attributed to the activity of supernatural forces— gods, demons, the dead—a crooked view of the living person or merely "they came from outside." These causes were faced mainly through magical formulas, which appear in the whole range of cases devoted to internal diseases. Some formulas refer to the treatment of a specific disease or its symptom, a certain organ, physical region, or a certain physiological function, and these cases are presented in the relevant subsequent sections. In contrast, other formulas are connected thematically with internal medicine, but are not specific in any way in their focus. We therefore summarize them all together in this section.

It seems that the recitation of magical texts usually accompanied the preparation of the medications as well as their applications. Magic thus comprised an indelible part of the treatment at that time. With illnesses hidden in the body, it was entirely natural for the ancient healers with medical experience tested by empirical methods to combine treatment, religious beliefs, and magic as their instruments, and these aspects, which we view separately today, complemented one another very well. The purpose of the formula recited in applying the medicine was to strengthen its effectiveness, which could strongly influence the mental state of the ill in favor of his recovery. It is necessary to keep in mind that ancient Egyptian medical papyri are the product of the time when medicine was first emerging. They represent the beginning of a long and complicated path that has led all the way to the high level of contemporary medicine.

Ebers 1–3—formulas for administering medicine
In the introduction to the Ebers Papyrus, we find three magical formulas which were recited in the application of medicinal remedies to strengthen their efficacy. The physician reciting the formula of Ebers 1 adds authority by deriving his magical knowledge from the important deities of Heliopolis and Sais, where important temples and apparently also a famous House of Life, connected with the medical arts, were located (Vymazalová and Coppens 2010, 35–43). These gods and knowledge, which they handed down, could provide protection against the undesirable influence of a god or the dead which may be manifested by a disease of any part of the human body. The main role in the provision of protection for the ill, however, was played by the creator god Re and along with him the god of wisdom Thoth (Janák 2005, 175–78), who is highlighted here as the author of medical books and the teacher of physicians. The postscript at the very end of the case indicates that the recitation of this protective formula during the treatment of the ill was truly effective and had significant merit in their recovery. There is no doubt that the faith and trust of the populace in the magical processes could have played an important role in healing, but the claimed effectiveness of the formula failed if the recovery was contrary to the wishes of the god.

Another effective formula of case Ebers 2 was to release from the body of the ill person the evil caused by a god, the dead, or an adversary. The text refers to the ancient Egyptian myth of Osiris and Isis and their son Horus, according to which the king of Egypt Osiris was murdered by his brother Seth, who took control of the land. The goddess Isis revived Osiris magically for a moment to conceive their son Horus, whom she raised in secret after his birth and with

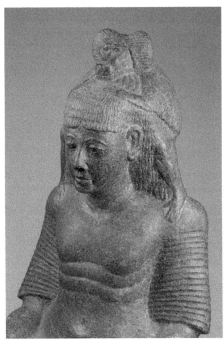

Fig. 15. The god Thoth, patron of scribes and the educated, who had immense secret knowledge, was considered the real author of medical treatises. He was depicted with the head of an ibis or in the form of a baboon, and sometimes as if whispering straight into the ear of the scribes. (Twentieth Dynasty, statue of the scribe Ramessenakht, Egyptian Museum in Cairo JE 36582, photo © Mohamed Megahed)

great power protected him from any danger. Horus subsequently overcame Seth in battle and acquired the position which belonged to him, whereas his father became the ruler of the underworld (Janák 2005, 83–85 and 166–67; Janák 2009, 98–102). The power by which Isis managed to protect the young Horus was to also help to protect the ill. This myth was often used in the treatment of small children, who were compared to her son Horus (Strouhal et al. 2014, 186–203), but it was also possible to use this method with an adult patient.

The following formula of Ebers 3 was intended for recitation when administering the medicine to the patient. The main motif again refers to the battle of Horus with Seth, from which the rightful heir to the throne came out as the victor. The formula highlights a specific moment of the battle, when Horus overcomes an eye injury caused by Seth and subsequently deprives his opponent of his testicles (Janák 2005, 167).

Berlin 189—formula for administering medicine
In the Berlin papyrus we find a spell which was to be recited when administering medicine in liquid form. The preparation, along with the formula, was to help against a weakness not more closely described and a problem caused by a

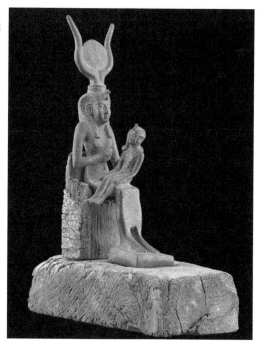

Fig. 16. The goddess Isis with the young Horus on her lap was venerated for millennia in Egypt as the goddess of protective magical power (Late Period, Imhotep Museum in Saqqara, photo © Sandro Vannini)

dead person or his seed, or even to release whoever is in their abdomen, which, based on a parallel in the case of Ebers 61, could be a stomach parasite. The formula refers to the gods Ptah and Sokar and also to Isis, her devoted sister and helper Nephthys, the falcon of Horus, and the god Seth, Nephthys's husband. The formula was adapted to the individual patients in that the physician placed the name of the ill and his mother in it. This individualizing feature was common and we also encounter it in many other formulas.

Ebers 242–47—divine healing means

These six cases from another part of the Ebers Papyrus do not comprise magical formulas—they are six recipes for the preparation of medicinal mixtures. Their magical effectiveness was ensured by the headings that claim them to be the work of the gods. Some headings state that this medicine was prepared by the god himself for himself: Re (Eb 242) or Shu (Eb 243). Another time, another god prepared the mixture for Re: Tefnut (Eb 244), Geb (Eb 245), Nut (Eb 246), and Isis (Eb 247). They are among the most important Egyptian gods and members of the Ennead of Heliopolis. Tefnut and Shu were the first created divine couple, personifying air and humidity, their children Geb and Nut were gods of the earth and heavens, and Isis had great magical and healing power (Janák 2005, 54, 58, 131, 171, and 174). For the Egyptian ill, the medicines associated with these gods thus had to have acquired great healing power.

The actual healing mixtures in question were intended against the harmful activity of gods, demons, and the dead in any part of the human body, which is connected with a lack of knowledge of the real causes of the given disease. These medicinal mixtures were prepared mainly from plant raw materials and were intended for external use as ointments for dressings. It is not clear from the text whether it was unexplained pain or another type of problem manifesting itself in the body.

The first mixture described in detail of Re comprised equal amounts (15 ml) of carob, yellow nutsedge, bryony, the *ibu* plant, *sar* plant fruits, coriander, resinous pellets of juniper and cedar, wild rue seeds, the *shasha* fruits, fresh mash, lukewarm honey, wax, incense pellets, high-quality incense, and red clay. The affected area should be bandaged with this mixture (Eb 242). A mixture for bandaging, for which 15 ml each of an herbal decoction; wheat, coriander, carob, and bean flours; the *qesentet* plant; incense; sea salt; oil; ocher; and soot removed from the wall were needed, was associated with the name of the god Shu (Eb 243). Geb was to prepare for Re a mixture for bandaging that assured rapid convalescence, which included 15 ml each of pea, carob, and myrtle flours, which was combined in fermented date juice (Eb 245). Rapid healing was also to be assured by a medicinal mixture from Tefnut for Re, which could be used on any place of the body and was composed of the equal amounts (15 ml) of flour from the *amaa* grain, *shenfet* fruits, and goose fat (Eb 244). Nut's medicine for Re, which was to be cooked before use, contained 15 ml each of fresh mash, *shenes* bread, cedar oil, roots of the *Cynodon*, honey, oil, sea salt, natron, and a coastal stone (Eb 246).

The last remedy from the hand of the goddess Isis was intended for Re's headache and was to assure quick relief of any ill person who suffered from this problem. It contained 15 ml each of chaste tree, bryony fruit, seeds of coriander and *Anacyclus*, pine nuts, and honey (Eb 247).

Hearst 71–75—divine healing means

This group contains parallels to the cases of Ebers 243–47, but the precise wording of the texts differs slightly not only in minor details, such as the way of writing some of the names of the additives or their order (Eb 243 and H 71), but also in more fundamental data. For instance, the heading of one case states that it is the preparation made by Geb for Re (Eb 245) or for himself (H 73). Other times, they differ in the labeling of the originators of the disease, which were gods (Eb 244, Eb 245) or the dead (H 72, H 73, and H 74) or both (H 74)

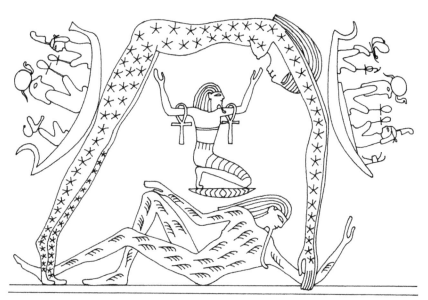

Fig. 17. The god of the earth Geb and goddess of the heavens Nut supported by the god of the air Shu and bearing the day and night solar barques (drawing © Archive of the Czech Institute of Egyptology, Faculty of Arts, Charles University, Jolana Malátková)

or other evil and harmful powers (Eb 246, Eb 247, and H 75). Moreover, the last case in the group specifies in more detail the place of the headache, which was to afflict the ill outside and/or inside the head (H 75). The composition of the prescriptions and their applications, however, are the same as with the group from the Ebers Papyrus.

Berlin 190—spell against the activity of an enemy

The formula in case Berlin 190 refers to a fever and health problems, the origin of which was a demon causing evil of all kinds, going against nature, health, and the divine order. This formula is told in the first person, as if the patient himself had to recite it, identifying himself with the god Horus. The formula thus naturally refers mainly to the goddess Isis, who protects the ill with the use of the healing art of the creator god Re. The physician acts here as their representative or authorized envoy, who "satisfies the god" *(netjer hotep)*. According to some experts, this phrase can be considered to be the name of the physician, who wrote down the case on papyrus (Nunn 1996, 38), but rather it is an attribute emphasizing that the physician in this case is acting according to the will of the god.

London 38—formula

The London papyrus contributes two more magical formulas, which are not focused on any specific malady or manifestation of the disease. The formula of L 38 is not presented with any heading, but it is clear from the text that it is intended for an unspecified problem caused by an enemy or the dead. Its main motif is again the god Horus, son of Osiris and Isis. Osiris appears here in the form of the "One who is Weak" (Imynehdef), hence Osiris, when he died and was revived for a short time to father a son with Isis-Mafdet (Westendorf 1999, 422). Egyptians often depicted the goddess Mafdet in the form of wild animals, such as wild cats, who managed to evade and render harmless the threatened danger (Janák 2005, 109). The formula also refers to the castration of Seth from the above-mentioned myth (see also Eb 3), where the seed of Osiris (hence his offspring Horus) is highly acclaimed. According to the case, the formula is to be said over bread in the shape of a donkey's penis, which is smeared with fat and fed to a cat, embodying Mafdet's protective power.

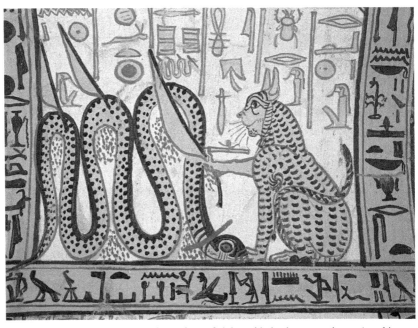

Fig. 18. The goddess Mafdet in the form of a cat fighting with the dangerous demon Apophis, which according to Egyptian beliefs threatened the order of the world (Nineteenth Dynasty, tomb of Nakhtamun in Deir el-Medina (TT 335), photo © Sandro Vannini)

London 25—the diseases *nesyt* and *temyt*

Another formula in the London papyrus was recommended in the case of the diseases *nesyt* and *temyt*, the precise meanings of which are unfortunately not known. The disease *temyt* also appears in the cases focused on the treatment of small children, for example in the formulas in the so-called Book for Mother and Child (Strouhal et al. 2014, 199), but they could apparently be suffered by adult patients as well. We find the disease *nesyt* in other cases which present the recipes for the preparation of medicinal mixtures for its treatment (e.g., Eb 752). It could also affect a person's eyes (Eb 751, see the forthcoming third volume in this series).

The authority of this magical spell is increased not only by the initial reference to the goddess Isis but also the claim that the knowledge of this goddess should have been transmitted in the form of a book sent in the night to the earth in the temple at Coptos for the lector priest there. This event was to have taken place during the reign of the pharaoh Khufu, the builder of the Great Pyramid at Giza, hence more than one thousand years before the London Papyrus BM 10059 was written down. The main motif of the formula is the myth of the battle of Horus with Seth, where Osiris allows his son Horus to speak (and act) on his behalf before the tribunal of the gods. Horus appears here in the form of Harnedjitef, thus "Horus, Savior (Avenger) of his Father" (Greek Harendotes, see Janák 2005, 85).

Chester Beatty VI verso—spell against the activity of demons and dead people

On the verso side of the Chester Beatty VI Papyrus, we find two formulas acting against a disease caused by demons. In the first spell (lines 2.2–2.5), it is necessary to drive away the demon Nesy or his female variant Nesyt. It is not clear from the text which demon it is about or what type of disease it caused. The formula directly addresses the demon and calls on him to retreat to keep him from reaching any place in the world or any creature. The second formula (lines 2.5–2.9), aimed at danger from an enemy or dead person, addresses the protectors and guards of the god Osiris, who are called upon to guard the ill just as carefully against danger.

Chester Beatty VIII—against the activity of gods, dead people, and all disease

The recto side of the Chester Beatty VIII Papyrus contains a magical formula which is to remove from the body of the ill problems coming from a malevolent god, dead person, or malicious seed. It is not only the formula itself, but also a recipe for the preparation of a liquid medicine from 37.5 ml of *Moringa* oil and the same amount of honey, wine, and incense.

Heart and Arteries

Currently, the medical internal subfield of cardiology includes illnesses of the heart and vascular circulation system (angiology), which was not discovered until the seventeenth century by William Harvey and which today is one of the cornerstones of medicine. Even in ancient Egypt, people knew of the importance of the beating heart for the maintenance of the life of the organism. The great significance of the heart in ancient Egyptian medicine is confirmed also by the fact that the cases and recipes for the treatment of the heart and arteries comprise the largest thematic group in the medical papyri in comparison with medicines for the diseases of other organs.

Characteristics of the Heart

The relationship between the heart and the pulse is mentioned already in Case 1 in the Smith Papyrus (Strouhal et al. 2014, 27) and in addition it is referred to by the name of the relevant group of cases in the Ebers Papyrus, beginning with the case of Ebers 854, which reads: "The beginning of the secret knowledge of the physician: knowledge of the operation of the heart (meaning) knowledge of the heart." In the case Ebers 854a, it is even written that the heart speaks through the blood vessels (Riedel 2009, 6). The author of the papyrus thus stood at the very beginning of the knowledge of the connection between the heart and the arterial part of blood circulation, but without then being able to reach the discovery of the network of capillaries nourishing and oxygenating all the body tissues and the venous return of deoxygenated blood to the lungs and from there oxygenated back into the heart.

According to the anatomical-physiological concept of that time, the human body was intertwined with an abundant system of tubes and canals generally designated in the ancient Egyptian language as *metu* (singular *met*, dual *metwy*). These were not only blood vessels but also various canals for the passage of tears, mucus, and saliva, by biliary ducts, urethras, sperm ducts, Fallopian tubes, and all of the respiratory and digestive tracts. Egyptian physicians included among the *metu* also other elongated thin bodies without cavities such as sinews, muscles, ligaments, and perhaps even nerves, whose importance they did not recognize (Nunn 1996, 44). Through these channels, life-sustaining substances, especially air and food, flowed into all parts of the body (Bardinet 1995, 94 and 102), besides the magical "breath of life" and "breath of death" (Riedel 2009, 6).

In this subchapter, we will discuss only the *metu* that start from the heart and branch in all directions to the distant places of the body, that is the arteries. During life, oxygenated blood flows through them from the pulsating heart,

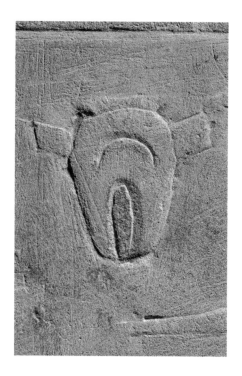

Fig. 19. Hieroglyph of a heart, Egyptian *ib* (Sixth Dynasty, tomb of Mehu in Saqqara, photo © Oxford Expedition to Egypt)

but after death they shrink, which pushes the blood out, so that in a cross-section they appear to be empty and filled only with air. It led Egyptians to the opinion that air flowed into the body through these *metu*, and this opinion prevailed until the times of Galen, a Greek physician active in Rome (Nunn 1996, 44–45).

Egyptians considered the heart not only as the center of human individuality, as mentioned above, but also as the organ of thought and intelligence, with which a person recognizes the will of the gods and the order of the world. In the heart, all of the good and bad acts were registered, which were then weighed in the last judgment against the principle of truth and justice *(maat)*. At the same time, the heart was considered as the seat of human feelings and emotions. This concept has essentially been preserved to this day in the sayings "he has a good heart," "his heart is cold," or "he has a heart of stone."

In contrast, Egyptian physicians considered the brain an unimportant organ in which mucus-like substances accumulated, which in their belief came from the head through seven orifices: tears poured out of the eyes, oily secretions through the ears, mucus through the nostrils, and saliva through the mouth. If the brain did not dissolve through the shining of the sun (colliquation), the embalmers took it out of the skull and discarded it along with the respectfully stored waste from their activity (see above). To a certain extent, physicians dealing with injuries to the head noticed the importance of the brain, as shown by cases 3–8 of the Smith Papyrus (Strouhal et al. 2014, 28–33 and 54–60), but we do not encounter this knowledge in medical texts written down later, so it seems that this observation did not lead to the correct explanation of the function of the brain.

Two ancient Egyptian expressions are known for the heart, namely *ib* and *haty*, which alternated in the medical papyri. Experts have presented a number of interpretations of these two expressions. The heart *ib* according to them could express the seat of emotions (Nunn 1996, 54), or the former could be the earlier and the latter a later name (Nunn 1996, 86). According to another interpretation, the heart as an anatomical organ was labelled as *haty*, within which the imaginary seat of individuality and the will of the person were located as the heart *ib* (Bardinet 1995, 70, 82, and 94; see also Janák 2012, 95–104). Egyptians imagined that breath, the breeze of life, was breathed through the nose and entered the lungs and from them to the heart *(haty)*, which divided it to all of the places in the body (Bardinet 1995, 102).

Five large sections are devoted to the heart and arteries in the Ebers Papyrus. The first is called "Beginning of the secret knowledge of a physician: knowledge of the operation of the heart (meaning) knowledge of the heart" (Eb 854a), the second "The beginning of the book on the spreading of the painful substances in any limb of a person, as was found in the writings under the feet (of the statue) of Anubis in Khem. And they were brought to the Majesty the King of Upper and Lower Egypt, Den, the justified" (Eb 856a). These groups are sometimes labeled collectively as the Books on the Tubes *(metu)* (Nunn 1996, 44). The third group is listed as "The beginning of a collection of remedies for making the heart accept food" (Eb 284–93). The fourth collection, not labelled with any special heading, contains the cases of heart failures (Eb 855a–z). The fifth group comprises the prescriptions for healing various heart ailments (Eb 217–40). In the following commentary, the cases will be discussed in this order with similar cases from the other preserved texts.

The theory of Egyptian pathophysiology relied on empirical evidence that if the tubes *(metu)* were freely passable, the body worked perfectly. Disease was caused by the tubes being blocked by poisonous agents causing a disease *(arut)* or pain *(wekhedu)*. At the same time, these substances were often to emerge in the rectum (e.g., Eb 138), caused by worms or the accumulation of congealed blood (e.g., Eb 198 or Eb 855 l). Ancient Egyptian physicians did not manage to reveal the life-giving role of blood *(senef)* in its physiological fluid form. They connected the spilling of blood in an injury with the production of a clot (*kefen* or baked blood), which aroused negative feelings of its harmfulness and the attempt to exude it from the body (more in the forthcoming third volume in this series).

In terms of the anatomic-physiological conception of the heart itself, we believe, especially based on the case Ebers 854, that ancient Egyptian physicians most likely were not able to investigate in detail cardiac activity by thumping (percussion) and listening (auscultation) as it was done by their later colleagues. However, physicians knew exactly where the heart was in the body and monitored its activity using touch (palpation) and the heart beat or pulse. They discovered that in many places of the body the *metu* type of arteries flowed, and they monitored the activity of the heart through palpation in the examination of the pulse in places where "the heart speaks in the arteries to of every limb" (Eb 854a). These arteries were thus suitable for evaluating the rhythm and speed of the patient's pulse by comparison with the pulse of the examiner, and it was easily possible to feel on the head, in the cardiac region, on the arm, wrist, and other places of the extremities, as shown not only by Ebers 854a, but also case 1 of the Smith Papyrus (Sm 1, Strouhal et al. 2014, 27). The text states that if the physician feels the pulse on these places, "he measures (directly) the heart."

Arteries

Egyptians thus knew that the heart distributes air from the lungs (Egyptian *wefa*) and food (from the stomach called *mendjer*) to the whole body through arteries *(metu)*. From experience acquired in disemboweling animals, they knew that they often contain air, whereas blood only rarely. Their stiff wall reminded them of the wall of the airways (larynx and trachea) leading to the lungs. In comparison, the Egyptians did not fully appreciate blood, the life-giving liquid, considered by other ancient civilizations as a valuable product of the liver, for example in the medicine of Mesopotamia (Haussperger 2012). They knew it mainly in its frequent form of coagulated blood, which they considered to be a substance causing pain *(wekhed)*, one of the obstacles to free movement in the system of *metu*, which could cause illness. Ancient Egyptian medical texts reveal to us what the ideas were on the system of *metu*, whence and where these tubes led, and what their function was.

The number of *metu* coming from the heart, thus arteries, is mentioned in cases 854 and 856 in the Ebers Papyrus and also case 163 in the Berlin Papyrus. Interestingly, the number of arteries given in the Ebers Papyrus is much higher than that in the Berlin Papyrus.

Egyptian physicians strictly distinguished between the right (favorable) and left (inauspicious) halves of the body, apparently as a consequence of the duality of the body and perhaps from the magical reasons inspired by the double nature of the Two Lands. According to Ebers 854, arteries led from the heart to twenty-seven places on each half of the body, whereas according to Ebers 856 and Berlin 163, there were only eleven places. However, in the literature we can encounter different sums of those arteries, for example forty-eight (Eb 854), thirty-two (Eb 856), and thirty (Bln 163) (Nunn 1996, 45), or forty-eight (Eb 854), twenty-two (Eb 856 and Bln 163) (Stephan 2001, 109). At the same time, the papyri with the descriptions of the individual arteries show possible pathological changes which could be connected with them, rarely also prescriptions for their treatment.

Ebers 854—knowledge of the heart and its operation

The individual subgroups of case Ebers 854 specify not only the numbers of *metu* in various parts of the body but often also their functions. According to them, four *metu* lead to both nostrils, of which two channels bring nasal mucus and two arteries blood, which was apparent particularly when injured (Eb 854b). Under the temple, four *metu* lead to the eyes, which promote blood circulation, but can also cause eye diseases, emerging with their opening. The water that flows from them (tears), is supposedly produced by either the iris or the pupil (pupilla) (Eb 854c). When the artery cannot be felt (or is deaf) and the person cannot open his mouth, it is clear that the extremities of the person were weakened by substances which have overwhelmed the heart (Eb 854c). At the head another four *metu* separate, which end in the crown of the head and cause loss of hair (capilli), baldness (alopecia), and festering (eczema) (Eb 854d). Two arteries on the temples, which supposedly lead to the roots of the eyes, are paradoxically the cause of deafness. They contain ear wax (cerumen), created by a demon called "Remover of Heads" (Eb 854e). Four *metu* lead in pairs to each ear, two in the right shoulder and two in the left shoulder of a person. According to the conceptions, the "breath of life" goes into the right ear, whereas the "breath of death" into the left ear (Eb 854f).

Three arteries lead into each arm, which reach all the way to the fingers (Eb 854g). It is similar in the lower extremities, where the arteries end in the feet (Eb 854h). Two *metu* supply both testicles, in which they create semen (sperm) (Eb 854i). Another two *metu* go to the buttocks (Eb 854k). Four arteries bring air and water to the liver, where, however, with the influence of blood congestion (hyperemia) symptoms of some of the diseases can emerge (Eb 854l). Four arteries supply water and air to the lungs and spleen (Eb 854m). In contrast, two *urethras*, also called *metu*, lead to the urinary bladder *(vesica urinaria)* (Eb 855n). The ancient author or scribe correctly did not confuse them with arteries (like Stephan 2001, 109).

Four arteries open into the *rectum*, supplying water and air and then taking both of them away. The rectum is also to be open for each of another pair of arteries from the right half of the abdomen, the left half of the abdomen, the arm, and the leg when they are full (Eb 854o). These eight arteries have to be counted with the others, so the sum of the arteries reaches fifty-four (instead of forty-eight according to Stephan and Nunn).

Ebers 856 and Berlin 163—substances causing pain

In the paragraphs of cases Ebers 856 and Berlin 163, individual groups of a total of twenty-two arteries on the head, neck, upper arms, and thighs are complemented by an explanation of their function and the illnesses that may arise in them, as well as the prescriptions to relieve the patient. In both of these texts, the cases are very similar and it is possible that they drew from the same models or built on the same medical tradition. In the Berlin case, nevertheless, some parts of cases Ebers 856d–e are lacking, as if the scribe skipped one paragraph by mistake. Case Berlin 163 also contains several prescriptions in the conclusion that are entirely missing in Ebers 856. It is, therefore, clear that in both cases they are copies of an early model from which each scribe drew slightly different information according to his own discretion.

The heading of both cases presents that it is a text to help the physicians fight against "painful substances," called in Egyptian *wekhedu* (Eb 856a, Bln 163a), and is to provide guidance "against all diseases" from which the ill could suffer (Bln 163b). The credibility of the cases is elevated by a reference to their antiquity and also divine origin, because according to their heading both were copied from a scroll found under the statue of the jackal god Anubis at the time of the First Dynasty during the reign of Pharaoh Den (twenty-ninth or thirtieth century BC) (Eb 856a, Bln 163a). Moreover, according to the Berlin papyrus, this old valuable scroll was taken to Pharaoh Senedj (Second Dynasty) and the effectiveness of the approaches written in it was proven (Bln 163a).

According to the text of this case, a person has twenty-two arteries in his body, which lead "to his heart," but correctly they lead from the heart. According to the ideas then, these arteries supplied air to all parts of the body (Eb 856b and Bln 163b).

Two arteries found in the chest and reminiscent of mesh (Eb 856c) could cause heat in a person's rectum (also Bln 163c). Against that undesirable heat, which could in fact be caused rather by an infection of widened rectal veins (hemorrhoids), they prescribed a drink prepared from fresh dates, the seeds of the sycomore tree, and *hemu* part of *Ricinus* (castor oil plant) pounded in water, which the sick person was to use for four days (Eb 856c and Bln 163c). It is noteworthy that the mentioned ingredients have a favorable effect on digestion; castor oil is used to this day for cleaning the intestines, and fresh dates and figs, rich in fiber, could work the same way. It is thus a question whether the phrase *metu* in this case could not mean even the intestine itself.

Two arteries lead to a person's thighs, where they can cause an arterial girdle causing pain, leg tremors, and also slackness (Eb 856d and Bln 163d). In this case, it might be an infection of the deep femoral arteries, but the typical manifestations of vasculitis are not mentioned here. A mixture of an herbal decoction with chaste tree and natron, which was used for four days, was to relieve the ill (Eb 856d).

The two arteries leading to a person's throat could cause pain in the throat and problems with vision (Eb 856e). It could be avoided by bandages applied on the throat and containing a mixture composed of myrtle, pine nuts, *Anacyclus* seeds, honey, and water for washing clothes (Eb 856e and Bln 163e).

The two arteries heading to the upper arm could cause pain of the shoulder and also tremors of the fingers. The cause was to be mucuses and the physician was to induce the patient to vomit through a mix of meat or fishes, beer, and wild rue. He was at the same time to spread watermelon on the fingers of the patient, possibly mixed with strong beer (Eb 856f and Bln 163f).

Another section names the seven pairs of arteries supplying the back of the head, the forehead, the eyes, the nose, and each of the ears separately. At the same time, it is explained here that the breath of life enters the body through the right ear, whereas the breath of death comes through the left ear (Eb 856g and Bln 163g).

The last paragraph of this case states that all of the arteries mentioned above come, according to the Egyptian belief, to the person's heart (in fact they come from the heart), they divide at the nose and join in the rectum, where they can—just like defecated ordure and excreted urine—cause disease. A disorder of some artery can even cause a person's death (Eb 856h), particularly the arteries in the lower extremities (Bln 163h). When a person was ill, various medicinal mixtures, which were used after one another, were recommended against the threatening danger. First, a drink was prepared from 600 ml of scalded cow's milk with vinegar, to which another 4 ml of honey was added after straining, which was recommended to be drunk for four days. Afterwards, the patient was to administer rectally for one night a mixture of

300 ml of sheep's or goat's milk scalded with 4 ml of honey and 37.5 ml of "milk fat oil" (perhaps an oil coagulum?) or human milk, which was itself considered a very effective remedy and was often used in pediatric medicine (Strouhal et al. 2014, 106). Subsequently, the patient was to be cured for four days with an enema from 225 ml of a fermented herbal decoction, 4 ml of *Moringa* oil, the same amount of honey, and a quarter amount of sea salt; and for another four days a similar mixture, where the amount of the individual ingredients was changed to 300 ml of herbal decoction, 37.5 ml of *Moringa* oil and honey, 2 ml of sea salt, and, moreover, 75 ml of strong beer was added. The next four days, it was a mixture with only 37.5 ml of *Moringa* oil, 375 ml of sweet beer, and 2 ml of sea salt; and as the last a mixture of 37.5 ml of honey, 4 ml of *Moringa* oil, and 150 ml of sweet beer was prescribed (Bln 163h). Although it is stated before each prescription that it is prepared "afterwards," it is not entirely clear whether all of these medicines were really used after one another, or whether they were mutually interchangeable remedies.

Illnesses of the Heart

We mainly find the cases that are devoted to illnesses of the heart in the Ebers Papyrus. The cases are of two types: one group describes various diseases, and the second group contains prescriptions for healing the heart, which we present in the next section. The first mentioned group contains cases of cardiac failures, which Nunn labeled as glosses (Nunn 1996, 85–86), but which alternate with pathophysiological knowledge. This group is not listed with any heading which would label the character of its original model.

Ebers 855—diseases of the heart

The entire section begins with a physiological statement, which essentially builds on the previous section on the arteries *(metu)*, namely that air enters the nose and continues further to the lungs and heart. Egyptian physicians moreover understood that the air from there was distributed by the arteries to the entire body (Eb 855a).

Different heart disorders are referred to using specific terms in Egypt, but they rarely indicate the real cause of the problem. It is therefore very difficult for us—and often impossible—to identify the Egyptian names with modern diagnoses. Moreover, the text only lists the heart defects, but not the methods for treating them, which could help us. It is possible that the treatment of these problems lay mainly in magical approaches, since the real cause was most likely unknown to physicians. In the cases, both labels are used for the heart, *haty* and *ib*, the second of which is more frequent here.

The idea of the flooding of the heart was connected with gastric juice and was manifested with the entirely limp extremities of a person (Eb 855b). These symptoms can be interpreted as insufficiency of the widened right heart with swelling of the limbs and enlargement of the liver. According to Nunn, it was a surplus of the oral fluid revealing the possibility of swelling (edema) of the lungs as a consequence of the insufficiency of the left heart (Nunn 1996, 86), which is, however, an unlikely construction.

The illness called "depression of the heart" could have been evoked by the artery called the "recipient," which according to the explication in the case passes water to the heart (Eb 855c). It could be a weakening heart.

Cardiac weakness (failure) emerged through deviation of the heart to the boundary of the lungs and liver, causing a "loss of hearing" of its arteries, or a failure all the way to discontinuation of the function of the cardiac arteries by the influence of increased temperature. However, according to the text, it was a situation which resolved itself (Eb 855d).

A flabby heart is described as "mute" and its arteries "do not speak" and cannot be felt. According to the concept, they were filled with air (Eb 855e). If the physician cannot feel the patient's pulse, as is presented here, it is the state of clinical death.

The rebelling heart, according to the text, is weakened by the heat of the rectum, for example in an inflammation of its veins (hemorrhoids). A strong indicator of this state can be the convulsive turning of the stomach, similar to the turning of the eyeball; in the text the author perhaps by mistake confused it with the word "iris" (Eb 855f).

If the heart, according to the physician, expands (dilates), it means that the cardiac arteries are under the influence of feces (Eb 855g). Here, it reflects the idea of the connection of the internal systems in the body and of the diseases caused by a failure of the circulation of their contents. However, the real cause could be rather intensive cardiac activity.

An unclear bitter disease *dehret*, whose name cannot be translated, was caused, according to the ideas of physicians then, by the magic activity of a priest (it was a *wab* priest, which means "pure"). It proves that its origin was unclear to the physicians. The disease could enter the body as a wind through the left eye and leave through the navel and cause the heart to be in a fever until it incinerates itself. Moreover, through the heart, the disease entered the arteries of the patient, which spread it to the entire body, which as a consequence also incinerated itself. At the same time, the arteries trembled. According to the conclusion of the text, it is possible that despite such a serious disability the arteries could overcome the disease—but if that was not managed, the arteries would overflow (Eb 855h). It is not clear what the cause of this illness was, but the high fever in the entire body of the patient was either overcome by the body itself or he was beyond help.

The failinge heart is a situation when the heart itself drowns or overflows, as a consequence of the liquid *(wiat)* which is found in it. The heart alternatively drops and rises up to the throat (Eb 855i). Problems described in this way correspond to the opinion that the internal organs are freely mobile. They can be caused by subjective feelings evoked by the movements of the body, anger, fear, or shock (Riedel 2009, 5).

The kneeling heart is a situation in which the heart remains in its place and is supplied by oxygenated blood from the lungs, but it is contracted and diminished emits heat, and tires out. Moreover, the patient lacks an appetite for food (Eb 855k). It could be a cardiac insufficiency. This case reveals that Egyptian physicians knew the functional connection of the heart and lungs, hence the small blood circulation (Stephan 2001, 78).

In a dry, or insufficiently perfused heart, blood clots could occur (Eb 855l). These could subsequently release and cause a blockage of one of the coronary arteries (thrombosis, myocardial infarction).

A kneeling heart was a phrase marking the reduction of the performance of the heart through the influence of substances causing pain (Egyptian *wekhedu*). These could cause a lowering of the volume of the heat and weaken the patient (Eb 855l bis).

Cardiac weakness, however, could also be caused by aging, when the heart could also be attacked by substances causing pain (Eb 855m). It is a reflection of a known fact that pain or shooting pain in the area of the heart often accompanies aging.

The dance of the heart was connected with the feeling that the heart shifted from its place in the left part of the chest towards the left shoulder (Eb 855n). It could be a manifestation of irregular cardiac activity (arrhythmia), but some experts reject that (Nunn 1996, 85).

Advanced bitterness of the heart or also submerged heart is explained in the text by the fall of the heart from its place in the body downwards (Eb 855o). The idea of the mobility of the internal organs again dominates here. It could be the result of the penetration of gastric juices into the esophagus or a characteristic bitter aftertaste caused by the outflow of bile to the stomach.

Another paragraph describes essentially the physiological position of the heart, which remains in its place and does not rise or fall (Eb 855p). The heart fat, which appears in several parts of the case, is most likely understood as the pericardium, under whose surface a layer of fat can be seen.

On the contrary, the permanently trembling heart is in its place in the body but suffers from a lack of declining movements, apparently a regular pulse (Eb 855q). It is a concise description of cardiac arrhythmia, when it could be the quivering of the auricle (fibrillation or flutter), which would cause unpleasant feelings and increase the suffering of a patient.

The next part (Eb 855r and 855s) came to be in the list of heart failures by the mistake of the author or the error of the scribe when he copied the text. It was very likely a disorder of the stomach, which is discussed on page 222.

The subsequent part of case Ebers 855 describes the failures of the function of the heart as the center of thought and feelings. The somber heart is associated with the heart of a man who eats ripe sycomore fruits (Eb 855t). The text might express the unhappy feelings of a person who overate figs.

The languishment and forgetfulness of the heart were attributed to the magically acting breath of a lector priest. His breath has to enter in various ways into the lungs, from which it acts subsequently on the heart *(ib)* (Eb 855u). Lector priests were very honored in ancient Egypt, since they had the knowledge of the religious rituals and incantations. According to the beliefs, they could abound in great power, which is described for instance in the stories of the miracles in the Westcar Papyrus (Khufu and the Magicians, see also Vymazalová and Coppens 2010, 40). However, in this case, it could be forgetfulness and confusion, low concentration, which could be triggered by a wide range of causes.

The constricted heart, which is manifested as a tightening by passion and is more often weak, is thought to be a consequence of the passion of anger. That can cause the heart to be filled with blood; the cause is considered to be drinking bad water and the consumption of heated spoiled food (Eb 855v). It is possible that in this case it was food poisoning accompanied by cramps in the abdomen.

The heart hidden by darkness, perhaps expressing insanity, is apprehensive, because the darkness caused by the passion of hate is scattered in the body. This acts in cases of absorption, or perhaps weakening of the heart (Eb 855w). It might be the feeling when a person is overcome by gloom or suffers from depression.

Another part of the case describes the situation when the person's whole body is hot and the heart exhausted, as if it were worn out by a long walk. According to the text, it means that his muscles are tired (perhaps the cardiac muscles are meant), as if the musculature of the person was exhausted after a long walk (Eb 855x).

When a patient is seized by an intense tremor, perhaps representing fury as a consequence of some external stimuli, according to the text it is a situation when the heart turns like a spindle because a malicious demon acts on it (Eb 855y). It is possible that it was a description of a high level of fury, when a person feels a tremor and anger in the heart.

The heart was flooded when it became forgetful like with a person who thinks about something else (Eb 855z). It could be an absent-minded patient.

Ebers 191 and 194—stomach disease (?), pain of the arms and on the breast

Two identical cases written in the Ebers Papyrus in "The book on the stomach" (we will discuss it on pages 212–23, where it belongs due to its contents) present a situation which apparently also concerned the heart. It describes the state here when a patient suffers pain of the arms and on the breast "on the side of the stomach" in addition to stomach problems, until the affected person's face turns green. The radiation of pain into the left arm was such a known symptom for the Egyptian physicians that they even labeled the forefinger of the left hand as the heart finger (Riedel 2009, 6). According to the text, this serious disease was caused by something that entered the ill through his mouth when some dead person went past. The dead were often considered as the origin of diseases, along with demons and enemies, as shown by the numerous magical incantations used for healing. However, this idea can also be expressed by the words that death approached the dead (Stephan 2001, 93).

In this case, the text recommends a stimulating healing drink prepared from herbs, namely from equal amounts (15 ml) of peas, bryony, thyme, an unknown plant called *niaia*, and barley flour. All of the ingredients were joined with oil or with beer and given to the sick to drink. During or after serving the drink, the physician was to place his bent hand on the stomach and most likely create pressure until the patient's arms relax and the pain receded to the intestines and rectum.

We agree with Nunn (1996, 87) and other authors that it was most likely an ischemic cardiomyopathy (angina pectoris or myocardial infarction). According to the text's conclusion, this treatment should never be repeated, apparently for the poor prognosis of this disease.

Whereas the text of the case designates a state explicable as the above-described heart disease, the treatment recommended could also have a connection with digestive problems (for a comparison, see also pages 223–48). An oil with peas, barley, and bryony, whose root was used in the past as a natural laxative, could effectively help clean the intestines. It is possible that the physicians in their ideas connected heart problems with the patency of the body, as we also find in other cases.

Ebers 197—sick stomach (?), shriveled body

The same part of the Ebers Papyrus contains still another case which appears related to the heart. The introduction of the text mentions that it is a case when the patient has a sick stomach and as a consequence of that the whole body is shriveled. At the same time, during the examination, the physician does not find any visible symptom of an illness on the patient's abdomen. It clearly is a long-lasting disease, which as a consequence of the loss of musculature and subcutaneous fat, has accentuated the bending creases of the body and wrinkles that the author of the text compares to the scoring of fruit pits. With this case, it is, according to the attached diagnosis, "a disquiet of your (that is, the patient's) home," hence an illness of the center of the organism, the heart. The text recommends a medicine prepared from an unstated amount of carob, flaxseed, honey, oil, and hematite, which the person was to drink for four days to completely get rid of the illness. Just as in the previous case, we encounter here the connection of a disease of the heart with the digestive tract. The recommended medicine contained an anti-inflammatory component (honey), a component for beneficial digestion (carob), which works against diarrhea, and oil, acting as a binder and lubricant. It is worth mentioning that hematite is used to this day in natural healing (naturopathy) because, thanks to the content of iron and its magnetic features, it supposedly helps improve the circulation of the blood.

Prescriptions for Treatment of the Heart

Besides the previous groups of cases, which describe various diseases of the heart and arteries, we also find in the Ebers Papyrus a wide range of cases which comprise only a recipe for the preparation of a medicine. Similar recipes

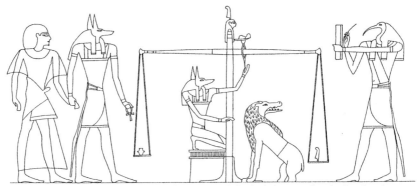

Fig. 20. The heart of a person played an important role in the judgment after death, when it was evaluated on the scales before the god Osiris and the tribunal of forty-two gods, against the symbol of justice, the feather *maat* (drawing © Archive of the Czech Institute of Egyptology, Faculty of Arts, Charles University, Jolana Malátková)

are also included in the Hearst and Berlin papyri. Although the text of the cases does not mention for which problems these medicinal mixtures were to be used, a closer look at their composition may allow their evaluation as a whole.

Hearst 51–52—healing the heart
In the Hearst Papyrus we find a group of two cases which are generally titled as means for the examination of the heart *(haty)*. The text presents the ingredients in precisely prescribed amounts. The first medicine comprised a drink from 300 ml of dark emmer wheat boiled in 2.4 l of water, which was then to be strained and reduced to 450 ml. The patient was to drink it for four days (H 51). The second concoction was prepared in the same way from 75 ml of earth almonds (tubers of yellow nutsedge), 2 ml milk, half the amount of goose fat, and juniper berries, which inter alia favorably affect digestion and the lymphatic system, and 300 ml of water (H 52).

Ebers 217–18 and 220—healing the heart
Another group of cases in the Ebers Papyrus deals with, as stated by the headings of two of them, the general treatment of the ill heart, without a closer specification of the diagnosis or manifestations of the disease. In 375 ml of sweet beer, 4 ml of date flour, 0.5 ml carob, 75 ml of the unknown fruits *amau* were to be cooked; after cooking, the mix was pressed through a sieve and reduced. The usage was prescribed for four days (Eb 217). Another preparation, used for the same period, comprised 150 ml of water, half the amount of milk, and 1 ml of honey (Eb 218).

For single use, a mix was intended of 300 ml of water, 75 ml of honey, the same amount of ripe sycomore fruits and fresh dates, 0.5 ml of honeydew melon and ocher, which was left to stand overnight without cooking, exposed to the dew, and then was strained (Eb 220).

Hearst 48–49—healing the heart
We find almost verbatim copied parallels to the cases Ebers 217 and 218 in the Hearst Papyrus. We find small differences in their headings. In the recipe Hearst 49, the scribe wrote down the wrong amount of honey.

Ebers 230—healing the heart
Before bedtime, the patient was to be given a medication that was prepared for the purpose of real healing of the heart and should provide immediate relief. It was a beverage prepared from 225 ml of water, 2 ml of figs, half the amount of ocher, and a quarter unit of a gum (mucilage).

Berlin 117—healing the heart

Similar to the previous recipe is a remedy made from 15 ml of figs, 0.5 ml ocher, the same amount of acacia leaves, half the amount of honey, and 375 ml of water. The mixture was to be pressed and left to stand overnight exposed to the dew. It was used as a healing drink.

Hearst 50—keeping down food

Another case in the Hearst Papyrus contains a recipe which was intended for the heart to accept food. It was prepared from 75 ml of water, 2 ml of figs and anise, and a fourth of the amount of honey and ocher, which was to be cooked, strained, and used for four days. It was apparently a medicine, which was to assure nutrition to the heart and benefit the organism, but the text does not present during which problems the patient should use it.

Ebers 284-93—accepting food

The group of ten cases in the Ebers Papyrus is listed with a common heading, according to which it was copied from the collection of medicines which were to ensure that the heart accept food. These mixtures were thus to serve this purpose as the previous case from the Hearst Papyrus, but none of them is entirely identical with it. They are again recipes with nutritious substances, administered for mostly undisclosed problems. The individual ingredients are prescribed in precisely set amounts.

The first medicine was prepared in the form of a beverage. Into the mixture of 375 ml of sweet and 75 ml of strong *djesret* beer were added 2 ml of figs, the *ished* fruits, goose fat, half the amount of juniper berries, the unknown *tiam* plant, fatty meat, 0.5 ml of red oche, a half share of cumin, garden cress, and incense (Eb 284). Some of the listed ingredients undoubtedly have beneficial effects on digestion. The length of use is not specified.

The majority of the medicines in the group were to be used regularly for a period of four days. The mixture, which was very similar to the first medicine, also contained sweet and strong *djesret* beer in the same amount of 75 ml, to which was added another 75 ml of an unknown beverage *sekh-pet*, further 2 ml of figs, date and wheat flours, raisins, and goose fat, half the amount of juniper berries, 0.25 ml of garden cress, and incense (Eb 285). Another beverage was prepared by mulling and then straining 375 ml of sweet beer with 2 ml of figs, earth almonds, and unpreserved parts of a willow, 0.5 ml of onion, and *wedja* of dates, half the amount of incense, and 4 ml of fatty meat (Eb 293).

A mixture with a similar composition was in 300 ml of wine instead of beer, with the addition of 2 ml of yellow nutsedge and the *tiam* plant, the same amount of beef marrow, 1 ml of ocher, and 0.25 ml of incense. The method of preparation and period of usage were the same (Eb 288). The healing mixture was made from 75 ml of wine and 375 ml of sweet beer with the addition of 1 ml of figs, raisins, celery, and fatty meat. After boiling and straining the mixture was used again for four days (Eb 291).

Instead of beer or wine, it was also possible to use water as the base. A concoction was prepared that way when 37.5 ml of water was mixed with 2 ml of earth almonds, the same amount of roasted bread, and a quarter of the amount of honey (Eb 290). A similar remedy was from 150 ml of water, 4 ml of earth almonds, 37.5 ml of roasted bread, 0.5 ml of honey, and the same amount of the stone *qesenty* (Eb 289). These two mixtures were not cooked, only strained and used for four days.

Other recommended mixtures were used only for a short time, for one day. They were therefore prepared in lesser quantities, as shown by the prescribed amounts of the individual ingredients. These medicines included, for instance, a drink which was made from 37.5 ml of sweet beer and 0.5 ml of the unknown fruits *shenfet*. After cooking it was strained and given to the patient to drink (Eb 286). In the same way, the mixture of 37.5 ml of wine and 2 ml of wheat semolina, which was left to stand overnight and collect dew and then strained before use, was recommended for short, one-day usage (Eb 287). Another mixture was to be cooked from 75 ml of wine, 2 ml of each of two types of bakery items, which were called *wetiu* and *heken*, the *wedja* part of dates, and a quarter of the amount of honey (Eb 292).

It would be very interesting to know whether the cardiac diets in the prescriptions in the given cases could strengthen the activity of the heart muscle, or whether they were rather harmful and with the influence of the fatty animal ingredients caused with more frequent usage coronary sclerosis of the (coronary) arteries or associated complications (angina pectoris, myocardial infarction).

Ebers 219 and 235—heat and cooling the heart

Another small group of recipes was intended against supposed fever of the heart. A healing mixture was to benefit in stopping heat on the heart. It was prepared from 300 ml of water, 15 ml of anise, 4 ml of honey, 2 ml of wheat semolina, and the *ished* fruits unknown to us, a quarter of the amount of the leaves of honeydew melon, of honey, of gum, and the stone *qesenty*. After mixing, the ingredients were left to stand overnight to collect dew and were administered to the patient for a period of four days (Eb 219).

The drink for cooling the heart comprised 150 ml of honey, in which there was mixed 2 ml each of anise, figs, and ocher (Eb 235), which were among the ingredients of many other prescriptions for healing the heart. The mixture was to be cooked and used as a beverage for four days.

Ebers 233–34—substances causing pain in the heart

A healing beverage was recommended against substances causing pain (Egyptian *wekhedu*) in the heart and was prepared from 375 ml of water, 2 ml each of figs, wheat semolina, and honey, and a quarter of the share of ocher (Eb 234). A very similar mixture, accompanied by a few more ingredients, could be cooked from 150 ml of water, 37.5 ml of wheat semolina, and also raisins, 2 ml each of figs and the *ished* fruits, a quarter of the amount of ocher and gum (Eb 233). Both drinks were used for four days.

Ebers 236–37—poisonous substances in the heart

Against poisonous substances which caused heart disease, a beverage was recommended made from 375 ml of sweet beer, 1 ml of celery, and a half amount of the unknown plant *ibu*, which were cooked together (Eb 236). Other times, the same ingredients were mixed in different amounts: 150 ml of sweet beer, 0.5 ml of celery, and a half amount of the plant *ibu*, to which peas were added. This mixture was left after cooking to stand overnight to collect dew and was strained before use (Eb 237). Both mixtures were used for a period of four days.

Ebers 221–24—poisonous substances in the abdomen and heart

Besides the heart, poisonous substances could also affect the abdomen, as shown by this group of cases, presented under a single heading. Before bedtime, they were to use a mixture of 37.5 ml (or perhaps 7.5 ml?) of honey, 0.25 ml of ocher, 1 ml seed of the *Anacyclus*, and a double measure of the *shasha* fruits (Eb 221); 37.5 ml (or perhaps 7.5 ml?) of honey, 2 ml each of yellow nutsedge and the *shasha* fruits, half of the amount of pine nuts, 0.5 ml of the fruits *pesedj*, amber, and a half amount of malachite (Eb 222); or 37.5 ml (or perhaps 7.5 ml?) of honey, 2 ml of the *shasha* fruits, half the amount each of *Anacyclus* and grapes, and 0.5 ml of gum (Eb 223).

On the contrary, a medicine was intended for immediate use prepared from 300 ml of water, into which 150 ml of fresh mash, 75 ml of ground earth almonds, and 2 ml each of fresh dates, part *hemu* of *Ricinus*, part *khesau* of the sycamore tree, and lotus leaves were mixed (Eb 224).

Hearst 79–82—poisonous substances in the abdomen and heart

This group of cases in the Hearst Papyrus represents parallels to Ebers 221–24 presented above. The wording of these cases is not, however, literal; we find differences in the headings and in other parts of the text.

Ebers 238–40—poisonous substances in the abdomen and heart

This group contains prescriptions for the preparation of further medicines which were to help expel from the patient poisonous substances which had settled in the abdomen as well as in the heart. The first medicine was a beverage which was to act immediately and was prepared from 75 ml of sweet beer, 1 ml of powdered coriander, and a quarter amount of a powder from the unknown plant *ibu*, which was administered to the patient for the evening before bedtime (Eb 238). Another used before bedtime was a cooked mash mixture from 7.5 ml of honey with 2 ml of the *shasha* fruits, a half amount of coriander, *Anacyclus*, and sorghum, and 0.25 ml of peas, and the unknown plant *ibu* (Eb 239). In contrast, a medicine was to be used for four days that was prepared from 75 ml of a decoction from ground and cooked barley mixed with 1 ml of honey and the plant *qesentet*, a half amount of carob, the tubers (?) of the plant *Astragalus*, and parts of the fig tree. Before use, the mixture was cooked, strained, and left to stand overnight to collect dew (Eb 240).

Ebers 241—poisonous substance

A preparation made to protect against a poisonous substance generally could also relate to the heart. A mixture of oil mulled with the sprouts of unspecified twigs was to be applied on the affected area.

Ebers 227–28—poisonous substance in the heart, cardiac weakness, faintness, shooting pain near the heart

This group of prescriptions contains the mixtures that should be strained and given to the patient for the night before he went to sleep. The first recommended mixture contained equal shares (2 ml) of anise, figs, and the unknown *shasha* fruits, a half amount of celery, and a quarter amount of honey and ocher, which was mixed in 150 ml of water (Eb 227). The second mixture included 2 ml of earth almonds, a half amount of anise, grapes, jujube bread, and the unknown *ibu* plant, and a quarter of the amount of celery, which was mixed in 150 ml of water (Eb 228).

It is interesting that these prescriptions were related to the heart according to their heading, but they follow the cases devoted to abdominal pain, and that a large part of the ingredients mentioned is the same for both of these groups (see Eb 226 on pages 231–32). That could again indicate the connection of the medical ideas on the diseases of the heart and digestive tract.

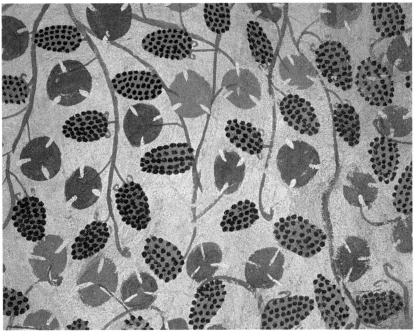

Fig. 21. Ripe grapes decorating tomb walls and ceilings indicate the popularity of the sweet fruit and wine with the ancient Egyptians (Eighteenth Dynasty, tomb of Sennefer in Sheikh Abd el-Qurna (TT 96), photo © Sandro Vannini)

Berlin 114—poisonous substances in the heart

The Berlin Papyrus recommends against the same problem a beverage made from cow's milk with honey, figs, grapes, and the cracked ripe fruits of the sycomore (the amounts are not specified). After scalding, the mixture was strained and administered to the patient.

Berlin 116—substances causing pain after being attacked by demons

According to another prescription, in which the undesirable substances in the heart are connected with the activity of spiteful dead people, the patient was to be relieved by a beverage prepared from human milk mixed with pine nuts, yellow nutsedge, the unknown *shasha* fruits, and a stone called in Egyptian "great protection." For the night, the treatment was to be complemented by mixtures of the same plant ingredients, that is pine nuts, yellow nutsedge, and the *shasha* fruits, but this time mixed in honey. The text does not provide the amounts of the ingredients. The use of human milk is interesting, as the milk of the mother of a male offspring is not demanded, as is often true in other cases.

Berlin 115—evil substances in the heart

The problems that affected the patient are described at the end of the text. He was to be helped by a prescription for a medicine prepared from pine nuts, the *shasha* fruits, *Anacyclus*, coriander, wild mint, peas, and sorghum, which was mulled in honey.

Berlin 77—the heart stung by a scorpion

Another case in the Berlin Papyrus might help a person who was stung by a scorpion so that his heart withstood the activity of the poison (?). The treatment lies in the fumigation of the person affected with a mixture of raisins, cracked ripe fruits of the sycomore, earth almonds, and the unknown plant *ineb*, wax, hematite, and orpiment. However, whether the inhalation of this mixture burnt on glowing coals can relieve the patient remains a question.

Heat of the Heart

Just like other problems with the heart, the cause of the heat was not usually mentioned in the cases and remains unknown. The heart can warm in fevers accompanying diverse internal diseases (Bardinet 1995, 171) or if it contains a hot substance *(kapu)* (Bardinet 1995, 284 and 458–59). In the prescriptions which the Egyptian texts recommend for these problems, we notice the striking similarities with the means for healing the abdomen (see pages 223–48). The cases thus reflect the conception of a welcome harmony between the perfect functioning of the heart, the abdomen, and the rectum for the health of the entire organism.

Berlin 185–86—heat of the heart

In the Berlin Papyrus, we find two cases intended for the treatment of the ill with whom a heat of the heart has occurred. The first case contains a detailed description of "red oil," which was created by mixing 2.85 l of water with 2 ml of oil, honey, and the plant *desher*, a quarter of the amount of the pulp of the carob pod, and an eighth of the amount of wheat semolina. The prescription precisely sets not only the necessary amounts of the ingredients but also the method and order of their usage. It was first necessary to bring the water with semolina to a boil, into which the plant *desher* was subsequently placed. Its name is related to the ancient Egyptian term for the color red, and thus this ingredient provided the subsequent mixture its color. The other ingredients, the carob pod pulp and oil, were added gradually, always when again reaching a boil. After reducing the entire mixture to the desired amount of 450 ml, the honey was added. The healing mixture was then to be left to stand overnight and collect dew and was to be strained before application. It was used for four days (Bln 185).

Another medicine for the same problems was prepared from 300 ml of water with the addition of 0.25 ml of yellow nutsedge, dates, and sorghum, and 2 ml of the unknown fruits *ihu*. The preparation this time was not cooked; the mixture was left overnight to stand and collect dew, then thoroughly mixed and strained, and again left for another night to stand and collect dew before being applied (Bln 186). It was used for a period of four days.

Chester Beatty VI

We find also in the Chester Beatty VI Papyrus a group of cases whose headings refer to the heart. They are prescriptions against cardiac heat (CB VI, 20–21) or prescriptions recommended for cooling the heart and also the rectum (CB VI, 18–19, 22, and 25–30). It seems likely that the expression for heart *(ib)* was confused in these cases with the expression for stomach *(ra-ib)*. According to the composition of the healing mixtures, they were rather medicines for the treatment of the digestive tract and rectum, comparable with other prescriptions in that text (see pages 255–57).

O.DeM 1091—heart

For completeness, we present that also the ostracon from Deir el-Medina (verso 1) contained a case concerning the heart, from which, however, only the beginning of the heading has been preserved. What is interesting is that the craftsmen who built the royal rock-cut tombs in the famous Valley of the Kings lived in Deir el-Medina. It thus seems that not even they were immune to cardiac problems.

Magical Healing of the Heart

Whereas the group of cases presented above dealt with the problems of the patient in a relatively rational way with the use of healing mixtures prepared from plant, animal, and mineral ingredients, other cases describe ingredients and methods which could indicate the somewhat magical activity of the healer. These methods are in accord with the heading of this group, which place the blame for problems with the heart on the activity of maleficent magical powers or poisons.

Berlin 58-65—poisonous substances, tiredness, and forgetfulness of the heart

The entire group of cases describes prescriptions for the preparation of medicinal mixtures against poisonous substances, fatigue, and forgetfulness of the heart, by which mainly the patient was fumigated. The required amounts of the ingredients are not presented in the text. The first mixture, which was to be cooked before application, included beans, fennel, carob, ricin seeds, and wild rue seeds (Bln 58). Another mixture contained myrtle, wild rue, hemp, bryony seeds, the unknown *wam* plant, a cockroach or a burying beetle (Westendorf 1999, 364), and a part of the mallet of a washer man, which could be the name of some unknown ingredient (Bln 59). From the myrtle and lichen another possible mixture was prepared, which was to be gradually placed on seven potter's wheels (or perhaps small balls of manure), then it was to be burned and the fire extinguished with an herbal decoction with girl's urine (Bln 60). Myrtle was also a component of another means, when Indian rubber was added to it, thus a stone for correction of papyrus scrolls, and a mineral called "great protection," which was mixed together with the fat of a goat or sheep (Bln 63). Myrtle with honey, thyme, *Moringa* oil, and salt could also be mixed with girl's urine and with the dung of a donkey, a tomcat, and a pig (Bln 64). Another two prescriptions described a medicinal mixture from reed and *Anacyclus*, either with pine nuts (Bln 61) or with thyme and honey (Bln 62).

A single case from the entire group contains a prescription for the preparation of a mix that was not intended for fumigation, but was smeared on the openings leading to the house, apparently to discourage malevolent demons who would want to enter and harm the inhabitants. The mixture contained *Moringa* oil mixed with the unknown *niaia* plant (Bln 65).

London 14—easing of what belongs to the heart
The London Papyrus, which contains a wide range of magical incantations, offers one case which was related to the heart. It is not entirely clear whether it was recommended in case of some specific problems or it was possible to also recite it when applying medicinal mixtures as their complement. The incantation repeatedly refers to the idea that internal problems and pains are caused by demons with their harmful activity. The incantation has not been preserved in its entirety; large parts of many lines of the text are missing, which significantly complicates their understanding. In the introduction, it refers to the myth of Isis saving her son Horus, whereas the second part of the incantation addresses the illness itself and names in which forms it is not to manifest itself on the patient. This description is reminiscent of many parasitic illnesses (see also pages 277–87).

Paleopathological Perspective
The modern field of paleopathology has recently brought new knowledge on diseases of the heart and arteries. A collection of forty-four mummies from the Middle Kingdom to the Ptolemaic and Roman periods with preserved cardiovascular structures showed atherosclerosis in twenty of them (that is, in 45.5

percent of the cases), clear in twelve of them, and likely in eight mummies. Calcification was found in the coronary arteries of the heart, in the carotid arteries in the neck, the iliac arteries in the pelvis, femoral in the thighs, and other peripheral arteries of the lower extremities. It is interesting that the people with ATS lived longer (45.1 ± 9.2 let) than people with healthy arteries (34.5 ± 11.8 let)—or rather we can say that this disease managed to develop in those who lived longer. The length of their lives naturally did not rely only on ATS, but also with lifestyle, diet, and other diseases. Higher-status individuals, who had themselves mummified, suffered from ATS much more often than was assumed before. The priests of the temples sacrificing to the gods three times a day fatty beef, poultry, bread, vegetables, fruits, cakes, wine, and beer took this food home with them after the services. It not only led to their obesity but also to ATS, so the heart and arteries of their mummies showed atheromatous plaques and calcifications, which blocked the arteries. Of the sixteen mummies with preserved heart or arteries from the collection of the University Museum in Manchester, nine were affected by this disease (56.3 percent) (David et al. 2010, 718).

We should also remember the case of Lady Rai—the wet nurse of Queen Ahmose Nefertari, mother of Pharaoh Amenhotep I (1514–1493 BC)—whose mummy in the Egyptian Museum in Cairo showed calcified ATS plaques in various arteries and signs of a past myocardial infarction (Abdelfattah et al. 2013). This case proves that not only men but also women suffered from cardiac and circulatory diseases.

Lungs and Chest
Pain in the Chest
In Egyptian, the lungs were known as *sema*, whereas the chest as a whole was known as *wef*. The most common symptom of lung diseases mentioned in the texts was a cough, in Egyptian *seryt*. According to the ancient Egyptian concept, the life-giving inhaled air, the Breath of Life, which kept him alive, flowed through the nose of a person into his body (Vymazalová and Coppens 2011, 195). According to case Ebers 855a, physicians were aware that air entered through the nose to the lungs and heart, from which arteries *(metu)* distributed it along with food to the entire body. The stopping of the breathing movements of the chest in a patient, like the disappearance of the heartbeat, meant death.

After death, during the mummification of the deceased, the lungs were removed and placed in a canopic jar which had a lid in the shape of the head of a baboon. This jar was connected with the god Hapi and was protected by the goddess Nephthys.

Ebers 187—pain in the chest

For prevention of pains in the chest, which are not more closely specified or described in the text, 2 ml of acacia leaves ground in 375 ml of sweet beer was prescribed. The mixture was to be left to stand overnight exposed to the dew and then strained to get only the liquid from it. The patient used the medicine repeatedly for four days.

Hearst 30—painful substances in the chest

Pains in the chest, which were attributed to the activity of harmful, painful substances *(wekhedu)*, were treated using a mixture of 75 ml of sweet beer with half that amount of milk, to which were added 2 ml of figs, earth almonds, and the *ished* fruits, half of the amount of peas, and a pinch of incense and *shenfet* fruits. The mixture was thickened to 75 ml and then further reduced to 1/30 (without units), which seems like an amount copied incorrectly.

Ebers 183-84—healing of the chest

Selected prescriptions were intended for healing the chest generally, and it is not clear from the texts for which problems they were recommended. A simple medicinal mixture could be prepared from 1 ml carob and four times the amount of cumin, which was mulled in wine (Eb 183). This mixture certainly had a calming effect and acted favorably also on digestion. Another, more complicated mixture included a number of ingredients, which were mixed in water. It was an aqueous solution from 4 ml of ground barley, the same amount of yellow nutsedge, half the amount of the *tiam* plant, a quarter of the amount of juniper berries, and an eighth of the amount of the inside of a carob pod, parts *(wetyt)* of a sycomore tree, and the plant *netjer* (Eb 184). With both medicinal mixtures, repeated use for a period of four days was recommended.

Ebers 35 and 185—healing of the chest, pain of the abdomen, and healing of the lung

The medicinal mixtures described in these two prescriptions were administered to patients who suffered from lung difficulties and also pains of the abdomen. Both cases appear in various parts of the Ebers Papyrus and are copied almost verbatim. They differ only in the heading, which in Ebers 35 does not mention healing of the chest, and in the conclusion when the same text lacks the recommended dosage. The actual text of the prescription is, however, identical. In the vessel *des*, warm, sweet beer was mixed with 150 ml of carob. The mixture was thoroughly stirred so that both components perfectly joined. The patient was to drink 1 *hin*, hence 480 ml of this beverage in the heated state, namely every day until there was an overall improvement of his state. The composition of this medicinal mixture is very similar to the remedies recommended for a cough (see below, pages 204–10).

Ebers 21—healing of the lung
In this prescription, it is the same medicinal mixture as in the cases of Ebers 35 and 185, but it provides a different amount of the ingredients and more precise period of usage. They were to mix 3.2 l of sweet beer with 75 ml of carob. After being left overnight to the dew, the mixture was used for a period of four days.

Hearst 57—healing of the lungs
According to this prescription, the lungs were to be benefited by a medicine prepared from 375 ml of water in which were mixed 2 ml of figs, the same amount of honey, and a quarter of the amount of gum and ocher. The mixture was left overnight to stand and collect dew. The sick person then used it for four days.

Ebers 186—fever and substances causing pain in the chest
If the patient suffered from pains in the chest and also had a high fever, the physician prepared for him a mixture from equal amounts (15 ml) of figs, garden cress, cumin, grape seeds, juniper berries, the *ished* fruits, the *wedja* part of dates, and incense. These ingredients were mulled in sweet beer and, after straining, the mixture was used for a period of four days.

Chester Beatty VI.14–15—driving away the disease *akhu* in the chest, cooling the rectum
The Chester Beatty Papyrus contains several cases devoted to treatment of respiratory diseases, which also manifested other symptoms in various parts of the body. According to this text, illness of the chest was connected with heat of other internal organs including the heart *(haty)* and the rectum.

The case, which cites "A comprehensive handbook of the medicines of a physician," deals with a disease unknown to us, which the Egyptian physicians called *akhu* and which according to the heading resided in the chest. At the same time, the side of the chest was to be treated (without presentation of the right favorable or left inauspicious) and cooling of the rectum assured. Westendorf (1992, 178) speculates that the disease *akhu* could be heat, apparently penetrating all the way to the rectum. It has not been ruled out that it was pneumonia (bronchopneumonia or pneumonia), which could not be recognized yet at that time. This complicated case (syndrome) required the preparation of

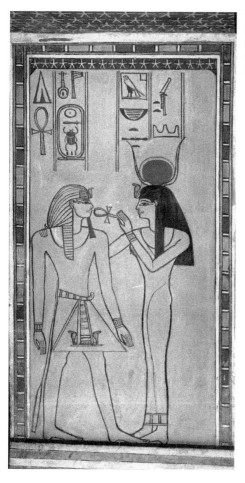

Fig. 22. Pharaoh Amenhotep II receives life in the form of the *ankh* symbol from the goddess Hathor (Eighteenth Dynasty, tomb of Amenhotep II in the Valley of the Kings (KV 35), photo © Sandro Vannini)

two medicines, one to be drunk and the other administered in the form of an intestinal enema.

The first preparation contained 75 ml of earth almonds, the same amount of fresh dates, 1 ml of anise, and half the amount of juniper berries, gum, honey, and ocher, which were mixed in 375 ml of water. The strained medicinal beverage was given to the ill person to drink for four days.

The second preparation was given afterwards as an enema and was to treat the heat of the rectum. It comprised 75 ml of old honey, half that amount of *Moringa* oil, and 2 ml of sea salt. The end of the text has not been preserved; the mixture could thus include other ingredients, and the method of preparation and number of applications are not known.

Chester Beatty VI.16–17—healing of the chest, cooling the heart and rectum, and driving away heat

This case again describes a prescription for a medicinal drink and subsequent enema. The beverage was prepared from 75 ml of fresh dates and earth almonds, half that amount of split ripe sycomore fruits and grapes, to which were added also 4 ml of sorghum and honey, and an unspecified amount of water. After being mixed, the ingredients were left to stand overnight and collect dew. The beverage was then strained and given to the patient to drink for four days.

The mixture intended for application in the form of an enema was produced from sheep's or goat's milk and honey. It was also applied for a period of four days. This case is interesting in that it was—according to the pronouns in its heading—intended explicitly for the treatment of women. The text does not explain in more detail in which ways the problems described were specific for female patients. The great care devoted to women is, however, attested also by the specialized texts and cases of a gynecological nature (see Strouhal et al. 2014, 97–185), which is fully in accord with the dignified position of women in ancient Egyptian society (Strouhal 1995, 51–61).

Treatment of a Cough

The main symptom of an illness of the upper airways and the lungs was clearly a cough (tussis), which is a component of an infection of the trachea (tracheitis), bronchial tubes (bronchitis) or pneumonia (brochopneumonia, pneumonia). It was also a symptom of pulmonary tuberculosis.

Some cases describe problems which, according to the headings, are seemingly related to the digestive system but in fact could be rather a consequence of an illness of the upper airways.

Worth attention is a case which describes the symptoms when the patient has constipation, a palpitation found under the ribs, and as a consequence he convulses "as if in a fit of coughing" (Eb 190). This case will be discussed on pages 240–41. Similarly, the cases combining vomiting with ocular and nasal inflammation (Eb 192–95) are addressed on pages 272–73.

Ebers 305–20—driving away a cough

Another extensive group of cases, entitled "Beginning (of a collection) of remedies for driving away a cough," shows that the cough was the center of the treatment efforts of ancient Egyptian physicians. We can thus judge that Egyptians were often bothered by or suffered from coughs. Unlike other often unnecessarily complicated prescriptions, we find in them mainly simple means utilizing particularly plant ingredients, herbs, spices, and also bonding agents. The amount of the ingredients is not always listed.

The first prescription for the preparation of a medicine for a cough recommends fresh carob in an aqueous solution. The medicine was to be prepared in a new *hin* vessel and used for four days (Eb 305). Other times, the same ingredients were used, but the method of preparation differed slightly. The same amount of water and carob was left to stand in the *hin* vessel for four days and nights, exposed to daily sunlight and evening dew. The patient was then given the beverage for four days, namely in an amount corresponding to approximately 18.75 ml (Eb 307). It was essentially a carob drink, which could have very favorable effects against a cough because it helped get rid of mucus.

According to another prescription, carob was mixed with sweet beer instead of with water, and the mixture was cooked. The medicine was used in an amount of 75 ml for a period of four days (Eb 306). Carob could also be combined with date purée, when 15 ml of each ingredient was mixed with 480 ml of milk (Eb 309). The dates gave the mixture greater sweetness and also energy.

In another prescription, flat cakes were prepared from dates. Two flat cakes were formed from 480 ml of date flour, and they were roasted on a fire in the *mehet* vessel. Fat and *Moringa* oil, which act as anti-inflammatory agents, were added on the finished flat cakes. The medicinal flat cakes were served warm (Eb 308). Another variation of the flat cake was prepared from 75 ml of date flour mixed with water. The mixture was kneaded into the dough and baked on a fire in two vessels called *pega*. The flat cake was then to be mixed with honey and fat and served to the sick person in one day (Eb 313).

A more complicated mixture was prepared from 300 ml of sweet beer, in which were mixed 0.5 ml of date flour and *shenfet* fruits and four times the amount of the *tiam* plant and the *sheny-ta* seeds, which were finely ground. The mixture was left overnight to collect dew, and after being strained the medicine was to be given for a period of four days (Eb 319). A fermented herbal decoction mixed with fat and beer in the same amount (4 ml), cooked together, was also to have a similar effect. Afterwards, 15 ml each of *Melilotus* and myrtle, which works as an astringent and an antiseptic, were then added. The mixture was scalded and strained and the ill person was to use it for a period of four days (Eb 312). A sorghum medicinal mixture, which could have an anti-inflammatory effect, was prepared from 75 ml of flour, which was mulled with the same amount of honey and goose fat. The sick person was to eat it for a period of four days (Eb 318).

A mixture prepared from milk was also suitable against a cough. According to one prescription, cow's milk was scalded and sour milk was added to it. The ill person was to sip the hot mixture for a period of four days (Eb 310). Cow's milk could also be scalded with earth almonds (the tubers of yellow nutsedge). The sick person was to drink milk and chew the tubers for four days (Eb 314). Another preparation against a cough included sour milk and honey, which was mixed and drunk with diluted beer for a period of four days. Warm milk with honey is given to this day even in Central Europe as a time-tested medicine for a cough (Eb 315). A mixture of sour milk and honey was other times mixed with a drink from date purée. The mixture was scalded and used for a period of four days. The ill person was to eat *feka* cakes with it, but their composition is not known (Eb 317).

A somewhat curious prescription described the production of a medicine from date seeds, which contain many beneficial antioxidants. According to this prescription, the seeds are to be ground and placed in grape juice inside a linen bag for a day and heated. The contents of the bag are subsequently mixed in water in a *hin* vessel and strained. It is to be used for four days (Eb 311).

A plant medicine for a cough was prepared from 0.5 ml of the *tiam* plant and the same amount of the *amau* plant. The ground ingredients were to be mixed and heated, and the sick person was to breath the smoke through a tube directly to the airways for one day. Unfortunately, we do not know which plants these terms labeled, so it is difficult to judge the effect of this medicinal mixture, but inhalation usage is not very common in Egyptian texts (Eb 320).

One prescription in the group of the treatment for a cough is somewhat curious, because it describes the preparation of a medicine with the usage of a pig's tooth. This was to be ground and placed in the *feka* cakes, whose composition is not specified. The effect of the pig's tooth against a cough was rather of a magical nature, but it cannot be ruled out that this label was used in Egyptian vernacular, for instance, for some medicinal herb (Eb 316).

Hearst 61—driving away a cough
Another prescription against a cough, written in the Hearst Papyrus, recommends a medicinal beverage from 375 ml of milk, 2 ml of marrow, half the amount of the *aam* plant, and the unknown substance *kerek*, a quarter of the amount of ocher, and an eighth of a pinch of incense. This mixture was cooked and served to the ill person for a period of four days.

Ebers 321-25—expelling a cough from the abdomen
A second, smaller group of cases in the Ebers Papyrus comprises prescriptions for "driving away a cough from the abdomen." This uncommon determination of the origin of a cough could have expressed a deep (sonorous) cough from the bronchioli of the lungs.

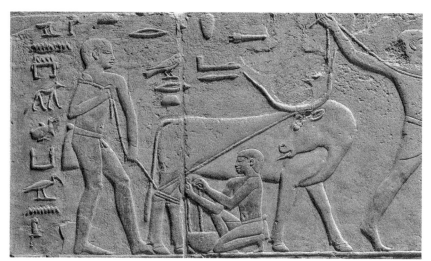
Fig. 23. Milkers and herders caring for livestock; cow's milk, as well as milk of smaller types of livestock, composed an important part of the diet and medicinal mixtures (Sixth Dynasty, tomb of Kagemni in Saqqara, photo © Archive of the Czech Institute of Egyptology, Faculty of Arts, Charles University, Martin Frouz)

Against such a cough, a medicinal beverage was prepared containing the same amount (2 ml) of figs, the *ished* fruits, and arugula, half the amount of raisins, a quarter of the amount of acacia leaves and the *niaia* plant, and an eighth of the amount of cumin and ocher. All of the ingredients were mixed in sweet beer, and the mixture was left to stand and collect dew overnight. The medicine, which could thanks to its composition have an astringent and laxative effect, and moreover could favorably influence the digestion, was drunk for a period of four days (Eb 321).

According to another prescription, a flat cake was to be baked in a *bedja* bread form from roasted sorghum mixed with beer. This was enough for two days (Eb 322). A more complicated prescription for the preparation of a medicinal mixture included 480 ml of honey and the same amount of beef fat and roasted sorghum, which was thoroughly mixed with twice the amount of date purée and acacia gum. The mix was cooked and was to be used at body temperature (Eb 323).

We also find in this group a prescription, which is very similar to cases Ebers 305 and 307 (see above), where carob in an aqueous solution was used for the treatment of a cough. The text specifies that the same amount of both ingredients was to be used so that the *hin* vessel contained half water and half carob. The patient was to drink 1 *hin* (480 ml) for a period of four days (Eb 324).

In the same group of cases, a prescription is also presented for the preparation of a medicinal remedy from 15 ml of red glass and the same amount of red chalk and the unknown *aam* plant, which were ground together. The physician was to apply the mentioned mixture gradually on seven stones, which were warmed on the fire. Every stone with the mixture was covered with a vessel with a hole in the bottom, and through this hole the patient breathed with the help of a straw or—as is written in the text—he swallowed the smoke. He was then to eat fatty meat or fat. We unfortunately do not know the medicinal effects of the *aam* plant or the other ingredients, but it is clear that the text describes the prototype of the earliest inhalator (Eb 325, see also Eb 320).

Berlin 29 and 31–34—driving away a cough

The Berlin Papyrus also contains an entire group of cases devoted to the treatment of a cough. Many of them are similar to the already presented prescriptions (see above Eb 310, and 314–17). The amount of the ingredients is listed in the text rather exceptionally; the period of usage was mainly four days.

The medicinal mixture from fresh cow's milk, sour milk, and honey, the amounts of which are not specified in the prescription, had a simple composition (Bln 29). Another medicine was made from sour milk and honey, to which was added cumin (Bln 31), or 75 ml of sour milk was mixed with the same amount of honey and 150 ml of squeezed dates (Bln 34). This prescription is very similar to case Ebers 317, but provides more precise amounts of the individual ingredients. Another preparation was made from 2 ml of wormwood, half the amount of peas and *shenfet* fruits, and double the amount of herbal decoction (Bln 32).

In contrast, a single-use medicine without more precise specification was made from the same amount (4 ml) of gum and honey, which was simmered and given to the patient to eat (Bln 33).

Berlin 44–46—driving away a cough

In this group of prescriptions, we again find lists of ingredients but not their amounts. The first prescription was an instruction on the preparation of a mixture from peas, wormwood, an herbal decoction, and the *shenfet* fruits, which were to be cooked together and used for four days (Bln 44). It is the same medicine as in case Berlin 32, but in more concise form. Another mixture for the same problems could be prepared from carob, which was mixed with barley flour and unknown ingredient *meqret*, which was to be found near water, perhaps on the banks of a pond, a water canal, or river. The mixture was to be gently ground and given to the patient (Bln 45). The text states that it is truly an excellent remedy, but the lack of knowledge of the third ingredient keeps us from judging its medicinal effect today.

Other than the medicines given orally (perorally), the group also included instruction for inhalation. A mixture of alum with crushed wormwood and another ingredient unknown to us was to be prepared. It was spread on seven potter's wheels into a bowl covered by another bowl, of which the upper one had an opening drilled in it. A tube from yellow nutsedge, the second end of which the patient had in his mouth, was placed in this opening. He was alternatingly to inhale it and drink a beer called *peseg*. The author of the text added in the conclusion encouragement that when this is done, the result will be very visible (Bln 46).

Berlin 37—good remedy for a cough
In this text, a remedy against cough labeled as "good" was made from 75 ml of milk, into which 2 ml of honey, half that amount of carob, and a quarter of the amount of white gum was mixed. The medicine was given to the patient for four days.

Berlin 47—good remedy for a cough
Another "good" medicine was prepared according to this prescription from sour milk with cumin and honey. It is a parallel to case Berlin 31 (see above), but the wordings of the text are not entirely identical. Moreover, they differ in their headings.

Berlin 36—mitigating a fit of coughing
If a sick person suffered from a fit of coughing, a medicine was prepared for him of equal amounts (15 ml) of *Melilotus*, myrtle, oil, sweet beer, and a fermented herbal decoction. All of the ingredients were mixed; the subsequent procedure of preparation has not been preserved in the text. It was to be used for four days.

Berlin 38-43—a fit of coughing
A mixture of cow's milk with sour milk and milk fat was also prepared to overcome a fit of coughing. According to the text, this medicine could be used by men and women, so any sick person with a cough, namely for a period of four days (Bln 38). Wine with sea salt, which was drunk for a period of four days was also to work for the same problems (Bln 39).

As a one-off, the patient could be given sweet beer mixed with honey and acacia leaf (Bln 40). This preparation is a bit similar to case Ebers 187, where, however, honey was not part of the mixture. Another remedy for a coughing fit was prepared by mixing cumin in sour milk (Bln 41). It is a variation of case Berlin 31, but without the honey. What could be effective against a cough and the fits associated with it was also a mixture prepared from the juice of carob with honey, which was to be given to the sick person to drink (Bln 43).

We also find in the group a more complicated prescription, the components of which were 75 ml of pork lard and the same amount of goose fat and barley. The prepared mixture was to be cooked and left overnight to stand and collect dew. It was given to the sick person for a period of four days. According to the conclusion of the text, the medicine was suitable for men and women who suffered with the cough and heat (an infection) of one of the abdominal organs (Bln 42). With this symptom, the case is somewhat reminiscent of some cases from the Ebers Papyrus which deal with pulmonary diseases and abdominal pains.

Cough in the Mirror of Paleopathology

The large number of the cases concerning the treatment of respiratory illnesses and particularly a cough proves that Egyptians apparently suffered from diseases of the lungs often. Due to the favorable climate that dominates in Egypt, they were not only infections of the upper respiratory tract, caused by common colds, and therefore it is necessary to consider also a cough accompanying tuberculosis.

The appearance of tuberculosis is proven already in the Predynastic Period (4500–3150 BC) (Dabernat and Crubézy 2010, 719–730). Recent research has proven that tuberculosis appeared more often in ancient Egypt than was assumed up to now (Strouhal 2006a; Donoghue et al. 2010). Using new molecular methods (analysis of the spoligotype of DNA with amplification), 118 mummies and skeletons from the time from the Middle Kingdom to the Late Period (2050–500 BC) were investigated on the west bank of the Nile in Luxor, hence from the area of ancient Waset (Thebes) (Zink et al. 2004). Of them, twenty-six (that is, 22 percent) showed the presence of *Mycobacterium tuberculosis*, where with a number of individuals from the Middle Kingdom *Mycobacterium africanum* also appeared. It is noteworthy that *Mycobacterium bovis*, affecting cattle, was not found with any case (Zink et al. 2004, 405). With another Egyptian set, an even higher appearance of tuberculosis was identified using the method of PCR DNA with almost every third group of investigated mummies (Ziskind and Halioua 2007). Tuberculosis was also recently found with the first women affected by cancer, whose mummies were investigated by Granville in 1824 (Donoghue et al. 2010; Granville 1825). The results of these studies independent of one another reveal an unexpectedly high sickness rate (morbidity) with tuberculosis in the Egyptian population of that time, from which also death frequently occurs (mortality).

The frequent occurrence of cough was also caused by the high levels of dust in the Egyptian air, which was triggered (and still is today) by the desert surrounding the fertile and populated area of the Nile Valley and Delta. The dustiness culminated every year with the sudden sandstorms in the spring months (Arabic *khamāsīn*), which bring the rounded sand and dust particles from the scorched Sahara. In breathing, they were deposited in the interstitial tissues between the pulmonary air sacs and their lymphatic capillaries, where they mainly do not irritate. This finding is labeled as a disease caused by inhalation of dust (pneumoconiosis). In connection with this disease, it is possible to mention the famous case of the mummy of Khar from the University Museum in Manchester, whose lungs were investigated endoscopically. It was shown that the lungs partially collapsed and, in some places, had grown together with the pleura, which testifies to an occurrence of pneumonia and pleuritis. The biopsy of the pulmonary air sacs in it showed the presence of an amount of dust. It was possible to make a similar finding with the mummy of a sixty-year-old man Nakhtankh from the same museum (Tapp and Wildsmith 1986, 353).

A more serious disease affected the stonemasons and sculptors in Egypt, who worked for long days with stone. The inhaled dust particles contain silicates with sharp edges that irritate the pulmonary air sacs (alveoli), which are pushed by the fast-growing interstitial tissue. The microscopic image is reminiscent of liver tissue (hepatization). With longer exposure, the patient is threatened for life with silicosis with the reduction of the breathing surface of the pulmonary air sacs.

Stomach and Liver
The Stomach as the Mouth of the Heart
Common Egyptians knew of the existence of the stomach and liver from their own experience in animal evisceration. The liver was called *miset*, whereas the name of the stomach in Egyptian was *r-ib*, which means "the mouth of the heart" (Nunn 1996, 88). This expression shows the close relationship of these two important organs that are anatomically close to one another, between which a connection was logically supposed. The food chewed in the mouth (*stoma* in Greek) descended through the esophageal tube (esophagus, another type of the tubes *metu*) for further processing in the stomach. From there, it was to get in an undocumented way directly to the heart so that it could then penetrate all of the regions of the body from the heart through the arteries along with air. This simple theory influenced Greco-Roman medicine across the millennia, so much so that the English term *stomach* is derived from *stoma* (Nunn 1996, 54). The undigested remnants of the food then descended all the way to the rectum, where they were expelled from the body.

During mummification, the stomach was separated from the intestine and placed in a canopic jar with a lid in the form of a jackal's head—the god Duamutef—which was protected by the goddess Neith. Another canopic jar was intended for the liver with a lid in the shape of a human head—the god Amset—over which the goddess Isis watched.

The tie between the stomach and heart is illustrated by a group of ten prescriptions of the Ebers Papyrus (Eb 284–93), adopted from the "Beginning (of a collection) of remedies for making the heart accept food" (this group of cases was discussed in detail above on pages 192–93). They are medicines containing common substances of plant origin, animal components (mainly fat), and also mineral substances. Other ingredients can be added to them, but we do not know their importance. It was prepared from the ingredients by mixing, grinding, cooking, and straining a drink, mainly dissolved in sweet and strong beer, wine, or water. The resulting mixture was to be drunk for one to four days.

Examination and Healing of the Stomach and Liver

The cases of the Ebers Papyrus 188–208 are aimed at illnesses of the stomach and their heading is sometimes translated as "The book on the stomach" (Nunn 1996, 88), but more often as "Instruction (or treatise) on stomach disease" (see also Bardinet 1995, 275). It is clear from the form of these cases that it was a guide for medical practice, because they are presented with the instruction "When you examine someone who has . . . ." There follows in the text a thorough and for us valuable description of the disease and also the recommended approach of treatment. The text of these cases in the second person singular addresses the physician, just like the cases of the Smith Surgical Papyrus (see Strouhal et al. 2014, 27–95). By this formulation, the entire group of cases strikingly differs from the other cases of the Ebers Papyrus devoted to internal diseases, where prescriptions without similar descriptions and instructions predominate.

Although the mentioned cases were connected with the stomach and digestive tract, some of them attributed the described diseases to the stomach incorrectly. That could be partially from not understanding the causes, but partly also the similarity of the Egyptian words for heart *(ib)* and stomach *(r-ib)*. We have included these cases into the sections where they fit thematically—to the heart (see pages 189–90; Eb 191, 194, and 197), to the lungs and upper respiratory tract (see pages 272–73; Eb 192 and 195), or to the abdomen (see page 218; Eb 193).

In the translations concerning the stomach, the term "constipation of the stomach" (Egyptian *shena*) is often repeated, which we consider to be a label of an obstacle (obstruction) or pressures of various origin, only sometimes determinable according to the context. Real constipation (obstipation) emerges only in the large intestine. With the cases of the "Examination of pains/diseases of stomach," it is also striking that the recommended medicines were used exclusively orally (perorally), not using enemas or suppositories into the rectum (Nunn 1996, 88–89), which distinguishes them from the prescriptions of our other two sections (pages 223–63).

In connection with the previous cases, we can present also a group of cases devoted to illnesses of the liver (Eb 477–81), which are preceded by the heading "Beginning (of the collection) of remedies for the treatment of the liver." In these cases, the clinical symptoms or diagnoses or even the approach to the examination are not in any way specified; it is only the recipes for the preparation of the medicines. It is possible that it was from a lack of knowledge of the liver, but it could be medicines recommended for cases described elsewhere.

Ebers 477–81—healing of the liver

The group of five prescriptions includes mixtures based mainly of plant ingredients; sometimes products of mineral origin were added to them. For the digestive tract, a mixture of the same portion (2 ml) of figs, ripe sycamore fruits, and the *ished* fruits, half the amount of grapes and bryony fruit, and an eighth of the amount of cress, gum, and incense was beneficial, which were mixed and ground in 225 ml of water. The mixture was left overnight to stand and collect dew, then it was strained and administered for four days (Eb 477).

The other medicines in this group were prepared in the same way, which were all given to the patient also for four days. A simpler medicine was composed of 2 ml of figs and raisins with half the amount of pine nuts and reed, a quarter the amount of ocher, and an eighth of the amount of incense, which was bound in water (Eb 478). According to another prescription, a mixture of 2 ml of figs and ripe sycamore fruits with the same amount of the unknown stone *sia,* and half the amount of the juniper berries, which were ground in 300 ml of water, could help. The medicine was left to stand and collect dew overnight and was used for four days (Eb 481).

At other times, 2 ml of figs, jujube flour, and lotus leaf were mixed with half the amount of milk and juniper berries, and with an eighth of the amount of incense, and it was all ground in 300 ml of sweet beer and 300 ml of wine; the mixture was strained after a night of collecting dew (Eb 479). Another remedy was prepared the same way, which is similar to the mixture from the first prescription, produced from the same amount (2 ml) of figs, the *ished* fruits and jujube bread, a double amount of anise, half the amount of ripe sycamore fruits, grape seeds, and a little carob, cress, and incense, which were mixed in 300 ml of sweet beer (Eb 480).

It is noteworthy that none of the prescriptions in this group contained the same ingredients as the subsequent cases intended for problems connected with the stomach itself. It could reflect the empirical experience of Egyptian physicians, who even without a precise distinction between the diagnoses knew how to suitably relieve the ill.

Ebers 189—the ill stomach

This case, belonging to the above-mentioned instructions on the stomach, describes the ill person with stomach upset (nausea) with the feeling of pressure throughout the body as if fatigue had fallen on him. The physician was to examine the ill person by touch (palpation) to discover whether the stomach was moving under his fingers. In this way, he apparently perceived gastric contractions. The diagnosis was clear, fatigue from the amount of food (binge eating, bulimia), which prevented the ill person from the further intake of foodstuffs.

The medicine which it was necessary to prepare comprised ground date seeds and the sediments of beer, which were to ensure the purging of the stomach so that the appetite of the patient was restored. During the control examination, the physician assured a warm hypochondrium and cool abdomen, where he could state the retreat of the disease, but the patient was to continue to avoid eating roasted meat; he was thus to observe some diet.

Ebers 200—the ill stomach

In this strange case, the symptom of the sick stomach was manifested as an intensive radiating pain in the back as if stung by a scorpion. The cause naturally was not precisely known, because according to the presented diagnosis it is a manifestation of substances causing pain. The author of the treatise emphatically exhorts the examining physician to not even deal with such a difficult-to-treat case, to give up on the use of "means of additional treatment." He was first to concoct a preparation unknown to us, labeled as *khemtu* from *djesfu*. To that was added a mixture of equal amounts (15 ml) of myrtle, acacia leaf, mason's gypsum, and the unknown *niaia* plant, mulled in the sediment of sweet beer, which undoubtedly had an antiseptic and astringent effect. The medicine was not used internally, but was applied to a certain place for four days.

With this case, it was apparently not a disease of the stomach but a biliary colic (cholelithiasis) (Miller and Ritner 1994, 71–76) or a stabbing pain from renal colic (nephralgia) (Stephan 2001, 102). It is not possible to rule out even lumbago or ischialgia.

Ebers 188—"constipation" of the stomach

The first case in this group describes a sick stomach complicated by an obstruction which caused the patient a long-term lack of appetite (anorexia), so that he is emaciated, has a weak pulse, and at the same time has a hot abdomen. The symptoms reveal a chronic infection of the stomach (chronic gastritis), sometimes newly flaring up (exacerbating). After examining the ill lying down, the physician diagnoses the cause of these problems as an illness of the liver *(miset)*, for which a medicinal mixture was to be prepared from herbs. According to the text, the physician himself was to prepare this medicine, since it was a secret remedy. It is clear that other, simpler prescriptions from commonly accessible ingredients could be prepared for the ill person and given by his relatives according to the instructions. The personal preparation by the physician might have been connected with the necessity of a precise and limited dosage of the medicine.

The medicinal mixture contained the *pakh-serit* plant and date seeds ground in water. We cannot judge its effect, because the mentioned plant is not known to us. It apparently was a mixture with a purgative effect, because it was to be used for four mornings and was to empty the abdomen.

Afterwards, the physician looked over and examined the sick person again and continued further according to the current finding. If the right half of the abdomen was hot, while the left was not, the physician stated that it was a persisting disease, which through its "gluttony" limits the patient's intake of food. In the next examination, the physician should discover with satisfaction that the patient's abdomen was already cool, which meant that his body had reacted to the treatment and his liver had absorbed the received medicine.

The symptoms described in this case allow consideration also of other diagnostic possibilities than the already mentioned infection of the stomach. It could also be an obstruction of the lower end of the esophagus, a stomach carcinoma, the narrowing of the end of the stomach (pyloric stenosis) with a gastric ulcer, less likely an obstruction of the lower part of the digestive tract (Nunn 1996, 88–89), which would have had to be revealed by vomiting, but an ancient Egyptian physician could only distinguish among the mentioned possibilities with difficulty. It is not possible to assume realistically the knowledge of an infection of the liver (hepatitis).

Ebers 198—"constipation" of the stomach

This is another case of stomach obstruction from the one described above in Ebers 188. It was manifested with blockage and constriction around the convolute of the congealed blood, which had not settled. The disease was to be removed by a medicinal beverage from the same amount of wormwood, the unknown *ished* and *shasha* fruits, and half the amount of pine nuts, which were mulled with offering beer. The ill person was to drink the strained mixture so that a substance similar to boiled pig's blood came out either from the mouth or from the rectum. In the meantime, the physician himself was to prepare a bandage, which he applied on the stomach area of the sick person. The bandage was smeared with a ground unguent from beef fat, celery seeds, myrrh, resin, and the unknown plant *shawyt*. According to the text, it was to be a "real best" ointment.

Ebers 199—"constipation" of the stomach

Another case described in Egyptian as "constipation," thus from our perspective rather an obstruction, was connected with the movements of the stomach under the fingers of the physician, which are similar to oil in a water skin. In that, the case is similar to case Ebers 189, but the cause here is not specified in any way and was apparently a different one. We can consider it to be spasmodic contractions when overcoming some obstacles. The problems were to subside through coughing or vomiting after using a mixture of sorghum and ground date seeds, which were cooked in oil and honey and used for the usual period of four days. The stomach region was also to be covered with a bandage with the pulverized *mikat* stone. Nunn (1996, 88) considers rather increased mobility of the intestine (peristalsis) in the effort to overcome obstacles, which, however, could be clear by observation rather than the mentioned palpation. The cited palpation finding could correspond to the narrowing of the exit of the stomach (pyloric stenosis) only with small children.

Ebers 201—"constipation" of the stomach

Another case describes the situation when the sick person felt a bitter taste apparently during belching (ructus) or throwing up (vomiting). Instead of identifying the likely inflammation of the gall bladder (cholecystitis) as the origin of the problem, the physician labeled the female demons called Hayt and Nesyt, who were said to have settled in the patient's abdomen. It was possible to remove their activity with a medicinal mixture prepared from equal amounts (15 ml) of carob, garden nutsedge and also wildly growing yellow nutsedge, the *tiam* plant, and *shasha* fruits, mulled in sweet beer. The period of usage is not prescribed.

Case Ebers 201 allows consideration of other diagnostic possibilities, for example an obstacle (obstruction) of the lower end of the esophagus, stomach carcinoma, narrowing of the end of the stomach (pyloric stenosis) at a gastric ulcer, less likely an obstruction of the lower part of the digestive tract (Nunn 1996, 88–89).

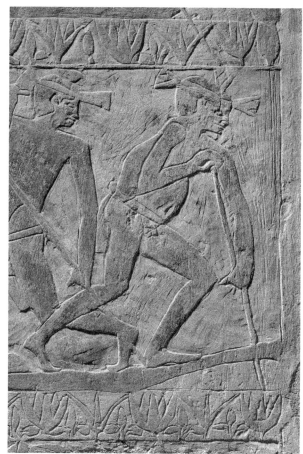

Fig. 24. In tomb scenes there sometimes appear figures with a swollen abdomen, apparently indicating a state of health whose cause is unknown to us—as it was to many Egyptian physicians (Sixth Dynasty, tomb of Ankhmahor in Saqqara, photo © Oxford Expedition to Egypt)

Ebers 196—immediate "constipation" of the stomach

This case describes an acute obstruction in the stomach, which was common with gluttons capable of eating spoiled foodstuffs (even feces). The patient felt weakness (fatigue), as if he were breathing heavily after running. As for the diagnosis, the text determines the accumulation of food which the patient cannot get up, which indicates difficulty or inability to vomit. There was also a mental manifestation, when the patient suffered his bad health unwillingly, and if, moreover, swelling occurred, it was a sign of the rotting of food in the body. The medicine, which according to the text the physician was to prepare, however, is not presented. It is possible that this case was not fully copied from the original model of the text or the physician could have prepared the medicine according to one of the prescriptions shown elsewhere in the papyrus.

Ebers 202—"constipation" of the stomach, vomiting

This case describes a more serious situation, when "constipation" (that is, an obstruction in the stomach) presents a gastric content comprising an "accumulation of feces, which had not yet settled," so that the patient vomited very painfully. We find the same justification, although with other manifestations, also in case Ebers 193 (see page 241). According to the text of the case, this obstruction was to be removed by frequent drinking of a beverage from the same amount (2 ml) of figs and ripe sycomore fruits with half of the amount of milk, which were left to stand overnight in 150 ml of sweet beer. According to Stephan (2001, 303), it could be a gastric ulcer (ulcus ventriculi), or even the pre-death fecal vomiting.

Ebers 205—illness of the stomach, constipation, pains, impairment of the heart

Another case presents an ill stomach with the feeling of a placed obstruction and pain on both sides of the body. The patient suffers anorexia and heart problems. In the text, the physician is first warned that it is an incurable disease, but the text continues and presents a recommended approach if he decides to fight the disease nevertheless. He is to prepare for the sick person an effective medicine based on a barley decoction. The physician was then to palpitate the stomach again and prepare another medicinal mixture, which was given for four mornings to strengthen the patient. It is a preparation called *djesfu*, comprising 7.5 ml of earth almonds, 2 ml of balls of gum, and half that amount of ocher, mulled in oil and honey.

If the physician then feels movements in the stomach as grains of sand and the body of the ill person was affected by a fever, it was a disease called "bitterness," which was caused by demons. The only things that could help anymore were magical means like moldy bread, contaminants, and food from poultry, which the physician was urgently encouraged by the author of the book to use and which were apparently to expel a demon.

It was a complicated case with a concise description and instructions to act, despite the unfavorable (infaust) prognosis, and to give pain-relieving (palliative), perhaps magical treatment. Nunn (1996, 88–90) does not speak on the case, nor does Westendorf (1992) nor Bardinet (1995). Stephan (2001, 101) suspects a stoppage of the intestine (ileus). We think it could have been a chronic inflammation of the stomach (chronic gastritis), a peptic ulcer, or stomach cancer in the final phase affecting also the bile ducts.

Ebers 206—"constipation" of the stomach, pain of the leg and hips

In this case, the patient suffered with a sick stomach after the usage of unsuitable food. He is stressed by that so that he shakes and refuses to have the physician palpate his painful and shriveled stomach. The situation is complicated by pain in the hips and leg but not the thigh. Through an examination, the physician found a stomach clogged with mucus and the shriveled face of the sick person. The author of the treatise emphatically calls on the physician to act using a preparation which was so secret that the physician could reveal it only to his son (or successor) but not his assistants. It was undried green barley heated in water so that it did not come to a boil. It was mixed with date seeds and strained. The beverage was given for four days, during which an improvement should happen. Green barley acts in a base-forming way and is therefore recommended in digestive problems including hyperacidity and constipation. Date seeds are also used to this day for cleaning the intestine. In this case, the existence of a medicinal professional secret, preserved in the family succession, is revealed.

Ebers 207—"constipation" of the stomach, paleness, heart palpitations, hotness, and flatulence

A similar case is devoted to patients who, moreover, suffer from flatulence (tympanites, meteorism), accelerated heart rate, and paleness. According to the text, it was a deep-lying accumulation of food as a consequence of the use of roasted meat. The physician was to conduct a cleansing of the stomach and duodenum to remove the roasted meat and open the passages to the intestinal tract. It was to be handled by a beverage left to stand overnight made of ripe sycomore fruits in sweet beer, used for the usual four days.

Furthermore, it was necessary for the physician to check early in the morning every day what the sick person had passed from the rectum, and according to that he adjusted the further approach. On that description, Nunn (1996, 89) correctly states that it is the earliest attested evidence of the medicinal examination of a patient's stool in the history of mankind. When black-colored feces came from him, compared to the unknown substance *arut*, the physician said that the meat had already passed, but the whole abdomen was affected. When he subsequently discovered that something like a mash of beans with beads of dew had come from the rectum, it was clear that everything had already left the stomach. The physician was to prepare for the patient a cooling preparation, apparently according to one of the prescriptions in another part of the papyrus.

Ebers 302, 750—driving away the bitter disease

These two cases were recorded in other parts of the Ebers Papyrus, but from today's perspective they could refer to a similar medical problem.

The first case (Eb 302) was a component of the "Collection of remedies for driving away mucus from the pelvic area" (more on that on pages 274–77), and it is a prescription for driving away a bitter disease supposedly caused by demons, which reflects the limited understanding of Egyptian physicians of internal problems. The recommended medicine comprised carob mixed with honey and was to be washed down with beer. The text arouses the suspicion that it could be an inflammation of the gall bladder (cholecystitis) or gall stones in the gall bladder or bile ducts (cholelithiasis).

In the second case (Eb 750), which is presented with the heading "Collection of remedies for driving away the devastating bitter disease *(dehret)*," a medicine was prescribed made from 150 ml of date flour boiled with a greater amount of water. The mixture was to be left on a fire to reduce to the amount of 960 ml and when cooled to body temperature was to be drunk and then vomited. The usage of this medicine was to chase the disease away from the entire body.

Hearst 131—driving away the bitter disease

This prescription in the Hearst Papyrus is similar to the already presented case Ebers 302. The wording of both cases is not entirely identical, but it only differs a little. The sick person was to eat carob with honey and wash it down with sweet beer.

Recipes for Healing the Stomach

Nine other cases for the removal of "constipation" or obstacles (obstruction) of the stomach, or only generally "for the stomach" do not contain more specific data on the diagnosis, with the exception of supposed magical causes of one case in the form of the female demon Nesyt. In essence, it is a mere prescription containing lists (partially repeating) of rational medicines, mainly with the use of ingredients from the plant kingdom, sometimes with the addition of mineral substances and animal products, especially fat. Some of them were intended for consumption; others for external application.

Ebers 212 and 214–16—stomach

In the collection, we also find general prescriptions for the stomach, the use of which is not in any way specified in more detail. The recommended medicines, which could be used by a man and a woman, included for instance a mixture of 75 ml of earth almonds and the same amount of raisins, *sheny-ta* seeds, a few figs, ripe sycomore fruits, or carob. The ingredients were to be ground, mixed with sweet offering beer, and left to stand covered overnight. Then, 75 ml of honey and 75 ml of goose fat were mixed in and the mixture was drunk (Eb 212).

Flat *feka* cakes could also be prepared: they heated honey, then added an equal amount of sorghum flour and half the amount of *sheny-ta* seeds. For four days, the patient was to eat one flat cake a day (Eb 215).

Another remedy was produced from honey, *sheny-ta* seeds, a small amount of pine nuts, and incense, which was mixed with 75 ml of wine and 75 ml of goose fat. After cooking, the sick person was to eat this mixture for a period of one day (Eb 216). Another prescription contained honey, *Moringa* oil, wine, and incense in the same amounts. The mixture was cooked and the sick person was to eat it (Eb 214).

Ebers 208 and 213—chasing away "constipation" of the stomach
The mixtures recommended in these two cases for relieving the obstacles in the stomach were produced from equal amounts (15 ml) of jujube bread, watermelon, and crocodile dung, which were mixed in the same amount of wine and sweet beer. After thorough blending, the mixture was applied to the stomach (Eb 208). The other prescription contained the same ingredients and also red ocher in the same amount (Eb 213).

Ebers 211—chasing away of "constipation" and sanguinary nature of the stomach
Another case contains a mixture which was to be applied in the case of an obstruction of the stomach, which was moreover accompanied by unspecified manifestations of sanguinary nature. However, what was considered to be the "bloodshed in the stomach" is not clear from the text. The treatise recommended the use of 15 ml of grape juice mixed with the same amount of fermented herbal decoction and *Moringa* oil. The mixture was applied on the abdomen.

Ebers 209-10—constipation in the right half of the abdomen
According to this treatise, constipation in the right half of the abdomen was the consequence of the activity of the female demon Nesyt. This concept is related to the fact that Egyptian physicians did not entirely understand the causes of internal diseases. A medicine to help expel the demon was prepared from 75 ml of sweet beer, in which were mixed 2 ml of white and green barley, mountain and Lower Egyptian celery, lotus leaves, myrtle, boat verdigris, the *tjun*

plant, and duck fat, half the amount of the rootstocks of bryony, juniper berries, myrrh, cedar oil, and the unknown *shenfet* fruit, and a quarter of the amount of honey. The mixture was to be left overnight to stand and collect the dew, then was to be strained and given to the ill person to drink for four days (Eb 209).

If the condition of the sick person improved weakly, a beverage was given made from 75 ml of wine and 375 ml of beer along with 2 ml of figs, *ished* fruit, milk, honey, and incense, half that amount of raisins, anise, juniper berries, ripe sycomore fruits, and the *qesenty* stone, and a quarter of the amount of acacia, fig and jujube leaves, ocher, and gum (Eb 210). The preparation method and period of administration were the same as in the previous case.

Ebers 855r, s—constricted and spicy stomach

The author of the treatise on the Ebers Papyrus included these two cases in the group devoted to the heart (see above, pages 185–89), but according to their wording there was apparently a stomach disorder in them. From the first case, only the heading is recorded, which presents that the label of "constricted stomach" means that the stomach expanded (Eb 855r). This description seems to be significantly illogical, since a closed stomach should rather be smaller in size—perhaps it is a mistake in the original text. The undesirable situation might have been possible to remove after the application of some medicine, which, however, is not mentioned in the treatise, perhaps through an error of the scribe, who copied the text from some model.

The following case of a "spicy stomach" was described as a feeling when there is a stinging and burning in the heart, similar to the acute pain caused by a sting. This case can most likely be interpreted as severe heartburn (pyrosis) (Eb 855s). The prescription for the preparation of the medicine which would bring relief during the problems is again lacking.

Berlin 154—deposit of traveling heat, stomach ache, heaviness, heat, and stabbing pains around the heart

It is hard to categorize a complicated case (syndrome) of the Berlin Papyrus, the heading of which states that it is a "deposit of traveling heat" in the body of the sick person. The text describes that the sick person feels a sense of heaviness in the abdomen, stomach ache, and stabbing pains around the heart, the weight of his clothing bothers him, he cannot stand more of its layers, and he has bad feelings in the area of his heart. His muscles are tired like after physical exertion and he has considerable problems when having a bowel movement. It is a disease caused, according to the ideas then, by substances causing pain (Egyptian *wekhedu*), with which it was possible to fight, according to the text.

The physician was to prepare for the patient a medicine which cured and helped overcome the painful substances. It was necessary to grind earth almonds and mix them with 75 ml of water, add 4 ml of white dates and honey, half the amount of fresh mash, *ished* fruit, and milk, and a quarter of the amount of juniper berries and the unknown ingredient *djernet,* and 300 ml of foam (apparently beer foam). All of the ingredients were ground and mixed. The period of the application of the medicine is not specified, but he is to be healed quickly.

Berlin 155–56—deposit of traveling heat, stomach ache, heaviness, heat, and stabbing pains around the heart

The alternative was a prescription against diarrhea containing 4 ml of raw meat, half that amount of figs, grapes, thyme, both parts of the *pesedj* fruits, and goose fat, and a quarter of the amount of *Potentilla,* an eighth of the amount of juniper berries, the *wedja* part of dates, and the *ished* and *shenfet* fruits, and an even smaller amount of incense, which was mixed in 375 ml of sweet beer. The medicinal beverage was thoroughly mixed and pressed (Bln 155). A much more concise variation of the prescription includes 2 ml of both honey and *sheny-ta* seeds and 75 ml of sweet beer (Bln 156).

Abdomen and Intestines
Pains of the Abdomen

After a person's death, embalmers placed the intestines separated from the stomach into a canopic jar with a lid in the shape of the head of the falcon god Qebehsenuf, protected by the goddess Selket (Serqet).

Intestinal problems as a consequence of binge eating or inappropriately prepared or bad food were one of the common disorders in ancient Egypt, which is documented by the large number of prescriptions coming from various primary sources. One group devoted to the abdomen is found right in the introduction of the Ebers Papyrus, just behind several incantations for the applications of medicines, and is presented by its heading "Collection of remedies for driving away diseases of the abdomen." We find other cases in the Berlin and Hearst Papyri. They were mainly mixtures which were usually strained, sometimes left overnight exposed to the morning dew, other times boiled, and then were either drunk one time or used for a period of one to four days. Above on pages 201–202, a case was described in which the pain of the abdomen was accompanied by pulmonary problems (Eb 35 = Eb 185) and a mixture of sweet beer and carob was given as a medicine.

The strikingly rich list of medicines (polypragmasy) recommended in the prescriptions in this chapter reveals the lack of knowledge of the processes causing the abdominal pain.

Ebers 4—disease of the abdomen

The first of a whole series of cases describes a very simple medicinal mixture for diseases of the abdomen. It was a simple beverage containing peas mixed with beer, which could benefit the ill and cleanse him because of its contents of fiber and proteins.

Ebers 19—abdomen

Another prescription intended generally for the abdomen was composed of 37.5 ml of squeezed dates, 4 ml of the *hemu,* an unknown part, of *Ricinus,* a quarter of the amount of yellow nutsedge, roots of bryony and coriander, and an eighth amount of soured beer. The ingredients were mixed and left overnight to stand and collect the dew, then the mixture was strained and drunk for four days.

Ebers 38—proper operation of the abdomen

According to this prescription, the preparation for good digestion was prepared from 15 ml of honey, *Anacyclus,* the unknown fruits *shasha* and *djaa,* and a little malachite. It was all mixed and used before sleeping. It is not possible to judge the effects of the types of fruits unknown to us, but it could be a gentle laxative, because this case is written after two cases devoted to means for emptying the bowels (see page 238).

Hearst 28—left half of the abdomen

One case concerned a more specifically unidentified problem with the left half of the abdomen, for which a medicinal beverage was prepared from 300 ml of water, in which were mixed 37.5 ml of anise, 4 ml of figs, half the amount of raisins and *ished* fruit, an eighth of the amount of cress, cumin, cracked ripe sycomore fruits, ocher and gum, and a little incense. The mixture was left overnight to stand and collect the dew and then was strained. It was administered for four days.

Ebers 631–33—treatment of the blood vessels in the left half of the abdomen

The heading of the first case in this group refers to the blood vessels *(metu)* in the left (inauspicious) half of the abdomen, where the following case applies only to the left half of the abdomen. The prescriptions are, however, very similar, and therefore we summarize them together. The ingredients used and the method of the application in the form of a medicinal beverage indicate that these cases could be related rather with digestion than with the blood vessels of the abdomen.

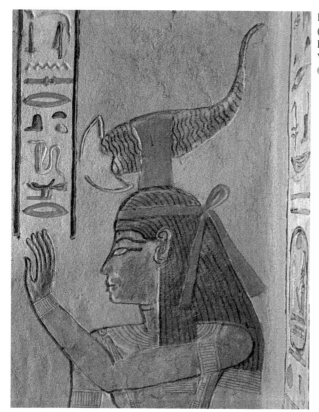

Fig. 25. The goddess Selket (Twentieth Dynasty, tomb of Khaemwaset (QV 44) in the Valley of the Queens, photo © Sandro Vannini)

The first of the recipes contained 2 ml each of figs, grapes, anise, *ished* fruit, leaves of a muskmelon, and jujube bread, further 0.5 ml each of reed, *Potentilla*, juniper berries, and ocher, half the amount of cumin, carob, and incense, 75 ml of wine, and 300 ml of sweet beer. The mixture was to be left to stand overnight exposed to the dew, then strained and used as a medicinal beverage for a period of four days (Eb 631).

The same method of preparation and period of usage was recommended with the following medicinal beverages, which were similar to the first one. It was a mixture containing 2 ml each of normally ripe and riper figs, raisins, anise, *ished* fruit, then 0.5 ml each of carob, ocher, and gum, and half the amount of cress, cumin, and incense, which were mixed in 75 ml of wine, the same amount of strong beer, and the *sekhpet* drink (Eb 632). Other times, only 2 ml of figs and carob, 0.5 ml of ocher and gum, half the amount of *ished* fruit, 37.5 ml of anise and grapes, and 300 ml of water (Eb 633) were used. The repetition of the same substances is striking that, with all three mixtures, they are in most cases demonstrably beneficial for digestion.

Ebers 5–6—pain of the abdomen
Pains of the abdomen with no specified cause were to be cured with a mixture of 300 ml of milk with 2 ml of goose fat and 0.25 ml of cumin (Eb 5) or a medicinal mixture from 2 ml of figs and *ished* fruit mulled with 300 ml of sweet beer (Eb 6). The mixtures were to be cooked, strained, and drunk one time.

Hearst 55–56—pains in the abdomen
When the abdomen of a person was suffering from an unspecified pain, the Hearst Papyrus recommended using a mixture of 300 ml of milk with 2 ml of goose fat and 0.5 ml of cumin (H 55). The other preparation contained 300 ml of sweet beer with a mixture of 2 ml of figs and *ished* fruit (H 56). It is similar to the cases Ebers 5–6.

Hearst 53—driving away pains in the abdomen
This simple case contains a recipe for a mixture which should help with any pains in the abdomen. It is the same medicine as in case Ebers 4, but with a different, more specific heading; it was made from peas and beer, which apparently caused relief by evacuation (by a laxative) of the intestines.

Berlin 191—pains of the abdomen
Since the cause of the pain in the abdomen was often unknown, Egyptian physicians sometimes proceeded to the use of magical methods (see also below). This case contains an incantation which compares the sick person to the god Horus, by which he was to be ensured protection. The incantation was pronounced over his abdomen after he drank a pomace ground in water. This method was to lead to rapid recuperation.

Ebers 40–43—driving away the pains of the abdomen
Several other prescriptions were to help against pain in the abdomen or its part. The first case is devoted to pain in the right (favorable) half of the abdomen, which could have had various causes. It was recommended to place on the abdomen a mixture of 15 ml of date juice and the same amount of *Melilotus*, which was cooked in oil (Eb 40). *Melilotus* is beneficial to digestion because it acts against flatulence and dampens the activity of smooth muscles. Despite the external application, this medicine could be somewhat effective.

Other times, a medicine was prepared from roasted figs, raisins, and pine nuts, which were soaked in advance in the oil of the *Moringa* tree. The sick person was to mix the ingredients, eat them, and then properly wash it down (Eb 41). Moreover, sometimes the same mixture was mixed with 480 ml of wine and the same amount of a beverage called *pa-ib* (Eb 42). For the entire day, a medicine could be used prepared from chaste tree and earth almonds, oil, honey, and crushed pearls (Eb 43).

O.DeM 1216—pain of the abdomen
On one of the ostraca from Deir el-Medina, we find the remnant of a magical incantation which was apparently intended against pains of the abdomen. Only a small part of the text has been preserved, which complicates understanding. In the introduction, the goddess Isis is called upon for help according to the conceptions then that the originator of the disease was most likely injurious beings.

Ebers 86—expulsion from the abdomen of the substances causing pain
A lengthier collection of cases in the Ebers Papyrus contained prescriptions for the expulsion or destruction of the substances *wekhedu*, which, according to the conceptions then, caused pain in the abdomen of the sick person. According to this prescription, the inauspicious substance causing pain in the abdomen of the patient was to be expelled by a preparation of 375 ml of sweet beer with 75 ml of fresh beef, 2 ml *Melilotus* and fresh bread, half the amount of juniper berries, and an eighth of the amount of incense. The ingredients were apparently mixed and most likely cooked. The patient used the strained medicine for a period of four days.

Ebers 87-89—protection from the substances causing pain in the abdomen
Other preparations were to protect the sick person from inauspicious substances. They thus might have worked as prevention or were used after the substances had been expelled from the body, against their return. A mixture could be prepared from 2 ml of *ished* fruit and the same amount of the *tiam* plant mixed with 75 ml of a drink called *sekhpet* and 150 ml of sweet beer. The mixture was to be cooked, strained, and drunk for a period of four days (Eb 87). The same method and use was recommended also with the other prescriptions, which had different compositions. The *ished* fruit in the amount of 2 ml could be mixed with half the amount of juniper berries and goose fat, a quarter of the amount of acacia leaves, and an eighth amount of cress, which were mixed in 375 ml of sweet beer (Eb 88). Other times to the 2 ml of *ished* fruit were added the same amount of figs, ripe sycamore fruits, half the amount of grapes,

juniper berries, goose fat, and an eighth of the amount of incense and cumin. All was again ground in 375 ml of sweet beer (Eb 89).

Ebers 97–101—expulsion and destruction of the substances causing pain in the abdomen

The first preparation in the group comprised the same amount (2 ml) of figs, *ished* fruits, *sheny-ta* seeds, and goose fat, half the amount of the *tiam* plant, a quarter of the amount of carob and the *aam* plant, an eighth of the amount of cumin, and 375 ml of sweet beer. The ingredients were mixed, strained, and boiled. The medicine was to be used for a period of four days (Eb 97). Another mixture was prepared in the same way, which comprised 2 ml of ripe sycomore fruits, half that amount of *pesedj* fruit, dates, 150 ml of stale beer, 75 ml of wine, and 300 ml of donkey's milk (Eb 98).

Other times, 75 ml of wheat and barley semolina were mixed with 4 ml of the *wedja* part of dates, date seeds, and *pesedj* fruit with half the amount of wormwood and *shenfet* fruit. The mixture was boiled and left overnight to stand and collect the dew. The period of usage was the usual four days (Eb 100). Another remedy contained 1.8 l of water, to which were added 1 ml of earth almonds, garden and wild yellow nutsedge, pine nuts, and juniper berries, half the amount of gum, and four times the amount of honey and goose fat (Eb 101).

In one case the substances causing pain in the abdomen were connected with the activity of poison of a dead person, which expressed the ancient Egyptian idea that the dead could influence the life and health of a person. The same amount (4 ml) of chaste tree, indigo, thyme, the plants *tia* and *niaia,* and raisins were to be mixed with 75 ml of acacia leaves, the same amount of bark, and part *kheru* of the acacia, *aru* tree leaves, its bark, and part of its *kheru*. The ingredients were mixed and were to be swallowed continuously for four days (Eb 99).

Ebers 103—destruction of the substances causing pain and a rash of the abdomen

In the case that in addition to pain in the abdomen a rash was found on the body of the person (man or woman), it was recommended to prepare a mixture of 4 ml of flour from earth almonds, the same amount of honey and goose fat, half that amount of date and sweet flour, and *sheny-ta* seeds. The ingredients were ground together and mixed, and the medicine was eaten all day.

Berlin 170—overcoming substances causing pain

In the Berlin Papyrus medicines are recommended against substances causing pain in the abdomen, which were not administered orally (perorally) but as an enema. When someone was having pains in the abdomen, an enema could be applied comprising 112.5 ml of herbal decoction and 4 ml of *Moringa* oil for a period of four days. We do not know the composition of this decoction, but *Moringa* oil acted as an anti-inflammatory agent.

Hearst 26, 29, and 47—overcoming/destroying the substances causing pain

According to the Hearst Papyrus, a mixture was prepared against the substances causing pain from the same amount (2 ml) of *shasha* fruit, the *aamu* plant, and *sheny-ta* seeds, which were mixed with 300 ml of sweet beer and 75 ml of date purée. The medicine was to be administered for a period of four days (H 26).

A similar medicine comprised 300 ml of sweet beer, in which were mixed 2 ml of figs, *ished* fruit, *sheny-ta* seeds and oil, half the amount of carob, twice the amount juniper berries and the *aamu* plant. The mixture was boiled, left overnight to collect the dew, strained, and then reduced to approximately 150 ml. It was to be administered for four days (H 29).

Other times, a preparation was produced from 150 ml of milk, 75 ml of goose fat, 37.5 ml of earth almonds, and the same amount of dates with 2 ml of acacia leaves, which were cooked together, left overnight to stand and collect the dew, and strained. The medicine was used for a period of four days (H 47).

Ebers 39—removal of swelling in the abdomen

For the removal of swelling in the abdomen (ascites), which could besides the accumulation of mucuses have a number of unspecified causes, a mixture was recommended from the same amount (2 ml) of figs, ripe sycomore fruits, raisins, bryony, *ished* fruit, and *shena*, ocher, and milk, and an eighth amount of incense, which was mixed with water. The mixture was left overnight to stand and collect the dew and used for a period of four days.

Berlin 204—digestive problems (?)

The beginning of this case has not been preserved; it is thus difficult to categorize it. The composition of the recommended medicine could, however, indicate digestive problems, because the recipe contains a number of plant ingredients that are beneficial to digestion. It describes the preparation of a mixture of 4 ml of juniper berries, the same amount of honey, twice the amount of the *ankh-imy* plant, which could be henna or perhaps a species of lotus (see Hannig 1995, 146; Germer 2008, 42–43), a quarter of the amount of *Melilotus* and acacia leaves, an eighth of the amount of cumin, pine nuts, and *Anacyclus* and wild rue seeds, which were mixed in 150 ml of sweet beer. The mixture was to be boiled on hot ash and given to the sick person to drink.

Treatment of Abdominal Problems Caused by the Activity of Magic

The frequent limitlessness of abdominal pains and lack of knowledge of the position and function of the individual organs is mirrored in the medical texts in a number of cases, when the causes of the health problems were attributed to the activity of inauspicious powers, demons, or the dead, who according to contemporary conceptions could intervene in life in this world. In the subsequent cases, neither the symptoms of the disease nor the method of the medical examination is described. They are collections of prescriptions which were to relieve the patient in unspecified problems of an unknown character. It is possible they were used also as a complement to another treatment.

Ebers 165–73—magical powers in the abdomen

Seven prescriptions of the Ebers Papyrus were intended for "Driving away magical powers from the abdomen of a man or woman." The cases do not describe the symptoms of the problem or the method of examination; they comprise only the recipes for the preparation of the medicinal mixtures. They are mixtures of plant and animal and sometimes also mineral ingredients, which were to be drunk or eaten usually before going to sleep. One of the cases contains a more detailed heading, according to which they are prescriptions against the evil activity of a god or dead person in the form of poisonous and magical substances. The medicine was a mixture of several types of plants including 0.25 ml of peas and four times the amount of *nehep* of yellow nutsedge, of the *shasha* fruit, and the *ibu* plant, which were ground into a flour and joined in beer (Eb 168). The peas and the *ibu* plant in the same amount (0.25 ml) were also possible to mull with four times the amount of *Anacyclus*, and eight times the amount of coriander (Eb 170), which undoubtedly acted favorably on digestion. Other times, 15 ml of incense, the same amount of *sheny-ta* seeds, and the inside of the *hemem* plant, along with the contents of a freshwater mussel were mixed in sweet beer (Eb 165). A mixture of 2 ml of *shasha* fruit, half the amount of *Anacyclus*, and an eighth of the amount of the *qesenty* stone, which was mixed with 37.5 ml of honey, could help in a similar way (Eb 171), or a mixture of 2 ml of *Anacyclus* with the same amount of grapes, and half the amount of the *shasha* fruit, honey, and gum (Eb 172). Other times, it was recommended to mix pine nuts with the same amount of thyme, *pesedj* fruit, a double amount of sorghum and chaste tree, and 75 ml of honey (Eb 173). Besides honey, the binding agent could be a product of honey fermentation, which was mixed with the same amount, that is 15 ml of pine nuts, wild rue, and natron (Eb 167). According to another recipe, a plant with the strange name "my hand seizes, my hand grasps" was to be left overnight to be infused in 300 ml of water. The patient was then to use 480 ml of it daily for a period of four days (Eb 166).

Hearst 83–87—poisonous substances in the abdomen

A group of cases in the Hearst Papyrus also shows, as their common heading states, abdominal problems caused by a deity or a dead person. Even for these magically caused diseases, the texts recommend natural medicines, which the sick person was to use either one time or over four days. Only in one case is a magical incantation also included.

Just as in the previous group, the symptoms of the problem are not described in the text. The simplest was a prescription for the preparation of a mixture of 0.5 ml of coriander seeds, half that amount of peas, and four times the amount of the unknown plant *ibu*, which was mixed in 150 ml of sweet beer. The mixture was strained and used before sleeping (H 87). Other times, 0.5 ml of coriander was mixed with the same amount of peas, pine nuts, yellow nutsedge, *shasha* fruit, and the *aamu* plant, half the amount of *Anacyclus*, bryony fruit, and ocher; four times the amount of honey was used as the binding agent. The mixture was also administered before sleeping (H 86). Another prescription recommended a mixture of 1 ml of coriander, earth almonds, grapes, and jujube bread with twice the amount of anise and figs, half the amount of the *ibu* plant, salt, ocher, and honey. The ingredients were mixed with 150 ml of water and left overnight to stand and collect the dew. The medicine was then to be used for a period of four days (H 84).

The sick person was given a boiled mixture containing 2 ml each of carob, grapes, peas, and *sheny-ta*, to which were added a double amount of *shasha* fruit, a quarter amount of the interior of a freshwater mussel, sea salt, honey, *aru* tree leaves, *kaa* (perhaps the bark?) of the *aru* tree, and an eighth of the amount of galenite. An herbal decoction in the amount of 375 ml served as the bonding agent. It was necessary to strain the mixture after boiling and use for a period of four days (H 83).

For the same problems, a dinner was also recommended prepared from the *abdju* fish, the mouth of which was supposed to be filled with incense before cooking. A component of this prescription was also an incantation, which was to be pronounced over the sick during the use of the medicinal fish. The incantation addresses directly the originator of the problems and calls on them to leave the body of the sick person. The phrase "look, I brought feces for you to eat" could mean that a fish prepared with incense did not taste good, or rather refers to disgusting food for the enemy (H 85).

Ebers 225–26—poisonous substances, the activity of demons in the abdomen

Substances harmful to the body of a person, which caused the disease in the abdomen, could be repelled with a mixture of 2 ml of carob, grapes, *shasha* fruit, and salt, half the amount of *Anacyclus*, a quarter of the amount of acacia leaves, the leaves and bark of the *aru* tree, and the inside of a freshwater mussel with 37.5 ml (or perhaps 7.5 ml?) of honey. This mixture was to be used before sleeping (Eb 225). Other times, a person was given to eat, also before sleeping, a strained mixture which comprised 300 ml of honey, 2 ml of figs and anise, half the amount of coriander, earth almonds, and jujube bread, a quarter of the amount of Lower Egyptian celery, grapes of the *ibu* plant, and the *qesenty* stone (Eb 226). It is worth noting that case Ebers 226 has a parallel in the Hearst Papyrus, namely the prescription Hearst 84, which we discussed above.

Ebers 229—poisonous substances, activity of demons

This prescription against poisonous substances did not provide the place of the pain of the sick person, but connects these substances again with the harmful activity of the gods or dead people. The composition of the prescription indicates that it could be against the detrimental activity of a demon in the abdomen of a person, as was the case with the previous and subsequent prescriptions. It was a mixture of 2 ml of figs and *ished* fruit, a quarter of the amount of wheat semolina and ocher, which were mixed in 75 ml of water. The mixture was to be strained and ingested before sleeping.

Ebers 231-32—the activity of a demon in the abdomen, poisonous substances, substances causing pain, evil things

Another group of cases against poisonous and painful substances contained prescriptions for the preparation of a mixture of 4 ml of earth almonds, half the amount of figs and ripe sycomore fruits, 0.5 ml of Lower Egyptian celery and honey, and half that amount of sorghum and *shasha* fruit, which were mixed in 150 ml of water. This medicinal mixture was to be strained and ingested before sleeping (Eb 231). A medicine with a slightly altered composition contained 2 ml each of figs, grapes, flour from earth almonds, and honey, half the amount of anise, pine nuts, a quarter of the amount of yellow nutsedge, an eighth of the amount of cumin, and 150 ml of water. The method of preparation and administration was the same as with the previous prescription (Eb 232).

Ebers 182—the activity of the dead in the abdomen

According to this prescription in the Ebers Papyrus, the usage of a medicinal mixture was to help against the harmful activity of a dead person in the body of the sick person. This mixture was made from equal amounts (15 ml) of peas, celery, *shasha* fruit, *kaa* (perhaps the bark) of the *aru* tree, and the insides of a freshwater mussel. The ingredients were to be ground, and it was recommended to eat this mixture with honey.

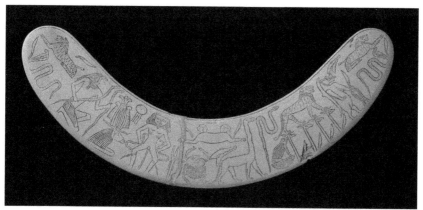

Fig. 26. The so-called magic wand, covered with depictions of Egyptian demons, protected against evil powers (Twelfth Dynasty, British Museum London EA18175, photo © The Trustees of the British Museum)

Hearst 16—driving away the dead

It is similar to the previous case Ebers 182, which differs in several details and contains scribal errors. The case's heading indicates the dead person as the cause of the problems, but it is not presented in connection with the sick person's abdomen. The composition of the recommended medicine, however, coincides with the prescription in Ebers 182; hence there is no doubt of its use for purging the abdomen.

Ebers 757–60—the disease *ruyt* in the right half of the abdomen

According to the heading, another group of cases was intended for the treatment of the unknown disease *ruyt*, which affected the right (favorable) half of the abdomen. The cases do not describe the symptoms of this disease, so that it is difficult today to judge what type of disease it could have been. Nevertheless, the term *ruyt* is related to the words "leave, move, stop," also "suspension" (Grapow 1958, 174–76), and thus could refer to symptoms of acute or temporary radiating and returning pains on the right side of the abdomen, which are characteristic of an infection of the gall bladder (cholecystitis) and could be very cruel in the case of a gallstone (cholelithiasis) wedged in the bile duct. The pain can radiate to the shoulder, the lower end of the right shoulder blade, and other places of the chest, abdomen, or back. This disease affects 10–15 percent of the adult population. Gallstones often form after rapid weight loss by dieting, namely also with wealthier individuals (Miller and Ritner 1994, 73–74). The constant, not returning pain rules out the possibility that it was an infection of the appendix (appendicitis).

Physicians fought against *ruyt* using natural medicines, which according to the texts were to be applied on the painful place on the abdomen, not used internally. It was recommended to use a mixture of 1 ml of barley with half the amount of fresh mash, which was mixed in strong beer and applied on the abdomen (Eb 757). Other times, 15 ml of honey, the same amount of goose fat, and the unknown *git* plant were used (Eb 760). More complicated to prepare was the medicine made from equal amounts (15 ml) of mash, raisins, sorghum, fenugreek, barley, the unknown plant *qesentet*, and the bindweed *senutet* (Eb 759). Another prescription refers to a mixture made of 1 ml juniper berries, mountain celery, and Lower Egyptian celery, *Potentilla*, *Juncus* (reed), white barley, green barley, the *git* plant, the Lower Egyptian *ibu* plant, the *tiam* and *khebu* plants, the *ibkhi* drink, and the stones *peshnet* and *rudj*. A double amount of myrtle, half the amount of honey, and a quarter share of incense, 75 ml of cedar resin and *pesedj* fruit also belonged to that (Eb 758). A large number of these ingredients are not known to us; we thus cannot judge the possible effects of the medicinal mixture, which was applied on the painful abdomen, but the number of ingredients could indicate that the physicians did not know much about how to deal with the disease.

Berlin 109–13—the disease *nesyt*

The disease *nesyt* is difficult to identify today because its symptoms are not specified in the preserved texts. Case London 25 (see page 177) contains a magical incantation against the disease *nesyt* and also another unknown disease *temyt*. However, besides this purely magical method, we also find prescriptions for the preparation of medicines in the preserved texts.

One of the cases in this group shows that, according to contemporary conceptions, the disease *nesyt* was caused by something from outside, perhaps a demon, which entered the body of the sick person to cause damage in him (Bln 112). Ointments could be prepared as a medicine, which were smeared over the body of the affected person, apparently the whole body, not just the painful place. The prescriptions recommend an ointment from pork lard with a girl's urine (Bln 109), an ointment from the best sheep's or goat's fat with fresh *Moringa* oil (Bln 113), or an ointment from the roots of the unknown *shas* plant, and dust from a horse's thigh (Bln 112). It seems that several of the mentioned ingredients were to act with magical power, but we cannot rule out the possibility that these terms were vernacular names of plants, unknown to us.

Another two cases in this group recommend the preparation of a medicinal beverage against the disease *nesyt*. It was a drink from goat's blood with wine (Bln 110) or from watermelon with wine (Bln 111).

Hearst 206–11—the disease *nesyt*

We find the same disease also in the Hearst Papyrus, where, however, different medicines are recommended, made from natural substances and used internally. A medicinal mixture against *nesyt* could be prepared from carob, fennel, *ihu* fruit, and sweet beer (H 211), or similarly from fennel, *Melilotus*, wild rue, garlic, and beer (H 209). Other times, an herbal decoction was prepared mixed with *hemayt* seeds, which might have been bitter almonds (H 210). An unappetizing prescription refers to a mixture of 75 ml of wine with crushed donkey feces, which was to be drunk for a period of four days (H 208).

Another two prescriptions present more precise measurements. According to one of them, a mixture was prepared from 2 ml of six-row green barley, the same amount of six-row white barley, and half the amount juniper berries, offshoots of bryony, and *shenfet* fruits, which the sick person was to drink for a period of four days (H 206). Another prescription describes a mixture for one-off use, which was prepared from 1 ml raisins and juniper berries, a double amount of *ished* fruit and white oil, half that amount of honey, 75 ml of figs, and 375 ml of sweet beer. Before consumption, the mixture was to be boiled and strained into the form of a curative drink (H 207). The last two cases are the same as cases Ebers 752 and 754 (see below).

London 5—the disease *nesyt*

The unknown cause of the disease *nesyt* was related to the concept that the problems were caused by evil powers. We, therefore, also find in the texts magical incantations which were to act against this disease. Unfortunately, its text is very badly preserved, and it is difficult to understand this incantation. We find a reference here to the activity of the disease in the body of the affected person that "you destroy his bones," and also to Nesy and Nesyt, the male and female forms of the demon who caused the disease in the body of the sick person. The text also refers to powerful deities who were to help protect the ill person. The sun god Re is mentioned here and his city of Heliopolis, and also the god or demon Bebi, who prevented unsuitable people from achieving a happy life in the afterlife while he protected the good ones from dangerous creatures (Janák 2005, 41).

Ebers 752–56—the disease *nesyt*

Although the heading of this group of prescriptions does not specify in which part of the body the disease *nesyt* was, the prescriptions indicate that the problems were in the abdomen, because some of the prescriptions have a very similar composition to some of the medicinal mixtures in the previous group.

An herbal decoction mixed and cooked with bitter almonds (Eb 753) is a medicine almost identical with the one in case Hearst 210. Case Hearst 208 is similar to the medicinal mixture prepared from donkey testicles, which were finely ground and mixed into wine (Eb 756). This medicine was to relieve the person quickly.

Another case recommends against the disease *nesyt* a medicinal mixture of 2 ml of white six-row barley, half the amount of juniper berries, offshoots of bryony, and *shenfet* fruit, which were to be mixed and drunk (Eb 752). It is similar to case Hearst 206, where, however, green barley was also used and the medicine was to be administered for four days.

A similar case, Hearst 207, but with a slightly different amount of some ingredients, is a prescription for a medicinal mixture of 4 ml of figs and *ished* fruit, 2 ml of white oil, 1 ml of raisins and juniper berries, and 0.5 ml of honey, which was to be cooked with 75 ml of sweet beer and then strained and drunk (Eb 754).

Another case in this group recommends preparing a medicine from equal amounts (15 ml) of dates, fermented date juice, carob, mint, sea salt, and honey. The end of the case has, unfortunately, not been preserved (Eb 755).

Hearst 36—magic in the abdomen

According to ancient Egyptian ideas, unspecified problems of the abdomen were caused by magic. Many times, it was the activity of a demon or a dead person, but in this case the originator of the problem is not specified. The usage of a mixture of pine nuts, incense, and a freshwater mussel was to help.

Hearst 54—magic in the abdomen

Other times, it was recommended to mix equal amounts (15 ml) of pine nuts, the part of dates called *wedja*, incense, and probably bitter almonds (?). During the usage, this medicinal mixture was to be washed down with beer.

Constipation

Ancient Egyptians and their physicians were almost fascinated with the correct functioning of the digestive tract. The members of the highest classes of ancient Egyptian society often happily ate well and abundantly at feasts, as captured by polychrome reliefs and paintings. They sit convivially at long tables weighted with vegetables, fruit, meat of domestic or game animals, while musicians, often blind harpists, play music for them to accompany the food. According to it all, many of the participants of the banquets did not know their limits and some are depicted even vomiting. This way of life led to overweight in them; the feared problems undoubtedly included constipation.

The Greek historian and geographer Herodotus (fifth century BC) pointed out this fact and reports to us that the (wealthy) Egyptians fast for three days every month and often use emetics and enemas to maintain their health (Herodotus 1972, II, §77). According to the Greek historian Diodorus of Sicily (first century BC) people tried "using drenches, fastings and emetics, sometimes every day and sometimes at intervals of three or four days. For they say that the larger part of the food taken into the body is superfluous and that it is from this superfluous part that diseases are engendered" (Diodorus of Sicily 1933, I.82).

We already encountered the term constipation (obstipation), called *shena* in Egyptian, in the previous part of the text in the incorrected phrase "constipation of the stomach" on the level of the upper part of the digestive tract (see above, pages 212–23). When it was a real constipation, the term was usually accompanied by references to the opening or cleansing of the abdomen and prescriptions for the preparation of laxatives to remove the feces from the large intestine, which was, according to contemporary conceptions, the largest tube *(metu)* of the human body. In the medical texts we find numerous groups of cases and recipes designed to have a laxative effect on the abdomen or facilitate excretion or emptying.

Ebers 7 and 9–18—a laxative medicine

A large group of prescriptions describe the preparation of laxatives, which were used orally. A very effective one was undoubtedly a mixture of 375 ml of milk scalded with 4 ml of ripe sycomore fruits and the same amount of honey, which was to be strained and used for a period of four days (Eb 7). Other times, the same ingredients were mixed in equal amounts of 15 ml each (Eb 18). A medicine prepared from 15 ml of *Avicennia* fruit, honey, *wam* fruit, *shenfet* fruit, and the *ineb* plant, which were thoroughly mixed before being administered, was also recommended for four days (Eb 16). It is not possible to judge the effectiveness, because we do not know the majority of the mentioned plant ingredients. Other times equal amounts (15 ml) of figs, carob, cumin, *ished* fruit, the *tiam* plant, and oil were mixed; this mixture undoubtedly helped cleanse the intestine (Eb 17).

The ill person could also consume a mixture of 15 ml of honey, *sheny-ta* seeds, and wine, which were strained before use (Eb 12). According to another set of instructions, it was possible to use a mixture of 2 ml of honey and *sheny-ta* seeds and drink 150 ml of beer or 75 ml of wine (Eb 9), or mix 4 ml of honey with half the amount of ground *sheny-ta* seeds, then eat and wash it down with sweet beer (Eb 14). Other times, 2 ml of carob was mixed with the same amount of *sheny-ta* seeds and the *aamu* plant, and in addition a quarter of the amount of honey (Eb 10). According to another prescription, 2 ml of honey was added to the same amount of arugula, an eighth of the amount of *sheny-ta* seeds, 75 ml of date juice, and 75 ml of oil, which was boiled before use (Eb 11). All of these mixtures were used once for a single day. Their composition indicated that the effects could have been quite reliable.

What was more complicated was the preparation of a mixture from equal amounts (15 ml) of fresh dates, sea salt, and grape juice, which was mixed in water, then chopped arugula was added and the mixture was simmered. The medicine was to be used while it was still warm and washed down with sweet beer (Eb 13).

One of the prescriptions uses a mineral ingredient: it recommends preparing pills from 15 ml of pulverized malachite, which was mixed with a bread pancake so that the sick person could consume it and wash it down with sweet beer (Eb 15).

Ebers 34—purging of the abdomen
A laxative could be prepared from sweet beer, in which were mixed 15 ml each of honey, goose fat, and *shena* and *sheny-ta* seeds. The sick person was to drink it for a period of four days.

Ebers 36–37—facilitation of evacuation
Problems with evacuation could be resolved with the help of a mixture of 375 ml of sweet beer, 2 ml of *ished* fruit, half that amount of *shenfet* fruit, and sea salt. The mixture was left overnight to stand and collect the dew and was drunk for four days (Eb 36). Another medicine with the same effect was prepared from 480 ml of barley, which was first roasted and then a bread called *feka* in Egyptian was prepared from it. A person suffering from constipation was to pour oil on it and eat it (Eb 37). Through roasting, the barley became more digestible, and the oil worked as a lubricant.

Ebers 20 and 22–24—emptying the stomach and expelling impurities
For the cleansing of the abdomen, a mixture of milk or sweet beer could also be made, which was then cooked with 15 ml of thyme and used until the abdomen was fully emptied (Eb 20). All of the bad and harmful influences could be removed from the body of a person by a mixture of 2 ml of honey and the same amount of *sheny-ta* seeds mixed with 75 ml of dates and 75 ml of earth almonds (Eb 22). A medicine from the same amount (4 ml) of *sheny-ta* seeds, arugula, and wormwood, which was mixed with 225 ml of sweet beer, boiled and strained, also acted favorably (Eb 24). In both cases, they are similar to

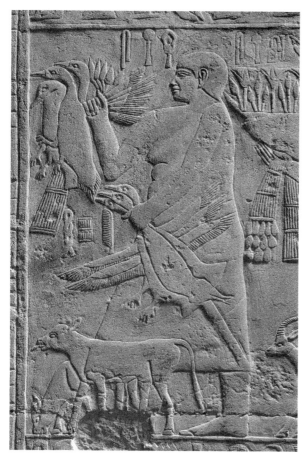

Fig. 27. An offering bearer depicted as an obese man, bringing offerings to the tomb owner. In tomb owners, obesity refers to a prosperous life, but in this case the relief could reflect the health condition of the depicted inspector of funerary priests, named Hepi (Sixth Dynasty, tomb of Ankhmahor in Saqqara, photo © Oxford Expedition to Egypt)

the above-mentioned prescriptions for a laxative. In the prescription Eb 24, this fact is mentioned in the conclusion, not in the more generally formulated heading.

Other times, a mixture was prepared from 1 ml of pine nuts and *shena* seeds, half the amount of chaste tree, yellow nutsedge, the *aam* plant, the *tiam* plant, sea salt, and a quarter of the amount of incense, and 7.5 ml of an herbal decoction. The amount of the decoction as a binding agent seems to be very little considering the other ingredients; it is therefore possible that it was incorrectly written down in the text, or possibly another binding agent is missing as an ingredient. Everything was mixed and put to boil, until the mixture was reduced to 225 ml. Then honey was added, and the mixture was removed from the fire. It was served warm for the period of one day (Eb 23).

Ramesseum III.A, I. 10–11 and 26–27—expulsion of impurities in the abdomen

These two cases written on one of the papyri from the Ramesseum represent a parallel to case Ebers 20, but they are very badly preserved. Only the part of the prescription mentioning milk and thyme has been preserved of them.

Ebers 25—evacuation and suppression of putrefaction in the abdomen

Another remedy was made from *Ricinus* and *shena* seeds, which the person was to chew, swallow, and wash down with beer. Thanks to the laxative effect of the herbs included, it should have entirely cleansed the abdomen.

Ebers 8, 26—a laxative suppository

Two other means are different for their origin and method of preparation and administration. A mixture from equal amounts (15 ml) of honey, carob flour, and wormwood was pressed into the shape of a suppository and applied in the rectum (Eb 8). Thanks to the antibacterial effects of honey and the calming effects of carob along with the bitterness of wormwood, it could be successful and calming overall. Another prescription recommends a suppository prepared from many ingredients, namely equal amounts (15 ml) of honey, cumin, wormwood, pine nuts, *shasha* fruit, *shena* seeds, the *aam* plant, the *tiam* plant, and sea salt. Some of the ingredients are contained also in the above-mentioned laxatives (Eb 26).

Berlin 149—constipation in the abdomen

In order to get rid of constipation (obstipation) in the abdomen, which is manifested in that the contents of the intestines are not moving, the Berlin Papyrus recommends preparing the same amount of a "male" herbal decoction, pomace, beer, and *sheny-ta* fruit. It was enough to use the mixture for a period of one day.

Ebers 190—constipation

This case is a component of "The book on the stomach" of the Ebers Papyrus (see pages 212–23) and describes symptoms when the sick person suffers constipation, the palpation finding in the hypogastrium is similar to "a clod of feces," and as a consequence of the problems it writhes as in a coughing fit, but it is not clear if the patient also suffered from a cough knotting his stomach or whether it is only a description of the condition compared to a cough. According to Nunn, it could have been a severe case of putrefaction in the enlarged bronchi, in which pocket-shaped deposits emerge filled with mucus (bronchiectasis) (Nunn 1996, 88). However, we can rather compare this case to the prescriptions for improving digestion (see also Westendorf 1999, 189). According to the text, a medicinal beverage was to be prepared for the patient from fresh mash with oil and honey, which was boiled with 1 ml of pine nuts, half the amount wormwood, and twice the amount of *shasha* fruit. This mash could effectively help to cleanse the intestine, and thanks to wormwood and pine nuts, it acted favorably on digestion. After boiling, the mixture was used for a period of four days. Then, the physician examined the patient again and by palpation of the abdomen discovered whether the symptoms had ceased.

Ebers 193—"constipation" of the stomach
This case states "constipation" of the stomach, but it clearly was problems of other parts of the digestive tract. According to the text, the physician examined the patient and found that his abdomen is distended and trembled during palpation, because it is full of feces that had not yet solidified. This description reveals that it was constipation in the large intestine. The medicine was prepared from 1 ml of two types of nutsedge, pine nuts, and the *tiam* plant, twice the amount of *shasha* fruit, and 112.5 ml of nuts of the *mendji* fruits cooked in oil and honey, which were mixed with an unspecified amount of wine and milk. The sick person was to eat this mixture and wash it down with sweet beer to recuperate quickly (Eb 193).

Ebers 203—constipation in the right half of the abdomen
In the following case, the physician examined the patient through palpation and felt constipation in the right half of the abdomen, where the contents had contracted and formed a lump. It was a condition for which the physician recommended a fast-acting pressed drink from sorghum, which was used for four days. The physician then examined the patient again; if he found that the condition continued, he had to give the sick person a strong remedy from peas and bitter almonds (?) ground and boiled in sweet beer. He was then to use a strong medicine from barley and the *aat* stone, ground and cooked in oil and honey. Ebbell (1937, 52) considered this urgent case to be an infection of the vermiform appendix (appendicitis), whereas Nunn (1996, 89) and Stephan (2001, 105) consider a fatal wedging of the intestinal contents (fecal impaction or ileus, possibly partial obstruction or subileus).

Ebers 204—constipation in the left half of the abdomen
From the same papyrus there also comes a case of constipation in the left hypogastrium (hypochondrium), or in the unfavorable left half of the abdomen. The author of the text characterized its manifestation by a comparison to a river (the

Nile) which formed an obstacle—a bank or shoal. The treatment of such a case was complicated and comprised several steps. First, a mixture was prepared of 1 ml ground pine nuts, twice the amount of *shasha* fruit and the *tiam* plant, and four times the amount of *pesedj* fruits, which were mixed and mulled in 3.2 l of oil and half the amount of honey. The sick person was to use this mixture for a period of four days.

If this method did not help and, moreover the constipation advanced, it was necessary to prepare a beverage by boiling the *pesedj* fruit to a mush, which the patient had to use again for a period of four days. This was to fill the abdomen so much that the intestine was to writhe like a centipede, meaning perhaps that there was a strengthening of the movement of the intestines (peristalsis). The physician was to examine the patient repeatedly to determine his condition. When feces came from him crumbled like grains, the patient was to receive for four days a cooling, pressed beverage from equal amounts (15 ml) of sorghum and *iuhu* fruit mixed in water.

Berlin 157–60—sated, overfilled abdomen

The Berlin Papyrus contains a group of prescriptions which are intended to get the abdomen that is sated and heavy moving. According to the texts of these cases, the sick person could be helped by a medicine against substances causing pain *(wekhedu)*. In fact, if we compare the recommended medicinal mixtures from this group with those where the problems are attributed to the substances *wekhedu* without further explanation (see pages 223–29), we find a number of similarities between them.

The effective mixture comprised the same amount (2 ml) of figs, grapes, *Melilotus*, mountain celery, *ished* fruit, thyme, *pesedj* fruit, fresh bread, and goose fat, to which were also added twice the amount of the cracked fruits of the sycomore, half the amount of juniper berries, a quarter of the amount of *Potentilla* and Lower Egyptian celery, a little incense, fatty meat, a little of the *amau* plant, and 375 ml of sweet beer. All of the ingredients were to be ground and mixed and then strained. The patient was to use them for a period of four days. This mixture undoubtedly had a favorable effect on digestion thanks to the relieving *Melilotus* and *Potentilla*, the large amount of fiber and vitamins, and the lubricating effect of the fat (Bln 157).

The other cases contained a simpler version of the remedy, which helped the ill person suffering from flatulence (meteorism). A mixture was recommended from the same amount (2 ml) of goose fat, the *aam* plant, and *ished* fruit, which were ground and mixed with 375 ml of sweet beer. The pressed medicine was to be drunk for a period of four days (Bln 158). Other times, a mixture was made of 2 ml each of figs, *ished* fruit, *Potentilla*, and 375 ml of sweet beer (Bln 160).

In contrast, one of the cases presents the preparation of an enema which was to be applied to the rectum. It was a mixture of 2 ml of the leaves of the jujube, acacia, and myrtle with the same amount of honey and *Moringa* oil, which thanks to its ingredients had astringent and anti-inflammatory effects (Bln 159). The patient was to use the enema for one day.

Hearst 1-3—evacuation of the abdomen

A number of cases of the Hearst Papyrus, which contains prescriptions for the preparation of laxatives, are also connected with constipation in the abdomen, but the entire wording has only been preserved for a few of them. One incompletely preserved prescription recommends creating seven pellets from *shasha* fruit and an herbal decoction (and perhaps also ingredients), which was then to be dipped in honey and given to the ill person to swallow (H 2). Another remedy comprised bitter almonds (?) and honey (and perhaps also other ingredients); the sick person was to lick honey with that and apparently wash it down with sweet beer for a period of four days (H 3). It is possible that also the previous, partially preserved case could contain a laxative. The beginning has not been preserved; the prepared medicine was to be given on the *feka* cake with honey (H 1).

Hearst 25—expulsion of constipation

A better-preserved text is that of a prescription for constipation which describes the preparation of a medicine from ground six-row barley, which was to be washed and left overnight to collect the dew. In the morning, it was pressed through a sieve and mixed with honey, and the mixture was pressed through a cloth. It was to be used for a period of four days. The author of the papyrus did not refrain from adding "I saw that it is effective" to confirm the credibility of the prescription.

Hearst 58-60—purging, excretion

A simple but also reliable preparation for having a laxative effect on the abdomen comprised 4 ml of the cracked fruits of the sycomore and the same amount of honey, which was scalded with 375 ml of milk. After pressing, the mixture was to be drunk for four days (H 58). Another preparation, which was intended for achieving excretion, was a mixture of 15 ml of juniper berries and the same amount of honey, which was added to sweet beer. The method of preparation and period of use were the same as in the previous prescription (H 59). Another mixture was prepared from 15 ml of an unknown stone called *khershu-mat*, which was pulverized and mixed with sweet beer. After it was boiled and pressed through a sieve, the ill person was to drink the mixture (H 60). Unfortunately, the effect of this mixture remains unknown to us.

Ramesseum III.A: 29–30—difficult evacuation from the rectum
This case has been preserved only partially. Its heading testifies that it is a prescription for a preparation for constipation, but the actual text of the prescription has been lost for the most part. According to the preserved fragment, date seeds and perhaps a flat cake, on which the mixture was spread and eaten, was used for the preparation of the laxative mixture. It was to be washed down with diluted beer.

Ebers 30–31—removal of putrefied feces from the abdomen
To remove putrefied feces which had accumulated in the abdomen of a person, it was necessary to prepare a laxative mixture from 15 ml of gum and the same amount of red ink, which were mixed with human milk and given to the sick person to drink (Eb 30). Other times, a remedy was made from equal amounts (15 ml) of wheat flour, arugula, barley, the *tiam* plant, and *shena* and *sheny-ta* seeds. The ingredients were ground and mixed, and from the resulting dough the *shenes* cake was shaped, which the ill person was to eat (Eb 31).

Ebers 32–33—emptying of the abdomen, expulsion of feces
The same purpose was to be fulfilled by a mixture presented with a slightly altered heading. The prescription for the *feka* cakes from ground bitter almonds (?), which were spread with honey (Eb 32) is similar to case Hearst 1. Other times, a simple mixture was prepared from 0.25 ml of pulverized malachite with honey (Eb 33).

Berlin 148—driving away all the bad things from the abdomen
The Berlin Papyrus also offers a universal preparation for expelling all bad things which are in the abdomen, a mixture prepared from 300 ml of an herbal decoction, 2 ml of *sheny-ta* seeds, half that amount of juniper berries, a quarter of the amount of yellow nutsedge and the *aamu* plant, a little sea salt, and incense. All of the ingredients were to be boiled together, reduced to 37.5 ml and then drunk for one day.

Berlin 150—driving away blood from the abdomen
This case also concerns problems with the abdomen, but the cause is attributed to the retention of blood. That was among the body-damaging substances

included along with pain in the term *wekhedu*, although in the conception of modern medicine, it is the most valuable body fluid. The means of relief is a mixture which is very similar to the laxative beverages mentioned above. The prescription describes the preparation of a beverage from the same amounts (15 ml) of beer, oil, the *henen* part of a date (this expression can be translated literally as the "phallus of a date"), and the *aam* plant. According to the text, the effect was to be "really excellent."

Diarrhea

Ancient Egyptian physicians devoted substantially less attention to the opposite of constipation, diarrhea, than to support of the excretion of feces or other supposedly harmful substances from a person's abdomen. At the same time, it can be assumed that in the not very suitable hygienic conditions, diarrheas could have been relatively frequent illnesses of adults and children.

Ebers 44–48—halting evacuation

A group of cases in the Ebers Papyrus presents various prescriptions for preparations against diarrhea, which included a number of plant and mineral ingredients.

Some prescriptions are hardly comprehensible for us today, such as a mixture prepared from 1 ml of a flat bread called *shenes*, the same amount of the *sekhet* of a jug called *djiu,* and half that amount of ocher, which was combined in 375 ml of water and administered for a period of four days (Eb 45). Other times the same flat bread was recommended with twice the amount of *sekhet* and, instead of ocher, half the amount of carob was added. The ingredients were also mixed in 375 ml of water (Eb 47).

According to another prescription, 2 ml carob was mixed with the same amount of fresh mash, oil, twice the amount of honey, and 375 ml of water. The mixture was boiled and used for four days (Eb 44). It was possible to mix carob in the amount of 0.5 ml also with 2 ml of ripe sycomore fruits and gum, four times the amount of figs, grapes, and pine nuts, and half the amount ocher. This prescription moreover contained the text of an incantation, which needed to be pronounced after mixing the ingredients during the final addition of 75 ml of water, and which refers to a demon (male or female) as the originator of the illness. The medicine prepared was left overnight to stand and collect the dew and was administered for four days (Eb 48).

It is difficult to judge the efficacy of a plant mixture of 1 ml of honey, raisins, and anise, which was mixed with the *shena* fruits that are unknown to us, twice the amount of *shenfet* and *ished* fruits, and 375 ml of water. The mixture was left overnight to stand and collect the dew and was also used for a period of four days (Eb 46). What is striking is the inclusion of carob in three of the above-mentioned prescriptions, which had a suppressive effect on the irritated large intestine.

Ebers 251—diarrhea and so on
In the passage devoted to the knowledge of what was prepared from *Ricinus* (the castor rod bush), it states with many other references that chewing bits of *Ricinus* seeds with beer removes the pain from the abdomen during diarrhea. According to the text, it is explicitly a medicine for a man, but also women could certainly use it. We will discuss another use of the *Ricinus* shrub in connection with the hair and skin in the forthcoming third volume in this series.

Hearst 19-20—for diarrhea
According to the Hearst Papyrus, the ingredients for stopping diarrhea included the cooked blood of a cow (H 19). After this prescription, there is another for the preparation of a remedy for putting the demon Hayt to sleep, but the connection with diarrhea is not explicitly mentioned. The medicine was pig's blood mixed with wine (H 20).

Pains in the Sides
Only the Chester Beatty Papyrus presents special medicines which were to be prepared for patients suffering in the area of the sides. Neither the symptoms nor the causes of the disease are described in the text, so it is difficult today to judge which diagnosis it could have been. Unspecified pains in the sides could have had diverse origins—from pressure on the sensitive nerves coming from the spine to pains of the organs localized close to the sides (on the right, the appendix or the caecum, on the left, the descending part of the large intestine, the colon descendens). The medicinal mixtures comprise mainly (but not only) plant ingredients.

Chester Beatty VI.32-36—cooling of the sides
The incompletely preserved heading of this group of cases presents the connection of the medicines prepared with a cooling of the sides. According to the composition, they could have been medicines for digestion problems, since a number of the ingredients are the same as in the prescriptions described above, some of which have been preserved only in part. It was possible to prepare the medicinal mixture from the same amount (2 ml) of anise, figs, grapes, and *ished* fruit (CB VI.32); other times figs were mixed with 2 ml of grapes, a

quarter of that amount of carob, and an eighth amount of cress and incense in 375 ml of water (CB VI.36).

Other times, the mixture comprised 2 ml of barley semolina mixed with the same amount of pine nuts and honey and 375 ml of water (CB VI.34); earth almonds might have been added instead of nuts and, moreover, an additional quarter of the amount of ocher (CB VI.33). After being pressed through a sieve, the mixtures were used for four days. A preparation was used in the same way, but its wording has been preserved only in a reference to 2 ml of honey, 37.5 ml of grapes, and 375 ml of water (CB VI.35).

Chester Beatty VI.37–41—sides

The heading of another small group of prescriptions has been only partially preserved and mentions that they are also prescriptions for treating the side (or the area under the ribs, the hypochondrium, see Westendorf 1999, 177). The first mixture had a similar composition as some of the medicines in the previous group. It was prepared from 2 ml of the cracked ripe fruits of the sycomore with the same amount of grapes and the leaves of the sycomore, a quarter of the amount of carob, an eighth of the amount of cress and incense, and with cumin, which were mixed with 375 ml of sweet beer (CB VI.37). This mixture contained a great deal of fiber and undoubtedly had a calming effect as well as an antiflatulent (carminative) effect thanks to the spices.

Another prescription has been preserved only in part and contained two medicinal mixtures, of which the first was administered orally and the second in the form of an enema. The first medicine contained the gall bladder of an animal, the species of which has not been preserved in the text, salt, and perhaps also other ingredients. Pellets were to be formed, which the ill person swallowed. The enema, which was to be applied for four days, was prepared from 75 ml of an herbal decoction, 375 ml of sweet beer, and perhaps also from other ingredients (CB VI.38).

The subsequent cases present an alternative mixture containing 2 ml each of sycomore fruit, *ished* fruit, and an unpreserved species of seeds, and 300 ml of water (CB VI.39–40), which after being pressed through a sieve was to be drunk for four days. Another prescription contained acacia leaves, but the rest of the text has not been preserved (CB VI.41).

A Supposed Tumor in the Hypogastrium

In connection with illnesses of the abdomen, we present a short prescription from the Berlin Papyrus which is related to a tumor, a spheroid formation in the area of the hypogastrium (for the translation of the Egyptian term *hema*, see Westendorf 1999, 306 ["Ball-Geschwulst"]; Hannig 1995, 532 ["Geschwulst"]).

Berlin 56—against the lump *hema*

The text does not mention that the lump was accompanied by pain. Drinking a medicinal beverage was recommended; it was made from 225 ml of sweet beer with 2 ml of the cracked ripe fruits of the sycomore and the same amount of carob. Neither the cause nor the problems accompanying this lump are mentioned in the text. If it was a malignant tumor (for example, of the large intestine), it could only be palliative care. The composition of the mixture is quite similar to those described in the previous sections, which concerned difficult digestion.

Rectum

It is characteristic that the end of the digestive tract (rectum) did not escape the interest of ancient Egyptian physicians, because it was the most accessible for their sight and touch. A number of them boasted the specialization heading of physician of the rectum (proctologist), specialists in diseases of the final segment of the long intestine. One of them was the late Sixth Dynasty physician Irenakhty, who had his title inscribed on the false doors in his tomb in Giza (Nunn 1996, 127). The importance of this field within ancient Egyptian medicine is revealed by the great number of cases and recommended prescriptions which we can find in the preserved papyri. Many of them were recorded particularly in the Chester Beatty Papyrus, which is sometimes called the proctological papyrus. The importance which the author of this papyrus attributed to the cases of the disorders of the rectum is also clear from the fact that the texts of the papyrus begin with them. We encountered the participation of disorders of the rectum with the diseases of the heart or stomach already in several prescriptions in other sections.

The medicinal remedies which were recommended in medical texts for the treatment of the rectum were applied either as a beverage or flat cake orally (perorally), or as a rectal suppository (suppositorium) or an enema (clyster).

Smith 22—rectum

We begin this part with a unique case from the Smith Papyrus, which aptly describes the condition of a person with a sick rectum: "When you examine a person having pain (in) the rectum, when he gets up or sits down, he is having pain from an amassing in both of his legs." Here, it might have been a swelling of the lower extremities caused by the repeated efforts to push the stool out while

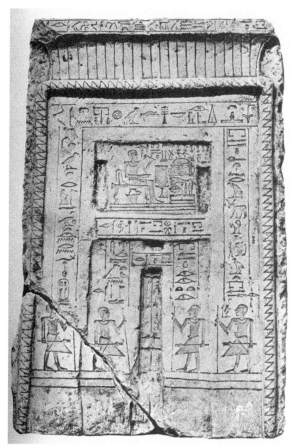

Fig. 28. The false door of Irenakhty Niankhpepy includes a number of medical titles, showing specializations of several medical fields; the title "physician of the abdomen of the royal palace attendants and guardian of the rear" is inscribed at the beginning of a vertical column of the text all the way to the right, and the title "physician of the eyes of the royal palace attendants" is in the short column right of the center (late Old Kingdom, Giza, after Junker 1928, Pl. II)

squatting, which was then common. The physician is called on to prepare an ointment for the patient from crushed acacia leaves boiled in oil with the stone called "great protection" in Egyptian. He was to apply this unguent on a bandage from the soft cloth *paqet*, which he placed in the rectum of the afflicted. It was a roll which, by irritating the mucous membrane, could relieve constipation like a suppository. Moreover, the leaves of the acacia have an astringent effect.

General Problems Connected with the Rectum

Some cases in the medical texts refer to treatment of the rectum, without specifying in any way which problems the patient suffered from. It is, therefore, very difficult from today's perspective to judge the seriousness of these cases or guess the relevant diagnosis. It is possible that at least some of them were related to intestinal problems described in the previous sections.

These two groups of cases from the Ebers Papyrus are written in different parts of the text, but contain the same prescriptions, copied with only minor modifications. The first group is presented with a heading which clarifies that they are prescriptions intended for the treatment of unspecified problems of the abdomen and rectum. In contrast, the heading of the second group presents only treatment of the rectum. They were mainly medicinal beverages which the patient was to take orally. They were prepared from ingredients which we already encountered above with the diseases and pains of the abdomen, during the treatment of constipation and diarrhea.

A simple preparation could be made from 150 ml of carob juice with 2 ml of honey, and after straining it, the patient was to use it for a period of four days (Eb 135). Another version of the same prescription presents the ratio of the ingredients as 15 ml of carob juice and 2 ml of honey (Eb 150).

A component of the majority of the other recommended beverages was *sheny-ta* seeds, which apparently played a crucial role in the treatment of the rectum, but we do not know its precise determination today. According to one prescription, 2 ml each of *sheny-ta* seeds and figs were mixed with half the amount of juniper berries and honey, twice the amount of sweet beer, an eighth of the amount incense, and 75 ml of raisins. The beverage was left overnight to stand and collect the dew; it was then to be strained through a sieve and used for one day (Eb 137). Another version of the prescription contained also 2 ml of *ished* fruit and was used for a period of four days (Eb 152).

Other times, a drink was recommended from the same amount (4 ml) of *sheny-ta* seeds, raisins, and flour from earth almonds, which along with half the amount of goose fat was mixed in 75 ml of milk (Eb 147). Another copy of the same prescription specifies the amount of the mash from earth almonds as 75 ml, and 150 ml of milk was to be used (Eb 132). The *sheny-ta* seeds were also to be mixed with the same amount of fresh bread and with a quarter of the amount of goose fat and honey (Eb 134 and 149). Other times, 7.5 ml of ripe sycomore fruits, half the amount of *sheny-ta* seeds, date and barley flours, a quarter of the amount of goose fat, and an eighth of the amount of honey were mixed (Eb 133), or 4 ml of *sheny-ta* seeds with the same amount of barley, wheat, and date flours, half the amount of fat (apparently goose), and a quarter of the amount of honey (Eb 148).

Besides beverages, the medicine could be administered in the form of baked goods as in the case when 2 ml of *sheny-ta* seeds were to be mixed with twice the amount of carob juice, cake dough, and goose fat, a quarter amount of honey, and 75 ml of wine. Later, the mixture was to be cooked into the form of a cake called a *shayt*, which the ill person was to eat every day and wash it down with hot beer (Eb 136). According to one version of the prescription, the hot beer was to be diluted with water in the ratio of 2:1 (Eb 151).

Cooling of an Inflammation of the Rectum
Specific problems of the rectum concerned predominantly prescriptions intended for cooling of the rectum or removal of heat in the rectum. The texts do not specify in any way how the problems were manifested with the patient and whether they could have been associated with or accompanied other issues, such as diarrhea or constipation. It is not possible to rule out that these remedies were prescribed for a wide range of difficulties. On the other hand, the heat, to which some of these prescriptions literally refer to, could also warn of a more serious problem. Such cases can be interpreted as treatment of an inflammation of the rectum (proctitis), possibly even enlarged inflamed veins (hemorrhoids). The medicines which the texts recommend mainly had the form of suppositories; only in a few cases was the medicine applied as an enema or exceptionally as a beverage.

Ebers 140—cooling of the rectum
This case recommends a suppository prepared from equal amounts (15 ml) of wild carrot, pine nuts, juniper berries, cumin, myrrh, camphor, incense, honey, and cuttlefish bones. Some of the mentioned ingredients could be accessible only to wealthier patients.

Ebers 143—cooling of the rectum
Elsewhere, a medicinal enema could also be used for cooling of the rectum, namely a mixture of 15 ml of a carob juice, *Moringa* and common oils, and 75 ml of honey. This mixture could have anti-inflammatory and calming effects.

Ebers 156-60—cooling of the rectum
Other medicinal remedies intended for cooling of the rectum were according to the common heading copied from a treatise called "Art of a Physician." According to the first prescription, 75 ml of wine was to be mixed with three times the amount of the beverage called *sedjer,* which is unknown to us; 7.5 ml of the brain of a fattened bull and a little onion were added, and the mixture was sweetened with honey. It was later strained and applied as an enema (Eb 156). Other times cow brain was mixed with the same amount of 75 ml of honey, half the amount of scalded milk, and 7.5 ml of milk fat. The

mixture was to be strained and applied to the rectum for the period of one day (Eb 157).

The next two prescriptions did not specify the period and method of application: 15 ml each of carob juice and thyme were to be mixed in water (Eb 158), or equal amounts (15 ml) of carob juice, acacia, and jujube leaves with milk fat (Eb 159). These mixtures could have calming and astringent effects.

According to another prescription, 0.5 ml of carob flour, the same amount of mallow, and 7.5 ml of honey were added to 75 ml of water. Unlike the previous mixtures, this one was administered orally as a medicinal drink, which the patient was to use for a period of four days (Eb 160).

Ebers 163—cooling of the rectum

The heading of this case indicated the preparation of a cooling suppository which was intended to be introduced into the rectum. The medicine comprised equal amounts (15 ml) of carob, date, and barley flours, wild carrot, the unknown *shasha* fruit, honey, sea salt, and wine sediment. The amounts of the ingredients listed indicates that it was possible to produce a greater amount of suppositories from the mixture and apply them repeatedly as needed.

Hearst 93—cooling of the rectum

According to the Hearst Papyrus, a medicinal beverage was used for the same purposes. It comprised 4 ml of crushed earth almonds with equal amounts of sorghum, the part of the dates called *wedja,* and half the amount of an unspecified mash, which was mixed in 300 ml of water. The mixture was then left overnight to stand and collect the dew, and the patient was to drink it for a period of four days.

Ebers 142—heat of the rectum

According to the Ebers Papyrus, medicines in the form of suppositories were also recommended for the removal of heat in the rectum. The suppository could be created from 15 ml of antelope fat mixed with the same amount of cumin, which was beneficial for digestive problems of various types.

Ebers 154-55—heat in the rectum

This group of prescriptions for expulsion of heat in the rectum describes the preparation of medicines for various methods of application. The patient was to take the first mixture orally (perorally). It was prepared from equal amounts (15 ml) of pine nuts, wormwood, onion, virgin dates, tubers (?) of *Astragalus,* sycomore seeds (?), *shasha* and *iuhu* fruits, gum, and ocher. The ingredients were to be ground and pressed until a juice was created, which the patient was to drink (Eb 154). The second medicine was applied as a suppository in the rectum. It was prepared by mixing equal amounts (15 ml) of carob flour, flour from beans, myrrh, resin, and galenite (Eb 155).

Chester Beatty VI.23-24—heat in the rectum
The text in the Chester Beatty papyrus also contains medicines for expelling heat, namely in the form of a drink and an enema. The first of them was prepared from 2 ml of fresh dates, half the amount of grape seeds, the same amount of the leaves (or perhaps roots) of a muskmelon, and a quarter of the amount of mash, which was mixed in 150 ml of water. The mixture was left overnight to collect the dew, and the patient was to sip it for a period of four days (CB VI.23). A mixture of 4 ml of hemp, an eighth of the amount of carob, and 375 ml of the unknown liquid *mesta* served as a complementary medicine in the form of an enema, which was also applied for four days (CB VI.24). Although we do not know the meaning of the last ingredient, carob acts beneficially in inflammations of the intestines. In the same context, the medicinal effects of hemp are currently being tested.

Chester Beatty VI.20-21—heat in the heart
In contrast, we find prescriptions in the previous and subsequent cases in the Chester Beatty VI Papyrus, the headings of which refer to heat in the heart and also in the rectum. It seems, however, that it was a disease of the abdomen and rectum rather than of the heart. These cases utilized the application rectally in the form of an enema (clyster).

First a medicinal mixture of 150 ml of sweet beer with 4 ml of honey and 0.25 ml of dates was to be used (CB 20), and then another enema prepared from 225 ml of sweet beer with the addition of 150 ml of juice from carob, 37.5 ml of milk fat, and 4 ml of sea salt (CB 21). Both mixtures were administered to the sick person for a period of four days.

Chester Beatty VI.18-19—cooling of the heart and rectum, revitalization of the arteries
In the summer, when great heat dominated in Egypt, the physicians recommended refreshment in the form of a drink or enema. The drink was prepared from 375 ml of water, in which 75 ml of crushed earth almonds, the same amount of fresh dates, and an unknown part of *Ricinus* (the castor rod bush), 4 ml of honey, and a quarter of the amount pine nuts were mixed (CB 18). After four days of use, an enema into the rectum was to follow prepared from

150 ml of sweet beer, 37.5 ml of honey, and 4 ml of fresh *Moringa* oil (CB 19), the effect of which was undoubtedly anti-inflammatory. These medicinal mixtures can be compared with the means for the abdomen, laxatives, and enemas, which are described in the relevant section (pages 223–48).

Chester Beatty VI.22—cooling of the heart, heat in the rectum
A drink prepared from 375 ml of water, in which were mixed 75 ml of grapes and earth almonds, 2 ml of honey, and half the amount of anise could serve a similar purpose, but it lacks specification of the season suitable for being applied. The beverage was strained and drunk for a period of four days.

Chester Beatty VI.25–30—heat in the heart, cooling of the rectum
Another group of cases contains prescriptions for the preparation of medical beverages and enemas, which were always applied for a period of four days. Since the prescriptions for drinks and enemas regularly alternate, it seems that the treatment usually comprised two connected steps. In the form of a beverage, a strained mixture was recommended that was prepared from 300 ml of water with 75 ml of grapes, the same amount of bryony seeds, and 0.5 ml each of honey and carob (CB 25); other times from 300 ml of water with 2 ml of figs, the same amount of wheat semolina, *ished* fruit, and a quarter of the amount of *qesenty* stone (CB 27), or 150 ml of water and 2 ml each of wheat semolina and *ished* fruit, and a quarter of the amount of *qesenty* stone and honey (CB 29).

After each of the drinks, there followed a prescription for the preparation of enemas, which comprised 75 ml of scalded milk with the same amount of honey, beef marrow, and 300 ml of *Moringa* oil (CB 26), or comprised 375 ml of sweet beer with 37.5 ml of oil, 4 ml of honey, an eighth of the amount of flour from beans, and salt (CB 28). The prescription has been preserved incompletely for a mixture of the cracked ripe sycomore fruits, 0.5 ml carob (in the text 1/12 is written by mistake), and the *shasha* fruit, 1 ml of pine nuts, and wild mint (CB 30).

Ebers 139—heat in the rectum and urinary bladder, flatulence
Even more-complicated cases appeared, such as the feeling of heat caused by an inflammation not only in the rectum, but also in the urinary bladder (cystitis) of the person, which was moreover accompanied by flatulence (meteorism). A suppository was to help made from equal amounts (15 ml) of watermelon, the unknown *ibu* plant, salt, and honey, which were ground and mixed.

Ebers 153—heat in the rectum, constipation, and stiffness of the leg
According to this case, the feeling of heat of the rectum could have been combined with constipation and stiffness of the lower extremities. The patient was to be relieved by a beverage prepared from 375 ml of water, 2 ml of fresh mash, and goose fat, half the amount of wax, and a quarter of the amount of carob. The mixture was to be left overnight to stand and collect the dew, and then used as a medicinal drink for a period of four days. This mixture could truly help cleanse the intestines.

Ebers 144—calming the rectum
Other prescriptions were intended more generally for calming the rectum, without the texts specifying what the cause of the problems were. One of the means was a mixture prepared from equal amounts (15 ml) of carob, juniper, cumin, *Moringa* oil, incense, fat, oil, sea salt, amber, balsam, galenite, and the unknown stone *sia*. All of the ingredients were to be ground and shaped into the form of a suppository. The application of this anti-inflammatory and calming mixture was to be repeated for a period of four days.

Ebers 164—calming the rectum and pubic area
According to the other cases, problems of the rectum could also be related to an illness of the entire pubic area. A medicinal mixture was to be prepared from equal amounts (15 ml) of carob flour and flour from beans, juniper berries, cumin, pine nuts, myrrh, incense, natron, honey, and balsam from Medja, the area of today's northern Sudan. All of the ingredients were ground and mixed, then suppositories were to be shaped from the mixture, which the patient used for a period of four days. Overall, this medicine was similar to the previous cases.

Ebers 161—calming the blood vessels of the rectum
Another prescription was intended literally for calming the blood vessels of the rectum. A mixture made from a small amount (0.25 ml) of acacia leaves, which act as an astringent, and beef fat was to be applied on the affected area. It was a calming ointment for hemorrhoids.

Pain of the Rectum
A number of cases in the medical texts refer to pains in the rectum, but their cause was not usually specified. It could have been pains accompanying another type of problem than hemorrhoids, or pains the cause of which was not precisely known by physicians then. They were therefore attributed sometimes to the activity of evil, pain-causing substances *(wekhedu)*.

Berlin 164—painful substances in the abdomen, their retention, and constipation in the rectum

This case comprises three parts and three prescriptions, each of which was provided with its own heading written in red ink. It is clear from the text that there were three steps to the treatment, which were applied one after the other. The treatment thus lasted for more days, which testifies to the persisting problems and pains. The reason for these problems was apparently unknown to physicians then; they therefore attributed it to pain-causing substances.

The first prescription describes the preparation of an enema which was to be injected into the patient's rectum for a period of four days. The medicine comprised 4 ml of honey and half the amount of *Moringa* oil, which were mixed with 150 ml of sweet beer. The same method and length of use was recommended with the second enema, which comprised 75 ml of honey, the same amount of *Moringa* oil, 300 ml of an herbal decoction, and a little sea salt. Both remedies were apparently intended for treatment of the internal environment in the rectum, and thanks to the honey and *Moringa* oil could act as an anti-inflammatory. The third enema, which was subsequently to act directly against the constipation, was prepared from 300 ml of hot water, in which 37.5 ml of sifted flour from beans was mixed. The effect of this medicine was supposedly immediate, apparently thanks to the high fiber content.

Ebers 141—substances causing pain in the rectum

According to this prescription, it was possible to prepare a medicine in a different form, such as a suppository, which was placed in the patient's rectum. It was made from equal amounts (15 ml) of figs, sea salt, incense, and beef spinal marrow.

Ebers 130—painful substances, wound (in the rectum?)

The heading of this case mentions wounds, by which they apparently meant very painful tears (rhagades) created in the walls of the rectum by violent pressure during defecation. A compress was to be applied on the affected place made from the softest cloth smeared with a mixture of equal amounts (15 ml) of sorghum flour, acacia leaves, aromatic myrrh, plant dye, and sweet beer and its sediments.

Ebers 138—poisonous substances, painful substances, harmful substances, cooling of the rectum

Against all the various types of harmful substances which could cause health problems in the area of the rectum, a beverage was recommended made from 2 ml of wormwood, half that amount of juniper berries, and a quarter of the amount of honey, which were mixed in 150 ml of sweet beer.

Hearst 4—agglomeration of the painful substances in the rectum

The remedy for expelling the obstacles, which were caused by the painful substances, was to be myrtle applied on the affected place.

Chester Beatty VI.31—burning sensation, substances causing pain

Although the text of this case does not explicitly mention any connection with the rectum, it was included in the group of the cases of Chester Beatty VI.18–30, which are devoted to the examination of the rectum and intestines during digestive difficulties (see pages 253–54). For this reason, it is possible to believe that the pain in this case also appeared precisely in the final segment of the digestive tract.

It is an incompletely preserved prescription for the preparation of a medicinal drink which was to act against harmful substances. It was made from 375 ml of water, in which 4 ml each of earth almonds and honey were mixed. The mixture was to be pressed through a sieve, and the patient used it for a period of four days.

Ebers 162—pain in the rectum

Another medicine against pain was to be prepared from equal amounts (15 ml) of beef spinal marrow and a coating from dried oil and wine sediments. The ingredients were mixed and made into the shape of a suppository. The period of use is not presented in the text.

Hearst 7—pain in the rectum

According to the Hearst Papyrus, it was possible to fumigate a painful rectum with a mixture prepared from limestone, sand, and an herbal decoction or beer.

Chester Beatty VI.1—pain in the rectum

This incompletely preserved case also refers to the treatment of a painful rectum. Milk fat was recommended mixed with herbs and perhaps also other ingredients which have not been preserved in the text. The ingredients were to be crushed in a mortar, strained through a cloth, and mixed with honey. The medicine was applied in the form of a suppository.

Ulcers in the Rectum

Ulcers could emerge from swollen veins (hemorrhoids) in the rectum through the influence of an infection clogged with scratching of the mucous membrane by a hard stool, which are a serious complication of its inflammation (proctitis). We can find a number of cases on this theme in the introductory passage of the

Chester Beatty Papyrus. However, some of these cases are very damaged, and it is not possible to correctly understand them today.

Chester Beatty VI.2–4—discharge, ulcers in the rectum, soothing the blood vessels, scratching

The text of the cases in this group have been only partially preserved. According to the incomplete heading, they are medicines for a number of problems caused by ulcers in the rectum and the scratching associated with them, which were able to give the patient a very hard time. The medicinal mixture was prepared from myrrh, incense, honey, goose fat, salt, human milk, and perhaps also other ingredients, which were to be mixed and apparently applied for a period of four days. The method of application has not been preserved in the text (CB VI.2). An accompanying treatment was to be assured by a medicine from goose fat, honey, a powder from frit, and many other ingredients, of which only the recommended amount has been preserved but not the names (CB VI.3). Only part of the heading written in red, mentioning the rectum, has been preserved of the last case (CB VI.4).

Chester Beatty VI.5–6—crushing ulcers

Another medicine intended for crushing ulcers contained linen leaves, yellow nutsedge imported from the area of the western oases, the scales of salt-water fish, and the liquid *mesta*. After a thorough mixing of the ingredients, twelve pellets were to be molded and, in sets of four, placed into the rectum of the sick person until he convalesced (CB VI.5). For a subsequent treatment, a suppository was suitable from equal amounts (15 ml) of fennel, goose fat, and honey. The mixture was molded with the help of a cloth pouch into the shape of four pellets, and one was placed into the rectum daily. If the patient bled from the rectum, juniper berries were to be crushed, left to collect the dew (apparently overnight), and then applied on the affected place. When he bled without stopping for a period of seven days, it was necessary to proceed to another treatment. A medical mixture was prepared of sorghum, ibex fat, and galenite, which was crushed, mixed, and left to collect the dew. Four pellets were molded from the mixture, which the patient was to introduce into the rectum one each day for relief (CB VI.6).

Chester Beatty VI. 7–8—anything in the rectum

Remedies intended for "any kind of thing" which could afflict a person in the area of the rectum were to have a wider effect. The first medicinal mixture was prepared from equal amounts (15 ml) of carob flour, natron, sea salt, and salt from the East, but the method of application is not specified (CB VI.7). The second prescription recommended a mixture of equal amounts (15 ml) of carob, natron, honey, and part of the unknown *ima* tree. The ingredients were to be mixed and applied on the affected place (CB VI.8).

Chester Beatty VI.10—crushing ulcers, heat in the rectum, and urinary bladder

This case contains a prescription which was to relieve not only ulcers but also expel heat in the rectum, urinary bladder, and in the area called in Egyptian *sak-mesha*, apparently it was a part of the pubic area (perineum). It could have an accompanying inflammation of the skin in the area. The medicinal ointment contained 15 ml each of dried and aromatic myrrh, almonds, pine nuts, reed, sweet gum, *tjun* plant seeds, the *qeneny* plant, and part of a tree the name of which has not been preserved in the text, further of honey, fine fat, cedar oil, natron, red ocher, and incense. The solid ingredients were crushed into a fine power and mixed with the other ingredients. The ointment was applied on the affected place until the patient was relieved of the discomfort.

Chester Beatty VI.13a and b—strain of the rectum including ulcers on the urinary bladder, mucus in the joints, heat of the limbs, discharge, and pain

It is a complicated case compared in the heading with the activity of demons, which indicates that it was a disease with an unknown cause. The description of the symptoms is quite detailed and includes alleged ulcers on the urinary bladder, which physicians could assume to be on its mucous membrane based on frequent purulent or bloody urination. Symptoms further included mucus in the joints, excretion of water between the buttocks (which might indicate excessive sweating), a rectum burdened by unending discharge (perhaps repeating diarrhea), further painful urination, and hot, painful limbs. The heading states that it was a disease with which the physician could fight, which by analogy to the Smith Surgical Papyrus (see Strouhal et al. 2014) means that the result of the treatment was uncertain. It was most likely an infection of the large intestine or rectum, which affected a wider area. First, a mixture was to be prepared from 75 ml of goose fat, the same amount of honey, and three times the amount of human milk. This mixture was to be applied as an enema for a period of the next four days and could help cleanse the large intestine. Later another medicine was prepared, comprising 15 ml of sorghum juice, hemp juice, juice from the unknown plant *kebu*, fresh mash, lotus offshoots, acacia leaves, and goose fat. The mixture was again poured into the rectum for a period of four days. It apparently acted as an anti-inflammatory and astringent.

Bleeding from the Rectum

Several cases from the preserved texts seemingly concern bleeding from the rectum, but the precise interpretation of the texts is often difficult because it is not always possible to distinguish clearly whether the cases are discussing bleeding in the excretion of urine or a stool. For this reason, we mention some cases in connection with the rectum and in the section devoted to urination (pages 269–70) in the commentary for completeness.

Ebers 49—excretion of blood

The heading of this case indicates excessive bleeding during excretion, probably of urine (see the commentary on page 269). However, it is also possible that it could have been bleeding from the swollen veins of the rectum (hemorrhoids). A drink was recommended as the medicine and was prepared from 75 ml of beaten earth almonds and 2 ml of fresh mash with the same amount of both oil and honey, which the sick person was to drink for four days.

Hearst 18—amount of blood

This case is a parallel to Ebers 49, but its heading does not mention a connection of blood with the excretion. The rest of the cases are identical.

Berlin 165—excretion of blood

Another case contains a prescription for a medicine for a case when the patient excretes a large amount of blood. While the place that was bleeding is not directly mentioned in the text, the method of application of the medicinal mixture indicates that it was rather swollen rectal veins (hemorrhoids) than a discharge from the urethra. The medicine was prepared from 150 ml of sweet beer mixed with 37.5 ml of honey and 4 ml of fresh *Moringa* oil and was to be poured into the rectum repeatedly for four days. This medicine is very similar to the enema from case Berlin 164, which focuses on pain in the abdomen and constipation (see page 256).

London 37—halting blood

This incantation, which is written down in the London Papyrus, was related to bleeding according to the heading. The place of the application of the medicinal amulet indicates that it was seemingly bleeding from the rectum. The text of the incantation attempts to stop the escape of the blood and calls on the gods Horus, Seth, and also the god of wisdom Thoth. At the same time, the person is to create a magically functioning barrier from a carnelian bead, which was placed in the rectum. Because of its color, carnelian was connected with blood and, according to the conceptions then, was to cleanse the blood and relieve pain.

Other Affections in the Rectum and Vicinity

Another group of cases describes further various problems associated with the rectum or pubic region. We include here also prescriptions for the treatment of two unidentified diseases, the causes and manifestations of which are unknown. It could concern any kind of complaint, but because the mixtures intended for their treatment were poured into the rectum, they were probably associated with it.

Ebers 175–81—heat in the pubic region

As we have already stated above, inflammation in the area of the rectum sometimes also influenced the vicinity and could cause problems in the entire pubic region. It was undoubtedly a skin inflammation (dermatitis). Medical ointments applied on the affected area were intended to expel such heat. They could be prepared from equal amounts (15 ml) of sorghum, cooked wheat, wheat and barley flours, myrtle, and honey (Eb 175). Another prescription describes an ointment made from 15 ml of figs, cumin, flour from earth almonds, honey, and beer sediment (Eb 176); other times it was the same amount of earth almonds with myrtle, the unknown *niaia* plant, honey, and oil (Eb 178); or equal amounts (15 ml) of juniper berries, dates, squeezed dates, *ished* fruit, incense, and oil (Eb 177).

According to the text, the ointments were intended for male patients (but could have been effective also for women) and were prepared from an herbal decoction with 15 ml of linen seeds (Eb 179), from oil collected from the edge of a cup called *des* (Eb 180), or from a mixture of mud with a liquid called *mesta* in Egyptian (Eb 181). The last ingredient may seem to be magical, but mud containing tannins and mineral substances could act favorably on inflamed skin, like peat in our spas.

Hearst 88—pain of the pubic region

A case from the Hearst Papyrus might possibly be attributed to the same problem. It contains a prescription for pain in a person's pubic region. It was a solution of 75 ml of water in which 4 ml of sorghum and an eighth of that amount of gum were mixed. The mixture was left overnight to stand exposed to the dew and then was given to the patient; surprisingly not as an ointment on the skin of the genitals, but as a beverage every day. It is not clear whether the text could be related to the pains connected with excretion or evacuation.

Ebers 145–46—displacement in the rectum

If there is a displacement (Egyptian *wenekh*) of the rectum, a fibrous suppository had to be prepared for the patient. It was prepared from equal amounts (15 ml) of myrrh, yellow nutsedge from the garden, and nutsedge from the shore, celery, coriander, salt, incense, and oil (Eb 145). Other times, it was enough to place a mixture of goose yolk and an unknown part of the goose called *amem* into the rectum (Eb 146). According to some specialists, the Egyptian term *amem* might indicate the brain (see Hannig 1995, 141).

With great likelihood it was a herniation of either all of the layers of the anus *(prolapsus ani)* or of the mucous membrane of the anus (*prolapsus mucosae ani* or *rectal ectropium*); more rarely it was a prolapse of the entire rectum *(prolapsus ani et recti)* in a length of 10–15 cm. After removal of the influences that caused the prolapse, today the prolapsed part is surgically pressed in place (reponation), so that there is not inflammation and other complications.

Chester Beatty VI.9—turning of the rectum

The remedy, which was to correct a reversal of the rectum, was a mixture of a barley decoction, flour from beans, sea salt, honey, and goose fat. Just like in the previous group of cases Ebers 145–46, it was probably a dangerous prolapse of the rectum from the anus *(prolapsus ani et recti).* However, the texts lack any mention of the necessity of immediately returning it to its place (reposition) in order to avoid serious complications.

Berlin 167—the illness *qesnet*

The text suggests that this was an evil, thus serious, disease, but the symptoms are not specified. It is therefore difficult to judge what diagnosis it could have been. A medicinal mixture was prepared from 75 ml of human milk, the same amount of *Moringa* oil, 375 ml of oil, 300 ml of herbal decoction, and a little sea salt. It was applied as an enema repeatedly for a period of four days. It was a mixture with indisputable anti-inflammatory and lubricating effects.

Berlin 173—the illness *qesnet*

Other times also an enema could be applied in the same way, prepared from 75 ml of sweet beer, the same amount of the "milk fat of oil," 150 ml of carob juice, and 2 ml of sea salt.

Berlin 172—the illness *khayt*

For another painful disease called *khayt* in Egyptian, an enema was prepared from 75 ml of sweet beer, the same amount of human milk and common oil,

375 ml of the "milk fat of oil," 2 ml of fresh *Moringa* oil, the same amount of honey, and half that amount of sea salt. It was applied into the rectum for a period of four days.

Urinary Tract

We are not certain about the Egyptian word for kidneys (perhaps *geget*?), which are hidden behind peritoneum, the wall lining the abdominal cavity, so that they might have escaped the notice of the embalmers (Nunn 1996, 54). They also apparently did not arouse greater attention when animals were disemboweled. Their function—excretion of urine with the body's waste products, expressed by the terms *wesesh, wekha,* and *khau*—however, did not escape the interest of Egyptian physicians. Nonetheless, the problem in working with the medical texts is posed by the fact that the same word sometimes also labels the evacuation of the stool (defecation), from which it is necessary to distinguish disorders of urination (micturition) according to the context (see pages 260–61). It is surprising, however, that, given the interest of Egyptian physicians in the appearance of the surface of the stool, not the least mention appears in the papyri of the examination of the characteristics of the excreted urine. Here, we do not find references to the evaluation of its appearance, color, density, smell, and so on, which received great attention from physicians in later periods and other lands.

In contrast to that, attention in Egypt was devoted to the prevention of urinary difficulties using various medicinal remedies. Another, special urological part of the texts can be divided according to the names of the symptoms listed in the headings into slowing urination, the accumulation of urine, usually with pain of the pubic region, frequent or abundant urination, impenetrable escape of urine, or bloody urination.

Prevention of Urinary Difficulties

In terms of the prevention and general remediation of urination, it is very difficult to distinguish between these cases and those of the evacuation of stools. In the Ebers Papyrus, it can help that the cases are divided into two separate wholes connected thematically (Eb 27–29 and Eb 261–83). We find several other prescriptions relating to them in the Hearst Papyrus.

Ebers 27–29—correction of urination, facilitation of excretion

To ease urination, a mixture was recommended of 75 ml of goose fat cooked with 0.5 ml of a stone called "great protection" in Egyptian. The mixture was to be left to cool to body temperature and then consumed and washed down with wine. Other times, a mixture was prepared from arugula, which according to the text is similar to a bean from Crete and the *menuh* plant, called here also *sheny-ta*. Both were finely ground and mixed with honey. When consuming this medicine, it was washed down with 75 ml of sweet date beer (Eb 28). Another prescription recommends a mixture of equal amounts (2 ml) of pine nuts and honey, which were boiled together. They were administered cooled to body temperature and washed down with hot, diluted beer (Eb 29).

All three cases (Bardinet 1995, 255) or at least the second two (Westendorf 1999, 209–10) are sometimes included in the section on defecation, where in the first prescription it is to correct both methods of evacuation. The ingredients used in the prescriptions are not very indicative.

Ebers 263 and 266—correction of urination
Another remedy for a person whose urination is not proper included equal amounts (4 ml) of juniper berries, fresh dates, and the roots of bryony, half the amount of an inflorescence of reed, 37.5 ml of honey, and 300 ml of water. The mixture was put through a sieve and administered to the sick person for a period of four days (Eb 263). Other times to the 0.5 ml juniper berries were added the same amount of date seeds, half the amount of fresh dates and earth almonds, twice the amount of *shasha* fruit and goose fat, and 75 ml of honey. The mixture was left overnight to stand and collect the dew, then it was strained and given to the sick person to drink for a period of four days (Eb 266).

Ebers 269-72—correction of urination
Other prescriptions for correction of urination were apparently intended for men, because the relevant medicinal mixtures were to be applied to the glans penis. They comprised 15 ml of antiseptic myrtle crushed in an herbal decoction (Eb 269), 15 ml of *Juncus* (reed) straw, and the same amount of roasted beans, which were mixed in oil (Eb 270); or jujube wood crushed into the diluted drink *mesta* (Eb 272). These mixtures applied or smeared on the glans penis could influence urination rather magically or psychotherapeutically.

The last case in this group describes a medicinal mixture which was administered in the form of a beverage. It was made from equal amounts (15 ml) of fresh dates, pine nuts, the twigs of bryony, the leaves of a muskmelon, an herbal decoction, and water from a fishpond in the *hin* vessel. The mixture was strained and given to the sick person for four days (Eb 271).

Hearst 62—correction of urination, treatment of the urinary bladder
Another form of medicinal beverage for the urinary tract comprised 4 ml of

crushed earth almonds, half the amount of newly-forming dates, and part of the *Ricinus* called *hemu*, a quarter of the amount of pomace, an eighth of the amount of pine nuts, the leaves of a muskmelon and bryony, and 375 ml of foam (or perhaps of water for washing). The mixture was left overnight to stand and collect the dew and given as a drink for a period of four days. According to the text, it should have a rapid effect.

Hearst 67—correction of urine

This case also helped to correct urination, as its brief heading indicates. It was a beverage prepared from equal amounts (4 ml) of juniper berries, honey, and milk, and half that amount of *Cynodon*, which was mixed in 3 l of sweet beer. The ill person was to drink the strained liquid for four days. The large amount of liquids along with diuretic, antiseptic, and astringent characteristics of the herbs added could certainly have a favorable effect on the urinary tract.

Congestion or Retention of Urine

We have already encountered one case concerning the retention of urine in the section devoted to the treatment of children (see Strouhal et al. 2014, 201–203). Apparently, it was a medicine acting magically, when an old book (a papyrus scroll) cooked in oil was applied on the abdomen of a child suffering from retention of urine (Eb 262). Other than that case, we find other cases concerning congestion or accumulation of urine in other texts.

The interpretation of some of them is relatively problematic. The difficulties were expressed using the Egyptian terms *tjesau* (Eb 261) and *henau* (Eb 267), the translation of which is quite unclear. According to Nunn (1996, 92) they could indicate the passage of kidney stones (nephro- or urethrolithiasis) through the urethra or the dropping of blood clots into the urinary bladder (vesica urinaria, urocystitis), which could evoke renal colic with unbearable pain. It is, however, noteworthy that kidney stones have so far been found only rarely in Egyptian mummies (for instance Smith and Dawson 1924; Brothwell 1972; Sandison 1972, 218–219). Nevertheless, it could other times be congestion to complete stoppage of urine (anuria) caused by an inflammation of the urinary bladder (urocystitis). Complete stoppage of urine production (anuria) was incompatible with life.

Ebers 267-68—cumulation *(henau)* of urine

In the case of the congestion of urine, a medicine was prepared for the sick person from 15 ml of anise and the same amount of cow's skin, from which a cake called *pat* was baked.

Another medicine for the same condition was prepared from 150 ml of water, in which were mixed 4 ml of crushed wheat, 2 ml of flax seeds, the same amount of the *ihu* plant, honey, and goose fat, and a quarter of the amount of carob. After boiling, the mixture was strained and given to the sick person to drink for a period of four days. The ingredients contained in these mixtures undoubtedly had favorable effects for the body. For instance anise, carob, and linen seed support digestion.

Ebers 261—accumulation *(tjesau)* of urine, pain of the pubic region

If during the problems with the congestion of the urine, the ill person suffered pains of the entire pubic region, it was recommended to prepare a mixture of 4 ml of dates and cooked earth almonds and half the amount of wheat. The ingredients were to be ground and mixed with 3.6 l of water. The patient used the medicine for four days.

Ebers 265—heat in the urinary bladder, retention of urine

This prescription for the removal of heat in the urinary bladder with patients suffering the retention of urine recommends preparing a mixture of 75 ml of milk fat, equal amounts (15 ml) of *Moringa* oil, honey, and sweet beer, and a pinch of sea salt. This medicine was intended as an enema. Nunn explains this case as a combination of an inflammation of the urinary bladder and strictures of the urethra or enlargement (hypertrophy) of the prostate (Nunn 1996, 92). The activity of the enema was expected based on the anatomical vicinity of the urinary bladder, urethra, and rectum.

Hearst 69-70—heat in the urinary bladder

According to the Hearst Papyrus, the penetration of heat into the urinary tract or also moving in it was to be prevented by a mixture prepared from 300 ml of water, in which 37.5 ml of cooked wheat, the same amount of *ihu* fruit, and 2 ml of goose fat were mixed. It was to be left overnight to stand and collect the dew, then was strained and given to the sick person as a drink for a period of four days (H 69). The same disease could also be cured by a drink prepared from 1.8 l of water, in which were mixed 75 ml each of cooked wheat and barley flours, sorghum, and figs, further 4 ml of juniper berries, pine nuts, earth almonds, goose fat, and honey, and 0.25 ml of incense and cumin. The mixture was to be left overnight to stand and collect the dew, then apparently reduced to 300 ml and given to the sick person to drink for a period of four days (H 70).

Frequent or Abundant Urination

The opposite of the previous cases was too frequent urination, which happens with an inflammation of the urinary bladder (urocystitis), in men also with enlargement (hypertrophy) of the prostate or its cancer *(carcinoma prostatis).* Abundant urination is also characteristic of diabetes. Drawing a distinction between these two diagnoses in Egyptian medical texts is difficult, because the crucial word *asha* can express both frequent and abundant urination in Egyptian (Nunn 1996, 91).

Ebers 264—frequent urination

According to this case, frequent urination was to be alleviated by equal amounts (15 ml) of yellow nutsedge, pine nuts, and the roots of the *beheh* plant, which were crushed together and left to steep overnight in sweet beer. The sick person was to drink the mixture with the sediments.

Ebers 274-75 and 277-80—abundant urination

More prescriptions were available for the treatment of abundant urination. According to one, a medicinal mixture was prepared from 75 ml of water, into which were added 2 ml each of wheat semolina and *ished* fruit, and a quarter of the amount of ocher. It was left to stand and collect the dew overnight and after straining was used for four days (Eb 274). Another variation of this medicine was also complemented with gum and mixed in a double amount, thus in 150 ml of water (Eb 279).

Other times, wheat semolina was mixed with equal amounts of fresh mash and gum; the mixture was strained and given to the patient to drink again for four days (Eb 275). The same mixture could sometimes be complemented with a little ocher, honey, and 225 ml of water, and only then left to stand overnight (Eb 277).

According to another prescription, 2 ml of grapes were mixed with twice the amount of honey and the roots of *Cynodon,* a quarter of the amount of juniper berries, and 112.5 ml of sweet beer (Eb 278). This mixture was first to be boiled and strained, then used for four days. Another prescription recommended a simple mixture of 2 ml of gum and 0.5 ml of honey, which was mixed with 75 ml of water. The mixture was strained and drunk for one day (Eb 280).

Hearst 63-66—excessive urination

This group of cases from the Hearst Papyrus contains several direct parallels to the above-mentioned cases from the Ebers Papyrus. Some of these cases are copied here almost verbatim (H 66 = Eb 279), but other times we find in the text prescription slight differences in the list of ingredients, for instance honey is lacking (H 63 = Eb 277), or in the instructions for the preparation and administration: sometimes the mixture was also to be boiled (H 65 = Eb 280) or the medicine was to be given only for one day instead of four (H 64 = Eb 278).

Imperceptible Leakage of Urine

Attention has already been devoted to the problem with incontinence in the section on the treatment of children (Strouhal et al. 2014, 201–203). Particularly, a powder from cooked faïence belongs here, which was given to older children to swallow, to young children in milk for four days (Eb 273). However, other times we also find in medical texts cases of the escape of urine that concerned adult patients. This disorder occurs in the irritation or inflammation of the urinary bladder, in men when the prostate is enlarged or is cancerous, in older women with the weakening of the urethral sphincters, and in children with bedwetting.

Ebers 276 and 281—leakage of urine

A mixture was prepared against the leakage of urine from equal amounts (15 ml) of pine nuts and yellow nutsedge, which were mixed in 480 ml of beer. The mixture was boiled, strained, and given to the sick person as a medicinal beverage. This case is written down twice in the Ebers Papyrus, entirely verbatim. The versions differ only in the recommended length of the use of the medicine, which could be one (Eb 481) or four (Eb 476) days.

Ebers 282—holding urine

For this problem, a drink was also prescribed prepared from 4 ml mountain celery, half the amount of Lower Egyptian celery and a fresh mash, and a quarter of the amount of juniper berries, the *ibu* plant from Upper Egypt, the *ibu* plant from Lower Egypt, the unknown plants *wam* and *duat*, 300 ml of water, and a stone called *peshnet* in Egyptian. The mixture was left to stand and collect the dew overnight and was then strained and used for four days.

Hearst 68—holding urine

We find a case similar to the previous one among the prescriptions in the Hearst Papyrus, but the wording of the text in the original is not entirely identical. The amount of the mountain celery is written here as 1/2 a measure, but it is undoubtedly a scribal error. The other ingredients and the method of preparation are exactly the same.

Painful Urination

Ebers 283—pain of the pubic region, correction of urination

At the first appearance of pain when urinating, a drink was prescribed made from 15 ml of pine nuts, the same amount of yellow nutsedge, fresh dates, the *khesau* part f the sycomore tree, the roots of the *Ricinus* and bryony, honey, baker's yeast, incense, and ocher, which was mixed in a mash. The mixture was to be heated at sunset in a vessel called a *tjab*, strained, and drunk. According to the text, this medicinal mixture was to be fast acting.

Berlin 166 and 171—pain during urination

A solution could be prepared against painful urination from 375 ml of an herbal decoction, in which 4 ml of *Moringa* oil and a quarter of the amount of salt were mixed. It was applied as an enema for a period of four days. This mixture acted osmotically and as an anti-inflammatory (Bln 166). A similar enema given for the same length of time was prepared from 300 ml of an herbal decoction, 4 ml of fresh *Moringa* oil, and a quarter of the amount of salt, to which half the amount of honey and the "milk fat of oil" was added (Bln 171).

Blood in the Urine

As we have already described, it is often hard to distinguish in medical texts when it is speaking about excreting urine and when stool (feces), because the Egyptian word *wesekh* means not only the excretion of urine, but also the excretion of the intestinal content. For this reason, some authors interpret these cases as blood in the urine (hematuria) (Ziskind 2009, 660), whereas others as bleeding from the rectum. The interpretation, however, is not clear, and some cases presented in the section on bleeding from the rectum (pages 260–61) could be discussed also here, for instance the prescription for stopping the excretion of blood in case Berlin 165 or the incantation in case London 37. While the medicinal mixtures presented above were applied to the rectum, other prescriptions described the preparation of medicinal beverages, which could be beneficial for the urinary tract.

Ebers 49 = Hearst 18—excretion of excessive blood

When the ill person passed blood (apparently in the urine), a mixture to help was made of 75 ml of beaten earth almonds and 2 ml of fresh mash, and the same amount of honey and oil. The mixture was strained and given to the patient to drink for a period of four days. According to the text, "any other remedy is less effective." The same text was written down in the Ebers and also in the Hearst Papyrus, only the formulation of the headings differs slightly. It could be hematuria or a manifestation of a severe inflammation of the urinary bladder. According to another interpretation, the problems described could refer to bleeding from expanded veins of the rectum (see pages 260–61).

Berlin 187–88—painful substances, excretion of blood

If the pain was accompanied moreover by the excretion of blood, a medicine was recommended that was prepared from 75 ml of goose fat, the same amount of the part of the date called *henen,* and 150 ml of sweet beer. The medicine was to be left overnight to stand and collect the dew and was administered for a period of four days, not into the rectum but as a beverage to drink (Bln 187). Another remedy contained 225 ml of sweet beer and 37.5 ml wormwood, 0.5 ml each of coriander and honey, and a double amount of the unknown *aru* tree seeds or perhaps juniper berries (Westendorf 1999, 335). It was also given as a medicinal beverage, after being left overnight to collect the dew and being strained through a cloth (Bln 188). Although neither of the cases describes the disease in detail, it could be painful, inflamed, and bleeding hemorrhoids. However, it is not possible to exclude bleeding in another place, such as after an injury.

Uncertain Diseases of the Urinary Tracts

In some cases, we encounter the Egyptian names of the diseases in the medical texts, the meaning of which remains unknown to us. The reason is that the cases do not describe the symptoms of the diseases in any way or the possible causes, and the prescriptions for the medicinal mixtures also do not indicate the nature of the illness. It is thus impossible to judge the diseases from the perspective of medicine today and compare them with modern diagnoses. We include in this group also the cases that refer to the secretion of mucuses.

Ebers 705–707—the disease *shepen*

For the unknown disease *shepen* the Ebers Papyrus recommends three different medicines. The first was prepared from 150 ml of an herbal decoction, to which were added 4 ml each of sea salt and incense, which could, however, be left out. This mixture was to be applied to the rectum of the sick person (Eb 705). The same administration was also used for a medicine prepared from 37.5 ml of carob, 75 ml of oil, and the same amount of urine (Eb 706), or the somewhat more complicated medicine prepared from 225 ml of an herbal decoction, 37.5 ml of *Moringa* oil, 2 ml of honey, and half the amount of galenite and copper grains, which undoubtedly must have been ground first (Eb 707). The last-mentioned medicine according to the text of the case could have been used also for curing pain, which was caused by painful substances *(wekhedu)* according to the conceptions of the time.

Berlin 183-84—the disease *shepen* in urine

The Berlin Papyrus recommended against this disease a simple enema and also a medicinal beverage. The former was prepared from 75 ml of wine and 0.5 ml each of sea salt and copper grains. The mixture was to be applied in the rectum for a period of four days (Bln 183).

A substantially more complicated issue was the preparation of the medicinal beverage, which immediately follows but is not explicitly connected with urinary problems. In the introduction, the necessary ingredients are named, which included 2.175 l of water, 75 ml wheat semolina, and equal amounts (2 ml) of oil and honey, then a description of the preparation follows as in modern cooking recipes. First, water was put on to boil. When it started to boil, it was mixed with semolina and the mixture was again brought to a boil. Then, oil was added. Only when this mixture had been reduced by boiling to 450 ml was honey added. The medicine was to be left overnight to stand and collect the dew before the ill person could drink it (Bln 184).

Chester Beatty VI.11-12—the disease *shenfet,* any kind of disease in the rectum

The Chester Beatty Papyrus offered a more generally useable prescription for problems in the area of the urinary tract and also the rectum. It was an enema from equal amounts (15 ml) of sesame and common oils, honey, human milk, and sea salt, which was applied to the rectum for four days (CB VI.11). According to the text, a bandage filled with a medicinal ointment from equal amounts (15 ml) of myrrh, cumin, goose fat, honey, and incense was placed after this enema, that is, it was applied repeatedly, until the sick person was entirely recovered (CB VI.12). The application of some medicines for urinary problems in the rectum came from knowledge of the anatomical and physiological proximity of the end of the digestive tract and the urinary tract, the direct influence of which was not accessible to the physician.

Berlin 143-47—driving away mucuses during urination

This group is presented with one common heading, which mentions mucuses during urination (or less likely during defecation). We will devote ourselves to mucuses in more detail on pages 272–77, but it seems more appropriate to present it along with other problems connected with urination.

A mixture could be drunk for one day that was prepared from 75 ml of sweet beer, in which 2 ml of *sheny-ta* seeds was mixed (Bln 143). Another prescription recommends a mixture of 75 ml of wine with 2 ml of honey and the same amount of *sheny-ta* seeds (Bln 147). Other times, a mixture was to be used during the day made from 4 ml of honey with 2 ml of *sheny-ta* seeds (Bln 144), possibly supplemented with 75 ml of milk (Bln 145).

A medicine was intended as food for one day made from 2 ml of carob flour, the same amount of honey, and *sheny-ta* seeds, to which were added 0.5 ml of the *aam* plant, which is unknown to us (Bln 146).

The ingredient *sheny-ta*, which plays a central role in this group of medicinal mixtures, is not known to us, so it is hard to judge the possible effectiveness of these medicines and their influence on the health.

Mucuses and Worms
The Supposed Origin of Mucus
Mucuses (slimes) and mucus-like substances played an unexpectedly important role in the conceptions of Egyptian physicians, as is shown by the number of prescriptions in which they are cited. They are labelled by the term *setet*, derived from the expression "to flow, to pour" and complemented by the determinative for a liquid (Stephan 2001, 130). Mucous substances could move through the entire body thanks to the network of blood vessels *(metu)*. Besides the pelvic area, where they were said to accummulate, they are alternately reported also in other parts of the body. They cannot be confused with the lymph, the fluid of the network of lymphatic vessels, which was only discovered by modern anatomy.

The origin of mucous substances was sought in a disorder of digestion (dyspepsia) or in the emptying of the gastric content and its subsequent putrefaction, supposedly connected with bad breath from the mouth (Stephan 2001, 133 and 135). In the pelvis, they transformed into worms, which is a peculiar ancient Egyptian hypothesis.

In the Ebers Papyrus, we find a reference to a special "Collection of remedies for leaving of mucuses from the pelvic area," assuming their origin and function in the human organism and gradual transformation into worms.

Ebers 192 = Ebers 195—disease of the stomach, vomiting, inflamed eyes, runny nose
A case repeats twice in the Ebers Papyrus of a sick person suffering from nausea and a cold. It would be possible to discuss them in the part devoted to a runny nose (pages 204–10) or nausea of the stomach (pages 211–23), but it rather fits in the section on the origin of mucuses. Both cases are copied almost verbatim, only with slight deviations in the writing, even in the same

part of the text as if the author of the text had forgotten that he had already copied the case once. The text is more detailed than other cases because it contains a description of the symptoms, determination of the diagnosis, and the method of the treatment including the prescription for the medicinal mixture. It is a case in which, according to the text, the patient frequently vomits and at the same time has inflamed eyes ("bloodshot," that is, conjunctivitis or blepharitis) and his nose is running (rhinitis). The physician considered the symptoms presented to be a manifestation of the release of mucuses, which for an unknown reason could not draw down into the pelvis, or be excreted in the natural way. According to Nunn, the mucuses in this case indicate pus (Nunn 1996, 88).

For the sick person a *shenes* wheat flat cake should be prepared, to which were added a large amount of anti-inflammatory wormwood, a *debeh* measure of onion, which is a natural antibiotic, and fatty beef meat. The sick person was to wash this food down with offering beer, until the cold in the form of mucuses withdrew and his eyes opened again. It could be a complication of a cold, perhaps even an acute inflammation of the upper respiratory tract (see pages 204–10).

Ebers 102 = Ebers 296—mucuses, sharp pain, stiff abdomen, pain of the stomach

This case is written down in two places in the papyrus, almost verbatim. The two copies differ only in small details. It shows the clinical conception then on the origin of mucuses and worms in the body of the sick person. The case describes a patient who suffered from mucuses and sharp pain, which led to a stiffness of the abdomen and pain in the area of the stomach. According to the text, the problems are caused by mucuses which cannot leave the body and therefore putrefy and change into worms. When that happens, the sick person throws up and is relieved. In the opposite case, the physician is to prepare a purgative remedy.

In this context, it is interesting that the increased production of mucuses from irritated mucous membranes of the respiratory and digestive tracts is also presented on the clay tablets of Mesopotamian medicine indicating a runny nose and cough (Haussperger 2012, 114–15) or an inflammation of the stomach (Haussperger 2012, 32–33, 204, 270, and 272). A frequent formulation of its presence went: "The inside is full of mucuses (slimes)." The treatments were rational and diagnostically took into account *colitis mucosa*, possibly mucoviscidosis (Haussperger 2012, 275). On the other hand, we do not find any mention of the production of worms in connection with mucuses.

Treatment of the Excessive Creation of Mucuses

Ebers 294—mucuses in the pelvic area

The sovereign medicine against the production of mucuses was the creeping plant *sem*, which is apparently bindweed (Germer 2008, 233–34, presents the transcription *sn-wtt*). The text moreover describes it as a plant growing "on its stomach," or a creeping plant, the flower of which is similar to the lotus and the flowers of white wood. This detailed description indicates that the plant *sem* was not used often and it was necessary to seek it out and bring it for this purpose. It was necessary to smear the pelvic area of the sick person with this plant and add its fruits to his food. The mucuses should quickly withdraw with such a method. Bindweed works as a natural laxative (see also Manniche 1989, 109), but its effect remains a question in external use.

Hearst 35—mucuses in the pelvic area

In the Hearst Papyrus, we find a parallel to the previous case Ebers 294, which differs slightly in the wording of the heading. We also find minor difference further in the text, when the title of the lotus or the expression labeling the leaf is written down incorrectly. The last sentence, referring to the fruits of the medicinal plant, is also left out here.

Ebers 297 and 300—mucuses in the abdomen

These cases were also related to the presence of mucuses in the abdomen of the ill person, but only contain the recipe for the preparation of the medicinal mixture. The symptoms of the sick person are not specified. The medicinal beverage was prepared from equal amounts (2 ml) of figs, *ished* fruit, and arugula, half that amount of raisins, a quarter of the amount of acacia leaves and the unknown *niaia* plant, and a little cumin and red ocher. The ingredients were to be mixed in sweet beer and left overnight to stand and collect the dew. The medicine was used for a period of four days (Eb 297). A similar prescription recommends mixing 2 ml each of figs, *ished* fruit, *sheny-ta* seeds, and honey, half the amount of raisins, and a little cumin and incense in 375 ml of sweet beer. The mixture was to be strained and then given to the sick person to drink (Eb 300).

Berlin 136-37—mucuses in the abdomen and any limb

If according to the ancient Egyptian physician there were mucuses in the abdomen or anywhere else in the body, he made a preparation against it from the equal amounts (2 ml) of figs, arugula, and sweet beer, half that amount of raisins, a quarter of the amount of the *niaia* plant, and a little acacia leaves and red ocher. It is a not quite identical parallel of the above-mentioned prescriptions from the Ebers papyrus. The mixture was to be left overnight to stand and collect the dew and then used for a period of four days (Bln 136). Another remedy for the same problem could be made simply from a barley drink, which was reduced to the amount of 450 ml. No other details of the preparation are presented in the text (Bln 137).

Berlin 48—mucuses in both sides
This case describes a two-phase approach against mucuses in the sides. First, the sick person had to use water boiled with carob (that is, a water solution of carob) for four days, for another four days he drank a boiled mixture of 375 ml of sweet beer in which were mixed 2 ml each of fermented herbal decoction and *pesedj* and *shasha* fruits, an unknown amount of wormwood, and a pinch of cumin.

Berlin 138—mucuses in the meat (muscles)
For all of the mucuses that wander around the body, it was necessary to prepare a medicine from 75 ml of crushed barley, half the amount of podded carob, further 0.5 ml of carob, pine nuts, wormwood, juniper berries, the *aam* plant, and resinous gum. The ingredients were to be mixed in 30 ml of water. According to some authors, it is a scribal error, because this amount seems quite nonstandard today (see also Westendorf 1999, 345, who states that it was to be 7.68 l of water). However, we cannot rule out that the ingredients were first mixed in a little binding agent and only then poured into a larger amount of water, because the mixture was to be left overnight to stand and collect the dew. Then early in the morning 2.4 l of water was added and it was put to boil and reduced. Another 5.28 l was gradually added and the mixture was again boiled and reduced. After being removed from a boil, it was strained through a cloth and administered as a medicinal drink for a period of four days. The large volume of liquid can indicate that the medicine was to properly hydrate the patient, thus the case could be related to a fever.

Berlin 139—mucuses and pain in any limb in the summer or winter
Another remedy was intended explicitly for the time of summer and winter. Sweet beer was to be mixed with crushed incense and fallow deer horn, and this ointment was to be smeared on the sides of the sick person. The prescription does not state the amount of the ingredients, but its nature indicates that the medicine could act rather by power of suggestion.

Berlin 140-41—mucuses and pain in any limb in the winter

An ointment intended only for the winter period was made from 75 ml of jujube bread and *ished* fruit and the same amount of oil and honey (Bln 140). Other times a similar mixture was prepared from 75 ml of jujube leaves, myrtle leaves, and cedar sawdust, half the amount of beef fat, and 4 ml of mash (Bln 141). Both ointments were placed on the affected area.

Ebers 295—mucuses in the throat, pain of the head and throat, stiffness of the neck

This case describes a wide range of symptoms which were related to pain and stiffness of the neck and pain of the head and were attributed to the presence of mucuses in the throat of the sick person. These problems could be treated by smearing the neck and head with aromatic ointments and beautifying with makeup. It might have essentially been a massage of the neck and back, which could relieve a person. According to Westendorf's translation, it was mucuses, pain, and stiffness of the neck, which could indicate a cold (Westendorf 1999, 602).

Ebers 298-99—runny nose in the head, mucuses in the throat

Two prescriptions state the medicinal means to help against a runny nose and mucuses that had settled in the throat (see also Westendorf 1999, 602). A mixture was made of 15 ml each of laudanum (an extract from immature poppy heads), balsam, incense, galenite, ocher, juniper twigs, and ibex fat. The ingredients were carefully ground and thoroughly mixed into the form of an ointment. This was smeared on the head of the sick person (Eb 298). Another prescription recommended equal amounts of *Potentilla*, cumin, juniper berries, myrrh, cedar resin, ibex fat, laudanum, and the stone *mehdet*. The ingredients were mixed, and the mixture was left to stand and collect the dew overnight. It was then strained and given to the sick person to drink (Eb 299).

Ebers 303-304—prevention of an inflammation

Two prescriptions that were intended for protection from an inflammation are curious in that both state the word inflammation rather than mucus (which could be caused by the inflammation) and prescribed similar, unusual animal ingredients. The first case recommends an ointment from frog boiled to mush in oil (Eb 303), whereas the second prescription, a compress, recommends the head of the *djedeb* fish boiled to mush in oil (Eb 304). Both were intended for spreading or placement using a compress. They were clearly medicines that acted magically.

Berlin 142—mucuses in the lower part of the breast

According to the heading, it is a case when mucuses accumulated in the lower part of the breast, whether the left or right. None of the other details or manifestations are specified. It is thus only possible to guess what the problems were related to, perhaps breastfeeding (see also Strouhal et al. 2014, 191–94), or an entirely unconnected disease. For the treatment, it recommends a compress of myrtle and mash. Because of its disinfection effects, myrtle is recommended for compresses today, for instance for the treatment of acne.

Parasitic Worms

Egyptian physicians were convinced that worms originate directly in the human body from the accumulation of mucuses. They understandably could not have any idea of the cycle of some parasitic worms from animals through possible interhosts to humans. Proctologists of that time, however, must have noticed that sometimes on the surface of their patient's stool something small and white was twisting (such as a roundworm) or shining (such as the released members of a tapeworm). Their frequent appearance and possible distinction then is clear already from the fact that medical papyri present a wide range of names for worms. Besides the general label of *pened* we often find also the name *hefat* and others such as *hesbet, betju, sa, sepy, shepet, fenet,* and *fenetj*. Unfortunately, we do not have any evidence in the texts for the identification of these individual names with the known types of worms today, with the exception of the tapeworm *(hefat)*.

The frequency of the cases related to worms in the preserved medical texts indicates that the infestation of worms was a truly common problem. In the Ebers Papyrus alone, we find more than thirty prescriptions for the expulsion of worms from the body! We distinguish between the commentaries on these cases according to the presented names of the types of worms in the following treatises. A number of plant means, the effectiveness of which is proven today, were used for the treatment of parasitic illnesses. The medications for the expulsion of parasitic worms (anthelmintic) are often water drinks, which were to be left overnight exposed to the dew, strained, and then drunk for one or four days. If is the medication was a dry mixture, it was necessary to eat it.

Ebers 62–63—remedy for the abdomen

These cases present medicinal means that were to benefit the abdomen if a person suffers as a consequence of worms which were impossible to expel otherwise. The first mixture was prepared from 15 ml of reed and the same amount of *Anacyclus*, which were finely ground and cooked with honey and

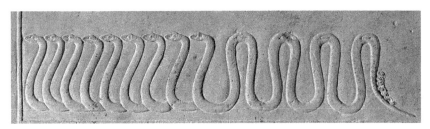

Fig. 29. Whereas snakes formed the model of many hieroglyphic signs and the outward appearance of Egyptian demons, worms and other parasites do not occur in depictions, even though the ancient Egyptians undoubtedly often encountered these in their lives. Wormwood in the medicinal mixtures could refer to their presence in the sick person (Twenty-seventh Dynasty, tomb of Iufaa in Abusir, photo © Archive of the Czech Institute of Egyptology, Faculty of Arts, Charles University, Martin Frouz)

given to the sick person to eat (Eb 62). A second remedy was made from the roots of the pomegranate tree, which was mixed in 75 ml of beer; the mixture was then joined with 225 ml of water and left overnight to stand and collect the dew. Early in the morning of the next day, it had to be strained and given to the patient to drink (Eb 63). *Anacyclus* is beneficial for digestion, and the bitter root or bark of the pomegranate tree is very effective against parasites.

Worms *(hefat)*

The term *hefat* in medical texts is mainly considered to be a label for the tapeworm (Erman and Grapow 1926–61, III: 72–73; Westendorf 1999, 197; Bardinet 1995, 161–162), which we also adopt, although we cannot exclude that it could be another species of internal parasite, for example the roundworm (see Hannig 1995, 525; Halioua 2004, 134).

Ebers 50-60—driving away of a tapeworm

The Ebers Papyrus includes an extensive group of cases with prescriptions for the preparation of medicines that were to work on the expulsion of a tapeworm from the abdomen of a person. The majority of them comprised a few ingredients and were administered exclusively orally in the form of a beverage or a meal.

It was possible to mix 150 ml of water with half the amount of the root of the pomegranate tree; the mixture was left overnight to stand and collect the dew and was strained. It was used for one day (Eb 50). A mixture with the same method of preparation and period of administration contained 150 ml of water, half the amount of Upper Egyptian barley, and a quarter of the amount sea salt (Eb 51), or 150 ml of water with half the amount of acacia leaves (Eb

52). Another possibility was to mix 225 ml of water with 75 ml of date purée and the same amount of the *Avicennia* tree fruit (Eb 54). Other times, the fruits of this tree were left to ripen for four days, they were exposed to the dew overnight, and then they were used for the production of another mixture, the description of which has unfortunately not been preserved in the text (Eb 57).

Other mixtures included 375 ml of sweet beer, into which carob and date seeds were added in equal amounts (2 ml). The mixture was to be boiled and strained before being drunk (Eb 55). Then 75 ml of chaste tree and the same amount of *Potamogeton* leaves, both properly ground, were mixed with 300 ml of sweet beer. The mixture was given directly after being strained (Eb 56).

Other medicines were given for four days. One mixture was prepared simply by boiling 75 ml of water with 0.5 ml of malachite and earth almonds (Eb 58). Another remedy was prepared by mixing 150 ml of water, possibly of beer, with 75 ml of the *wam* plant and left to stand overnight (Eb 60). Other times the same amount of the *wam* plant and *shenfet* were mixed with half the amount of the part of *Avicennia* called *kher* and honey. The ingredients were thoroughly ground and left overnight in honey, then in the early morning they were mixed with 75 ml of beer and given to the sick person to drink, where the period of administration is not specified (Eb 59).

One case describes the production of a medicine in the form of a flat cake. Pieces of malachite were baked into four flat cakes called *feka*. The sick person was to eat the flat cake (Eb 53).

Ebers 61—driving away of a tapeworm
This case contains a prescription for the preparation of a medicine and a magical spell that was to support its efficacy. The medicine was prepared from 75 ml of reed and 4 ml of *Anacyclus*, which were cooked in honey and given to the sick person to eat. They are the same ingredients as in case Ebers 62, but in a different amount (see above, page 277). During the administration of the medicine, it was recommended to deliver the incantation, which attributes the presence of the tapeworm to the work of an unfriendly god and curses it so that the sick person is rid of it.

Ebers 64-65 and 68—removal and expulsion of a tapeworm
Other means against tapeworms could be prepared from equal amounts (15 ml) of wormwood, the unknown *aba* plant, and natron. The ingredients were mixed and given to the sick person to eat (Eb 64). Other times, 15 ml of dates were mixed with the same amount of dried sycamore fruits that were thoroughly mashed and mixed with a thick beer, which the sick person drank (Eb 65).

A medicinal mixture from acacia leaves required a more complex preparation. They were first to be soaked in water in the vessel called *niu*, covered with a cloth and left to stand overnight. In the early morning, the mixture was to be pounded in a mortar and given to the sick person to drink. According to the text, the nose of the sick person was to be smeared with reed until he drinks it all (Eb 68).

Ebers 70-71—driving away of a tapeworm
Another remedy which worked against tapeworm comprised 2 ml of honey, the same amount of *wam* fruit, half the amount of *shenfet* fruit, and a quarter of the amount of sea salt, which was mixed and eaten for one day (Eb 70). Other times the dried bark of the fig tree and also fresh dates in equal amounts (15 ml) were crumbled into beer. This medicine was used for four days (Eb 71).

Berlin 1-4—tapeworm
The headings of this group of cases have not been preserved but it was most likely the treatment of tapeworm, because we find here two parallels to the already described cases from the Ebers Papyrus. The wordings of the cases differ slightly, but the ingredients and their amounts are the same. It was a mixture which included 375 ml of sweet beer, into which 2 ml each of carob flour and date seeds were added and the mixture was boiled and drunk (Bln 2). Another was a medicine from the same amount of *wam* and *shenfet* fruits, with half the amount of the part of *Avicennia* called *kher* and honey, and 75 ml of beer (Bln 4). Both mixtures were left to sit in honey overnight and administered for one day. These two prescriptions are not entirely verbatim parallels of cases Ebers 55 and 59. Other times the sick person was given sweet beer to drink, in which unspecified amounts of ground *Anacyclus* and the unknown *aam* plant were mixed (Bln 3).

The text of the first case is almost entirely destroyed; only a mention has been preserved that the parasite or its part comes out through the rectum (Bln 1).

Berlin 5-12—extermination of a tapeworm
According to another case, 75 ml of strong beer called *djesret* in Egyptian was mixed with the *kher* part of the *bekheb* tree, and the mixture was cooked and strained before the sick person drank it (Bln 5). Other times, it was mixed with an unspecified amount of the root of the pomegranate tree with the *kher* part of *Avicennia* and the *tjehu* part of the *Moringa*, which was crushed early in the morning in a mortar and mixed with water. The sick person was to drink this medicine on an empty stomach (Bln 6). Another prescription recommended

preparing a mixture of honey, wine, and fresh incense, which was used for one day (Bln 7). The other prescriptions in this group have been only partially preserved. Of two, almost nothing has been preserved (Bln 11–12), whereas in the other we find references to the root of the pomegranate tree (Bln 10) and *wam* fruit, which was to be mixed either with cumin and given early in the morning (Bln 8), or with a fermented herbal decoction (Bln 9).

Louvre E.4864—extermination of a tapeworm
Another prescription for the extermination of a tapeworm, which has been preserved only partially, recommends mixing sea salt and natron with bitter almonds (?). The rest of the text has been destroyed.

Ramesseum III.A, I. 28–29—extermination of a tapeworm
A case for the extermination of a tapeworm can also be found in the Ramesseum Papyrus, but its text is almost destroyed. Only the mention of some extremity of a person has been preserved.

The *pened* worm
The word *pened* could indicate in Egyptian a certain type of internal parasite, but its precise determination is not possible today (Erman and Grapow 1926–61, I: 511). Some specialists consider it to be the tapeworm (Hannig 1995, 278; Halioua 2004, 134), but it is not possible to verify this finding. It is clear from the cases in the medical texts that this worm caused a disease in the abdomen. It appears among the prescriptions in the Ebers Papyrus, whereas we do not encounter it in the other texts.

Ebers 66—illness from the tapeworm or the *pened* worm
In this case, a universal remedy was intended for the treatment of the disease, which is attributed to either of the two mentioned types of parasites. It was prepared from 15 ml of goose fat, the same amount of flour from ground *pesedj* fruit, and the best *amau* fruit, and after being strained was to be used as a drink for four days.

Ebers 67 and 69—illness from the *pened* worm
Against the disease which this internal parasite caused, a mixture was prepared from equal amounts (15 ml) of acacia leaves, *Melilotus*, wild rue, and offshoots of the *niaia* plant, which were mixed and applied on the abdomen of a person. Acacia and *Melilotus* could act as astringents and favorably affect digestion (Eb 67).

Another remedy was applied internally. The prescription describes a mixture of equal amounts (15 ml) of thyme, the *ineb* plant, and the *tjeset* part of *Juncus* (reed), which were mixed in honey. The sick person was to use the mixture for a period of four days (Eb 69).

Ebers 72–81—expulsion of the *pened* worm

The remedies by which the sick person was to get rid of the parasite named *pened* were relatively numerous. Their efficacy is difficult to judge because we do not know a large number of the ingredients. According to the first case in the group, it was possible to mix 75 ml of strong beer with the same amount of the *kher* part of *Avicennia*. The mixture was to be boiled, strained, and given to the sick person to drink (Eb 72). Other times equal amounts (15 ml) of strong beer, cumin, *Potentilla*, wild rue, the *tiam* plant, and *amau* and *ished* fruits were mixed with an unspecified amount of sweet beer. The mixture was to be boiled and given for a period of one day (Eb 79).

Another medicinal beverage was prepared from equal amounts (15 ml) of the *qesentet* plant, starch, red ocher, bitumen, and soft bread, which were ground and mixed in sweet beer. After it was strained, the patient was to use it for one day (Eb 76).

It was also recommended to drink a beverage from 75 ml of wine mixed with 2 ml of the thorny bush *bages* seeds and 75 ml of the *amau* fruit for a period of four days. Before use, this drink was to be heated (Eb 78). Other times, into wine were mixed 15 ml of carob tree fruit, the same amount of *sheny-ta* seeds, honey, and milk. The mixture was cooked and strained; it was also used for four days. According to the notes in the conclusion of the text, this medicinal beverage was to empty the abdomen (Eb 80).

Other times 4 ml of the ground *wam* fruit and an eighth of the amount of *shenfet* fruit were mixed in 75 ml of sweet beer. This medicinal beverage was used for one day (Eb 74). Another similar remedy was administered in the form of a pill, which was shaped from a thick mixture prepared from 37.5 ml of sweet beer, 2 ml of honey, the same amount of *wam* fruit, a quarter of the amount of *shenfet* fruit, and sea salt. This amount was enough for four pills, which the sick person was apparently to use for four days and wash down with the same amount of sweet beer (Eb 73).

A medicine was given in the form of a *feka* cake for one day. It contained 15 ml each of cedar oil, fat, bull bile, natron, and *sheny-ta* seeds (Eb 75). Other times the flat *feka* cake was prepared in a simpler form from 15 ml of cedar oil, the same amount of red natron, and *sheny-ta* seeds (Eb 78).

A curious remedy required the heart of the *mesha* bird mixed with *sheny-ta* seeds, thyme, honey, wine, and sweet beer in the same quantity of 15 ml. The prepared *feka* cakes from this mixture were used for one day (Eb 81).

Ebers 82–85—treating the *pened* worm

Another group of cases associated with the parasite called *pened* recommends other simpler and more complicated natural medicines. According to one prescription, 75 ml of juniper berries were mixed with the same amount of white oil, and this mixture was to be drunk for a period of one day (Eb 85). Other times, the medicine was prepared by mixing 37.5 ml of fermented herbal decoction and 375 ml of sweet beer with 2 ml of carob, the same amount of white oil, and 0.23 ml of red ocher. The mixture was first to be boiled and then drunk (Eb 84). A medicinal mixture from equal amounts (15 ml) of *niaia* and *nua* plants, *amau* fruit, and the *kemu* stone contained only ingredients unknown to us. A liquid was apparently also added, because after cooking, the mixture was to be strained and used as a drink for one day (Eb 82).

For a period of four days, it was recommended to drink a medicinal beverage prepared from 2 ml of wormwood, half that amount of date seeds and yellow nutsedge, 0.45 ml of *shenfet* fruit, and half the amount of cumin, *amau* fruit, and the great protection stone, 37.5 ml of bindweed, and 300 ml of sweet beer. The mixture was to be first cooked and then strained before use (Eb 83).

A great number of as-yet untranslated ingredients in these prescriptions reduce their testimonial value and do not allow judgment of their efficacy.

Other Worms and Evidence in Mummies

Other species of internal parasites can be determined only with difficulty based on the preserved texts. However, we encounter in the presented cases a wide range of other Egyptian terms indicating various types of worms.

Hearst 196—the *fenet* worm in fingers or toes

The Hearst Papyrus presents a prescription intended to remove the *fenet* worm from the fingers or toes. A mixture served for that was made from an unspecified amount of carob, the *henayt* stone, and red ocher. It is not clear whether the label *fenet* refers to a type of parasite or whether it can be the label of certain formations on the fingers of a person reminiscent of worms. If it was a parasite, we can put this case in the context of the cyst of the guinea worm (*Dracunculus medinensis*), which according to Miller (1989, 251–52) was likely hidden behind the description of the "tumor of tumors" (Eb 875, discussed already in Strouhal et al. 2014, 78).

Other than the text evidence in medical papyri, it is sometimes possible to identify the presence of parasitic worms in the microscopic examination of the tissues of ancient Egyptian mummies. The autopsies of the mummies conducted in the last decades using modern laboratory techniques have shown in almost every one of them the presence of one or more species of parasitic worms transmitted from person to person or animal, sometimes through an interhost. It shows that parasitical diseases were common in ancient Egypt. It was connected to the poor hygienic conditions in villagers' dwellings and the presence of parasites in the interhosts in the water.

The guinea worm was found in the mummy of a 13-year-old boy from the Ptolemaic or Roman Period (Manchester Museum Mummy Project No. 1770; dating after Tapp 1979a, 83). A dense knot containing calcified twisted microfilaria was formed in his front abdominal wall. The females of this parasite prefer to settle in the lower extremities, where they lay their eggs and form blisters from which ulcers form. They clog the lymphatic vessels, through which swellings emerge distally from the obstruction of the swelling, often reaching monstrous dimensions. The boy lacked the lower parts of both legs, which was originally connected with the infestations of this worm (Tapp 1986, 348; Tapp and Wildsmith 1992, 132–53). However, the ends of the bones are broken irregularly, so that surgical amputation has more recently been ruled out (Nunn and Tapp 2000, 147–53).

Another demonstrable parasitic disease is the mosquito-borne filariasis, which was found in the connective tissue of the mummy of Natsefamun, the priest of Amun of the temple in Karnak, from the museum in Leeds (Tapp and Wildsmith 1992, 132–53). In this context, we mention also the first proof of the presence of the microfilaria of the guinea worm in the lung tissue of the mummy of a 7- to 8-year-old boy from the Ptolemaic or Roman Period from the Senckenberg Museum in Frankfurt am Main (Schultz et al. 1995, 317–20).

Several authors also connect a parasitic disease with the cases dedicated to the excretion of a great deal of blood in the urine, which are described above on pages 269–70. Such symptoms could be correctly connected with schistosomiasis (previously called bilharzia), a parasitic disease discovered by Theodor Bilharz in 1851. Schistosomiasis has been proven in the Nile Valley since 3000 BC (Contis and David 1996, 253). It is caused by the worm *Schistosoma haematobium*, whose calcified egg was found in 1910 by Marc Armand Ruffer in the kidneys of two mummies from the period of the Twentieth Dynasty (Ruffer 1910, 16). Of the other findings of schistosomiasis, it is possible to mention the appearance of its antigen in fifteen of the twenty-three bodies examined from the Balana Culture (fourth to sixth centuries AD) in Nubia (Miller et al. 1992,

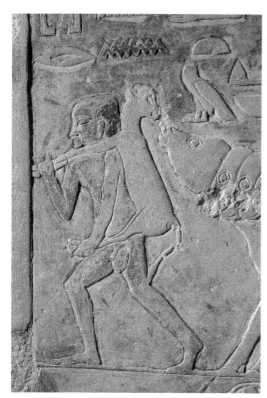

Fig. 30. A cattle herder with a swollen scrotum, a manifestation that is usually attributed to schistosomiasis (Sixth Dynasty, tomb of Mehu in Saqqara, photo © Oxford Expedition to Egypt)

555–56). The recent research using the ELISA (DNA) method found the presence of schistosomiasis in 45 percent of the examined Egyptian mummies from various dynastic periods (Ziskind 2009, 661). What is interesting is a comparison of the results from the areas of the Balana Culture at Wadi Halfa (4000 to 6000 BC) and from the area of Kulubnarti, settled by Christians (sixth to tenth century AD). In the first, the fields were cultivated using water wheels *(saqiya)* and the frequency of the occurrence of parasitic diseases in mature males was 66.7 percent, whereas in the second area the fields were hydrated by the annual floods and only 9.4 percent of the populace suffered from these problems. The difference documents the influence of the environment on the infestation of the population by this parasite (Hibbs et al. 2011, 293–97).

Many authors have tried to identify schistosomiasis with the disease *aaa* from the medical papyri (Ebbell 1927, 44–49; Jonckheere 1944; Lefebvre 1956, 153; Westendorf 1999, 469–71), where it is listed in them in twenty-two places of the body. This opinion is no longer accepted today. The reversal in the interpretation of the term *aaa* as a magical "poisonous seed" came from a

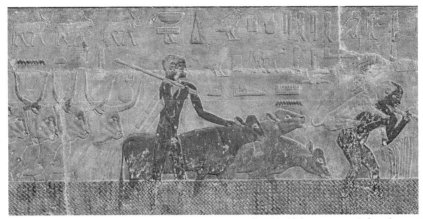

Fig. 31. Danger of infection by parasitic illnesses was particularly high near water. Infestation was common with fishermen, or when herding cattle in the river and standing in water canals (Fifth Dynasty, tomb of Ty in Saqqara, photo © Archive of the Czech Institute of Egyptology, Faculty of Arts, Charles University, Martin Frouz)

translation of the medical texts (Deines and Westendorf 1961, 129–33), and even Nunn agrees with it (1996, 63, 69, and 82) and Stephan (2001, 79, 144, and 147–48). It can be added that in an infestation of the parasite in question, there is not usually massive bleeding (hematuria), so the urine was not red, but pink as a consequence of slight bleeding (microhematuria). Moreover, the terms *senef* (blood) and *mewyt* (urine) are not presented at the same time in any of the preserved texts (Nunn and Tapp 2000, 149). This illness remains a health problem of some Egyptian villages to this day.

Other commonly identified worms include the large roundworm (*Ascaris lumbricoides*), whose egg appeared in the wall of the small intestine during the autopsy of the mummy PUM II from the University of Pennsylvania Museum of Archaeology and Anthropology in Philadelphia (Late Period) carried out in 1973 in Detroit (Cockburn et al. 1975, 1156–57; Tapp 1986, 348; Cockburn et al. 1998, 79; Jírovec 1954, 290–96).

A number of other parasitic worms were discovered by E. Tapp using X-ray, histopathology, and endoscopy in the mummies from the museum in Manchester, England. They included the bladder worm (larva stage) with hooks and suckers (scolices) of the hydatid worm *(Echinococcus granulosus)* in the cranial cavity of the isolated head of mummy No. 22,460. The growth of a cyst in the brain and its coverings can increase the intracranial pressure and cause pain, the gradual loss of sight, and unconsciousness (Tapp 1979b; Thompson et al. 1986, 375–78; Tapp and Wildsmith 1986, 351–54).

Interesting findings came from an examination of the mummy of the poor weaver Nakht from the period of the Twentieth Dynasty, which is found in the Royal Ontario Museum in Toronto. The internal organs remained in Nakht's body, apparently because his relatives did not have the money for proper, full mummification. Besides the eggs of *Schistosoma haematobium*, segments of a tapeworm (*Taenia* sp.) were also found in the body, and a cyst of a trichina worm *(Trichinella spiralis)* was found in the intercostal muscle (Hart et al. 1977 461–76; Tapp 1986, 349; Jírovec 1954, 309–14).

Another interesting finding was revealed by the mummy of Lady Asru from the Third Intermediate Period from the museum in Manchester. During mummification, a package was placed between her thighs containing her intestines, showing larvae of the parasite *Strongyloides stercoralis*, typical for the tropics and subtropics, in the walls of her intestines. Like larvae of the *Schistosoma*, they penetrate the intact skin into the veins, through which they travel to the right half of the heart and thus to the lungs. From there, they reach via the airways and again to the intestines in adult form (Jírovec 1954, 304–306; Tapp 1986, 348).

The first attestation of the occurrence of pinworm *(Enterobius vermicularis)* was published by Patrick D. Horne (2002).

Thanks to the autopsies of mummies, we today have a number of pieces of evidence that the thousand-year presence of worms in the bodies of the Egyptians (infestation) literally plagued the population there and contributed to the lowering of their resistance (immunity) and increased their morbidity.

The Head

The head with the skull, which protects one of the two organs most important for life—the brain—, was for ancient Egyptian physicians only a tank for mucous substances, which exited it through seven sacred apertures: the eyes as tears, the nostrils as mucus or a runny nose, the ears as earwax, and the mouth as saliva. The author of the Smith Papyrus was the only one who mentioned that an injury to the head could lead to severe neurological consequences (see Strouhal et al. 2014, cases Sm 3–8). It is interesting that this discovery did not change the original mistaken conception of the function of the brain in later Egyptian texts and later medicinal systems.

In the context of internal diseases, we are interested in pains and other problems of the head caused by inflammation of the nerves (neuritis), which were treated by the means then available. We will deal with diseases of the eyes, ears, nose, mouth, jaw, teeth, and skin in the third volume of this series.

The cases related to various pains and diseases of the head that we find in the Egyptian medical texts show that treatment of the head was predominantly

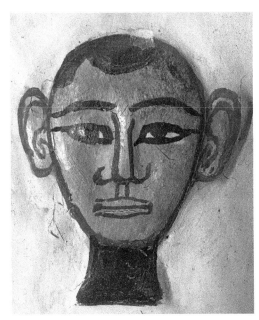

Fig. 32. The hieroglyphic sign *her*, "face," served in Egyptian as an ideogram indicating the relevant part of the body but also fulfilled, for instance, the function of the preposition "on" (Nineteenth Dynasty, tomb of Queen Nefertari in the Valley of the Queens (QV 66), photo © Mohamed Megahed)

magical, apparently for a lack of knowledge of its pathophysiology. Despite that, there is also a group of prescriptions in the Ebers Papyrus for the preparation of ointments which were to relieve the sick person during headaches. In seven cases, the basic ingredient was incense, which apparently played the main role in the treatment.

Other than a few cases mentioning pain in the middle of the head, the precise place of the pain is usually not presented in the texts, so that it could be various diagnoses, such as a blunt diffuse headache, sometimes drilling vasomotoric headache *(cephalalgia vasomotorica)*, and other times an inflammation of the trigeminal nerve *(neuralgia trigemina)*.

Chester Beatty V verso—migraine

In Chester Beatty Papyrus V, we find cases dedicated to the migraine, which is described as pain in the middle of the head. A migraine is marked by pain exclusively on one of the two temples. It tends to run in the family, is more frequent in women, is accompanied by photophobia, increased sensitivity to sound, and a loss of appetite, and begins with ocular symptoms (prodomes). It often lasts several hours and has a drilling, often unbearable character. The treatment process lay in a magical incantation, which indicates that Egyptian physicians did not know how to effectively resolve this unpleasant disease.

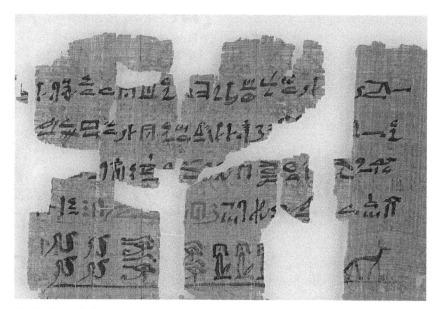

Fig. 33. The end of an incantation on the Papyrus Chester Beatty V (verso 4.10–6.4) with model images of deities for drawing on protective amulets (British Museum, London EA10685.2, photo © The Trustees of the British Museum)

The first incantation (4.1–4.9) calls individually on the gods of the Great and Small Ennead, the society of gods related to the Heliopolitan tradition of the creation myth (Janák 2005, 50–51; Janák 2009, 94–97), along with Anubis, one of the leading gods from the divine pantheon. These gods are asked to remove the pain from the face of the person, whose name was filled into the incantation. The pain was ascribed to the activity of harmful forces, and the originator could be any enemy or evil deceased person. The incantation was to be recited over a clay figure of a crocodile with faïence eyes and a grain of cereal in its mouth. This statuette was wrapped in a soft cloth painted with the images of the mentioned gods and placed on the head of the sick person. The treatment was to take place over statuettes of the mentioned gods of the Ennead, a statuette of the goddess Mehit, and a statuette of Horus standing on the back of an oryx. The translation of this part of the text is rather unclear.

Another incantation against a migraine (4.10–6.4) identifies the head of the sick person with the head of Osiris Wennefer, which protects the 377 divine uraei (rearing cobras) that spit flames. Afterwards, the incantation addresses the disease itself and threatens that if it does not leave the body of the sick person, the incantation will cause for it and the whole world a wide range of inauspicious things. The text names the severest punishments which the fantasy of the author of this incantation could imagine. The incantation was recited as in the previous case over drawings of the divinities on a soft cloth, which was placed on the temple of the sick person. After the end of the text of this incantation, the papyrus shows a drawing of the deities, which have the form of a jackal, a seated god, the divine eye, and the uraeus.

Ebers 250—pain in the middle of the head
Pains in the middle of the head apparently also referred to a migraine. The medicine was an ointment prepared from a catfish skull burned to ashes, the cinder of which was mixed with oil. It was undoubtedly another magical method that could serve as an accompaniment to some incantation.

Ebers 255-56—treatment of the head
Which problem of the head the sick person suffered from is not stated in this case, but most likely it was an unspecified pain. As a medicine 15 ml of the best incense was to help, which was to be smeared very often on the head of the affected person (Eb 256). Other times a mixture was prepared from equal amounts (15 ml) of incense, camphor, the soft part of balsam, and mint, which after mixing were smeared on the head repeatedly each day (Eb 255).

Ebers 260—treatment of the head and temple
This case is presented as a remedy for the head and temple, without the text specifying the symptoms of the pain. It cannot be ruled out that it was also a pain in one part of the head, possibly pulsing pain in the temples. An ointment was to help which was prepared from 1 ml of malachite, half that amount of galenite, hematite from Qus (near Qift, from which the expeditions set out to the Eastern Desert), the *netjerit* stone, and *senen* resin, a quarter of the amount of incense, common resin, and the *wah-nebet* stone. The ingredients were ground, mixed in 37.5 ml of water, and the mixture was spread on the patient's temple.

Ebers 253-54—pain of the head, substances causing pain
A number of other prescriptions were intended for headaches, which were attributed to the substances causing pain *(wekhedu)*. A mixture which was to help was prepared from equal amounts (15 ml) of incense, laudanum, reed, pulp of the *ibu* plant, and fat. The ingredients were ground, mixed, and cooked; the mixture was smeared on the head of the affected person (Eb

253). Other times, they mixed the equal amounts (15 ml) of incense, cumin, and goose fat and used the cooked mixture as an ointment to spread on the head (Eb 254).

Ebers 257-58—pain of the head
Other prescriptions intended for curing headaches recommended mixtures containing 15 ml each of incense, cedar resin, reed, juniper, laurel fruit, and fat (Eb 257) or 15 ml each of myrrh, resinous gum, cumin, *Moringa*, juniper berries, the *tentem* plant fruit, and lotus (Eb 258). In both cases the ingredients were ground and the mixture was applied to the head.

Ebers 259—cooling of the head, pain of the head
The last prescription in the group is intended for cooling a painful head. According to this, it was possible to prepare a healing ointment from equal amounts (15 ml) of incense, ocher, camphor, gum, the *netjerit* stone, stonemason's clay, petrified wood, carob, the *waneb* plant, a fallow deer's antler, and water. The ingredients were ground and mixed together; the ointment was then smeared on the head. It seems that some ingredients such as petrified wood, a fallow deer's antler, or stonemason's clay worked rather magically.

Ebers 252—trembling in the head
This case was dedicated to a sick person who felt trembling in the head and did not recognize when the physician put his hand on his head. He was to prepare for him an ointment from crushed natron, water, oil, honey, and wax. The amounts of the individual ingredients are not stated in the text.

Ebers 248-49—activity of demons in the head
The cause of a problem, probably a headache, which the ancient Egyptians attributed to the activity of demons, is unknown. It is interesting that in these cases they did not use a magical incantation against it, but medicinal mixtures, whose effects were undoubtedly verified empirically. It was a mixture containing 15 ml each of myrtle, thyme, and coriander, bryony, and dill seeds, which were mixed with the same amount of donkey fat (Eb 249). This ointment was to be spread on the head of the sick person. For a period of four days, a more complicated medicinal ointment was used. For its preparation it was necessary to have 15 ml each of carob, the *khesau* part of the *ima* tree, laudanum, honey, natron, mud, the cooked bones of the Nile perch and Nile tilapia, and the boiled skull of the *Synodontis* (Eb 248).

Hearst 76–77—the disease *seket* in the head

The unknown disease *seket*, the symptoms of which are not more closely described in the text, was attributed to the activity of demons. The cases in this group are parallels to the cases Ebers 248–49 (see above), but where the name of the disease is not presented.

Hearst 167—the disease *meshshut*

In this case, the physician struggles with a disease which was called *meshshut* in Egyptian. Nevertheless, the text does not present any symptoms or causes of this disease. According to the place of application of the medicine, it seems that it was an illness of the head. A mixture to help was made of camphor, sour milk, and snake skin, which was smeared on the head.

Chester Beatty V verso 6.5–6.7—the disease *hek* in the temple

Although the text of this case is preserved only in small part and is hard to understand, it seems that it concerned an illness of the head. It is a magical incantation which addressed the disease *hek* and calls on it to leave the left temple. The remainder of the text is destroyed unfortunately. In the conclusion, a recommendation has also been preserved that the incantation is to be recited seven times, with the left hand held in the right hand, but it is not clear if it refers to the hands of the one reciting or the hands of the ill.

Limbs

Pain of All the Extremities

Pains in the bones and joints of the upper and lower limbs, connected with the strenuous physical work of the farmers, and in contrast the lack of movement in people with sedentary occupations, caused the feelings of stiffness and rheumatic pain in the joints or swelling and cramps due to strained muscles. These problems also belonged to the sphere of ancient Egyptian internal doctors, who treated them with the only means available to them at that time.

Ebers 636—healing the bones

This prescription describes the preparation of an aromatic ointment which was to help in the treatment of the bones of the body and was to be very effective. It contained 15 ml each of honey, natron, black flint, the *weshbet* stone, and fat, which was to be applied on the limb. It is not entirely clear whether this mixture could influence the health of the bones. The Edwin Smith Surgical Papyrus, which presents the methods of examining injuries and fractures, does not contain this remedy. It is, however, worth mentioning that according to this papyrus, honey and oil or fat were often used to treat wounds and fractures (see Strouhal et al. 2014, 26–27).

Ebers 654–55—easing the joints of any extremity

Two cases for easing the joints recommended an ointment comprised of equal amounts (15 ml) of honey, high-quality incense, laudanum, wax, milk fat, carob flour, *shasha* fruit, and wild rue seeds. The ingredients were ground, mixed, and the painful joint was to be smeared with this ointment (Eb 654). Other times, a mixture was applied on the joint which was made from equal amounts (15 ml) of incense, beads of incense, red clay, juniper berries, juniper seeds (?), bryony, celery seeds, and tubers (?) of *Astragalus* (Eb 655).

Hearst 123–24—easing the joints of any extremity

We find parallels to the previous cases Ebers 645 and 655 in the Hearst Papyrus, but their wording is not entirely the same and the ingredients are named without their recommended amounts.

Berlin 153—painful substances in the extremities

The heading of the case describes the wandering of the painful substances in the extremities of a person, which indicates pains in various parts of the limbs, but the following instruction for the preparation of the medicine refers to substances causing pain in the abdomen. It could thus be pain in various parts of the whole body.

The medicine paradoxically was composed of 75 ml of fresh fatty meat, 2 ml of thyme and jujube bread, half the amount of mountain celery, bits of incense and fresh bread, and 300 ml of the beverage called *sekhpet*. The ingredients were to be ground finely, mixed to cook, and shaped into the form of the *shayt* cake. The sick person was to eat this medicinal cake for a period of four days and wash it down with sweet beer.

Hearst 42–46—painful substances in all extremities

The Hearst Papyrus offered a mixture for expelling the pain in all extremities prepared from 150 ml of fatty meat, the same amount of *Melilotus*, 1 ml of thyme, juniper berries, and incense, 112.5 ml of both halves of the *pesedj* fruit, which might have been some legume (Westendorf 1999, 336), further 225 ml of the strong beer *djeseret,* and 375 ml of sweet beer. The mixture was to be boiled and strained, reduced to 150 ml, and given to the sick person for a period of four days (H 42). Another prescription describes the preparation of a mixture of 75 ml of both halves of the *pesedj* fruit, 37.5 ml of sorted and crushed barley, 2 ml of yellow nutsedge and the *tiam* plant, half that amount of juniper berries, and 1.8 l of water, which was to be boiled and then left overnight to stand exposed to the dew and strained. The period of use was set at four days (H 46).

A simpler variation was to mix 2 ml of dates, the same amount of raisins, and a quarter of the amount of dill, which were mixed in 75 ml of wine, boiled, strained, and given to the sick person to drink for a period of four days (H 44). Another mixture contained 2 ml of fresh bread, half the amount of honey and *merhet-sa* oil, and 0.23 ml of incense and cumin in 300 ml of sweet beer. After boiling, this medicine was given for a period of four days (H 43). Other times, it was possible to take 300 ml of an ingredient unknown to us called *hemaret* (it could be the incorrect writing of the expression *hemayt*, so perhaps bitter almonds?), 300 ml of carob juice, 4 ml of honey, and the same amount of fat. The ingredients were ground, mixed, pressed through a cloth, and strained; when administered more honey was added (H 45).

Berlin 119—painful substances in the tips of the extremities
This case is devoted to pain in the final segments of all of the extremities of the patient. The causes of this pain were attributed to the substances causing pain, since the real cause was not revealed. The means for expelling the symptoms of these substances was a mixture of equal amounts (2 ml) of figs, dates, raisins, and wheat, and half the amount of gum, which were mixed in 75 ml of water. The mixture was left to stand overnight exposed to the dew and was to then be strained. It was to be used for a period of four days.

Ebers 696—painful substances in the arm, trembling
A trembling in the arm, most likely accompanied by pains, was attributed to the painful substances *wekhedu*. Against that, it was helpful to drink 2.88 l of a warm beverage from a fermented barley decoction, which caused vomiting. The application was to be repeated for a period of four days. The connection between the arm and vomiting is not clear; it could have been the result of some poisoning.

Leiden verso IX–X.2—illness of the arm
We find among the magical methods one incantation intended for removing the disease from the arm, which contrasts with a wide range of cases concerning the lower limbs. According to the text, the disease of the arm, which is not described in more detail, was caused by unfriendly forces, an unfriendly god, or a dead person. The incantation addresses these possible originators of the problem and calls on them to leave the arm of the sick person, and then it calls on a number of the gods of the Egyptian pantheon. The text of the incantation is, however, very

damaged, and so it is difficult to understand the parts that have been preserved. We find mentions here of the gods Atum and Horus, and also of Re and Apophis, who symbolized the order and disorder of the world (Janák 2005, 30–31), of the protective solar eye and sun, and of the god of immensity and infinity Heh (Janák 2005, 70). According to the partially preserved final passage of the case, this incantation was to be recited during the preparation of the medicinal mixture, which was to be applied on the affected arm. It was a mixture of myrrh, goat's blood, the unknown *nui* plant, the beverage called *mesta,* and something from the oryx (fat, blood, hair?).

Pain of the Legs

A greater number of cases in the preserved medical texts is connected with illnesses of the lower limbs. As with the previous group, their causes are not more closely specified, so it is hard from today's perspective to judge the medical severity, possible causes, and effectiveness of the recommended treatment. In some cases, it was pain in the lower limbs, which could have diverse causes. Other times, the heading of the text mentions swelling, which might have most often been related to exhaustion of the lower extremities, impairment with varicose veins (varicose syndrome), or clogging of the veins (thrombosis). Progressively rising swelling from the ankles up accompanies weakening activity of the heart.

Berlin 120-21—painful substances in both legs

According to the Berlin Papyrus, a medicinal beverage and a medicinal ointment were prepared for painful legs at the same time. The drink consisted of 300 ml of sweet beer, 75 ml of wine, 4 ml of dates, and both halves of the *pesedj* fruit, half the amount of thyme and fresh bread, 0.5 ml of juniper berries, half that amount of cumin and incense, and 37.5 ml of fatty meat. The mixture was first to be boiled and then drunk for four days. After its use, the patient was supposed to walk, apparently so that the medicine quickly penetrated the legs (Bln 120). An accompanying medicinal ointment was prepared from the sawdust of the *aru* tree and the *afed* part of a goat's leg, which was to be finely ground, mixed, and spread on both of the lower limbs of the sick person (Bln 121). The dissolving agent is lacking in the prescription, which was apparently magical.

Leiden verso XXIII—painful substances in the legs

This case contains an incantation against the painful substances in the lower extremities. The text is heavily damaged and therefore hard to understand. Moreover, it is not clear whether the incantation was accompanied by the preparation of some medicine as was usual in other similar cases. The incantation addresses the pain itself and calls on various gods such as Horus, Seth, or the god of wisdom Thoth. It also mentions Khentyirty, the local deity of the town of Khemu (in Greek Letopolis), who was the god of heavenly bodies and also the protector from snakes (Janák 2005, 90–91).

Ebers 561—painful swelling of the leg

A simple remedy, which was prepared when the legs swelled painfully (see Westendorf 1999, 643), comprised 15 ml of red natron mixed with fermented date juice. This mixture was applied on the affected place.

Berlin 125-35—swelling in both legs

We can find another eleven cases of the swelling of the lower limbs in the Berlin Papyrus. The remedies were mainly applied using compresses. They are very simple prescriptions, which name the individual ingredients without specifying their amounts or further conveying the method of preparation. We find here mixtures of honey and wine, which were mixed with sorghum (Bln 125) or with the *tekhu* plant seeds (Bln 127). Other times, the wine itself was mixed with the *tekhu* plant seeds and the *shebeb* plant (Bln 128). The honey itself was mixed with natron and the *shasha* plant, which might have been valerian (Bardinet 1995, 425) (Bln 129), with acacia and jujube leaves and ocher (Bln 131), with juniper berries and natron (Bln 133), or with juniper berries and peas (Bln 134). Other times oil was mixed with acacia leaves and ocher (Bln 132). Other remedies recommended mixing juice from date purée with natron and fine fat (Bln 130; literally sweet fat, see Hannig 1995, 166; Westendorf 1999, 291) or ground fennel with the *nesty* part of the *besha* grain (Bln 135). Other times an *aat* vessel of Palestinian wine was ground with vinegar (Bln 126). The last medicine was certainly not accessible to everyone because of the high price of imported wine.

Leiden recto XXVI 7–12—swelling in both legs

We find further cases of swelling of the lower extremities and other limbs in the Leiden Papyrus, which recommends various medicinal mixtures. The first of them was put on the affected place for a period of four days and comprised equal amounts (15 ml) of ink, carob flour, dates, and perhaps also other, unpreserved ingredients, which were mixed in honey (7–9). Other times a mixture was applied made from equal amounts (15 ml) of date seeds, natron, and pomace, which were ground until fine and mixed (11), or from an unspecified amount of an herbal decoction with sea salt and *shenfet* fruits (erroneously written as *menfet*, see also Westendorf 1999, 68) (11–12). The period of application is not specified. A medicine prepared from equal amounts of red ocher, pomace, fermented herbal decoction, and human feces seems disgusting (9–10).

Leiden recto XXVI 12–XXVIII 5—an inflammation in parts of the leg

This case deals with an inflammation (see Massart 1954, 96) in part of the lower extremity called *sedja*, but the cause or manifestations of it are not described in the text other than the usual consequence of the activity of inauspicious powers. Any inflammation was always dangerous for a patient in antiquity, because the natural medicines did not usually manage to fight it effectively. An inflammation was therefore magically exorcized, so the ill person would recuperate with the help of the gods. The incantation describes how chaos rules in the world, on earth, and in heaven, unless the gods are reconciled to cure the inflammation. Re (Ra) and Atum, Horus's protective eye, and also Seth's testicles are mentioned. The incantation was to be recited four times, which enhances its effect.

Hearst 27—the illness *henut* in both legs

The disease *henut*, which could affect the lower limbs, also had an unknown cause. Its interpretation is difficult; the Egyptian term *henut* labeled a wrinkling of the skin, but it could also be a clogging (of the blood vessels?) (Hannig 1995, 538). The means against this disease was a mixture prepared from 4 ml wheat semolina, half the amount of honey and oil, 75 ml of crushed earth almonds, the same amount of dried *ihu* fruits, and 1.2 l of water. The mixture was to be well mixed, strained, and used as a beverage for a period of four days.

Berlin 169—the lump *henhenet* in both legs

An unknown lump called in Egyptian *henhenet* could appear in both legs, and for its treatment it was recommended to apply an enema into the rectum made from 4 ml of honey, 0.5 ml of sea salt, 35.5 ml of *Moringa* oil, and 375 ml of sweet beer. The connection between the legs and the enema could possibly indicate a connection with hemorrhoids (see pages 257–59).

Pains of the Knee, Lower Leg, and Foot

Other cases devoted to the lower extremities focus on their certain parts, namely the knee, lower leg, and final segments of the lower extremities.

Ebers 603, 608, and 610—easing of the knee

Several prescriptions in the Ebers Papyrus, which are entitled "Collection of medicinal means for easing the knee" were intended for treating the knee

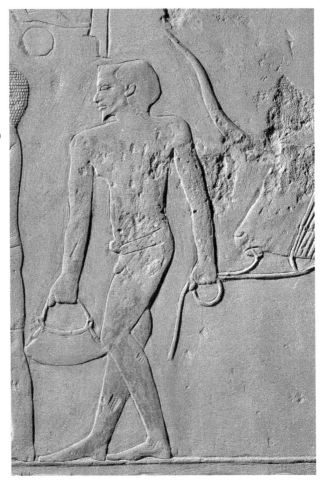

Fig. 34. Impairment of the lower extremities is often shown in depictions of cattle herders; here an elderly man with thinning hair, swollen stomach, and clearly sick leg leads a heavy sacrificial bull to the slaughter (Sixth Dynasty, tomb of Idut in Saqqara, photo © Oxford Expedition to Egypt)

joint. They were mainly compresses or bandages applied on the ill knee. The first prescription recommends a mixture containing 15 ml each of wheat flour, honey, fatty meat, and the unknown *git* plant, which were ground together and applied on the knee (Eb 603). Another case describes the preparation of an ointment from the same amount (15 ml) of *Melilotus*, myrtle, peas, fermented date juice, sediments of sweet beer, honey, beef, beef fat, beef marrow, beef spleen, the unknown substance *seska,* and sea salt (Eb 608). Another prescription includes 15 ml each of bryony fruit, peas, celery and *Anacyclus* seeds, the same amount of honey, oil, and red clay, which were thoroughly ground and mixed together (Eb 610).

Ebers 609—sick knee

For the treatment of unspecified problems of the knee, a mixture was prescribed that was prepared from the same amount (15 ml) of *Melilotus*, wild rue, the *iagut* fruits (?), flour from the threshing floor, red natron, sea salt, sediments of sweet beer, and the unknown substance *djat*. The ingredients were boiled together and used as a compress.

Ebers 604—dropped knee

According to this prescription, a simple medicine was to help against the knee which had dropped. It was made from sifted straw mixed with water, which was applied on the affected place. According to the text, this remedy could be used also on any other join with the same disease. It could only work thanks to suggestion or autosuggestion.

Ramesseum III.A, l. 3-4—knee

This case is preserved incompletely; a large part of its heading and also the end of the case have been lost. The recipe is identical with Ebers 604, but it differs with details in the heading and instruction.

Ebers 605-606—painful knee

Pain in the knee, the cause of which is not specified, was treated with a mixture of 15 ml of wild rue and the same amount of flour from *qaat*, which were ground together in sweet beer. The mixture was cooked and applied on the knee (Eb 605). Other times a small swamp hen was crushed in a mortar, namely whole, with everything that belonged to it. This medicine was also applied as a compress (Eb 606).

Ramesseum III.B: l. 1-2—hunger in both knees

A case for expelling the hunger of both knees sounds mysterious. "Hunger of both knees" could be meant as their creaking, pain, and slowing of the movement that accompanied arthrosis, a degenerative disease of ageing joints. The recommended method required placing the innards of the tilapia on the knee and then a halved salamander and bandaging it. Further, bull bile was to be crushed with a small swamp hen and also placed on the knee.

Ramesseum V.1—knee (?)

Another case related to an illness of the knee joint in the Ramesseum Papyri is very damaged. Of the case itself, only the reference to the knee and the concluding instruction for placement for a period of four days have been preserved.

Ebers 612—pain of the kneecap

For a painful kneecap, thus "knee apple or cap" (patella), a medicinal mixture of the ground *shasha* fruits mixed with water and the *mesta* drink was applied.

Hearst 247—pain of the kneecap (?)

This very poorly preserved case seems to be a parallel to the previous prescription Ebers 612, because it contains the same ingredients for the preparation of a medicinal mixture and also the length of application, which was to be four days.

Hearst 252—pain of the kneecap

A prescription for a painful kneecap was also written down in the Hearst Papyrus, but only a small part of its text has been preserved. Besides part of the heading, only a part of the title of the first ingredient is legible—an expression labeling the roots of some plant.

Ebers 128—tibial bone

This case contains preparation for treating the tibia, most likely after an injury, such as a collision with a bruise (contusion with a hematoma), which did not require a surgical examination. It recommends placing on the shin the *amem* part of a catfish, which can be found in its head (according to some specialists this could be its brain, see Hannig 1995, 141), soaked in honey.

Ebers 613-14—the disease of the calves

A medicine could serve to heal the calves, whose disease is not specified. It was made from the same amount (15 ml) of dried myrrh, incense, honey, beef fat, and pellets (Egyptian *khepa*) of malachite, which were cooked together and applied as a compress (Eb 613). Other times, a more complex medicine was prepared from many ingredients, namely from an amount (15 ml) of dried myrrh, bryony, fennel, yellow nutsedge, chaste tree, juniper berries, pine nuts, acacia leaves, the leaves of the *mafet* tree, cedar, and juniper resinous pellets, incense, acacia gum, wax, camphor, fresh *Moringa* oil, balsam, and the water of heavenly dew. The ingredients were ground finely, mixed, and applied on the calf (Eb 614).

Berlin 123-24—pain in the calf

A compress with a rare mixture of the bile of the royal antelope and bile of the tilapia was recommended for an unspecified pain in the calf (Bln 123), possibly a mixture of oil and the plant called in Egyptian *henen-aa*, literally "donkey phallus" (Bln 124).

Ebers 607—limping

Against limping, the cause of which remains unknown to us, there was a medicine available made from the same amount (15 ml) of peas, the *qenet* plant, and flour from the threshing floor, which was mixed with fermented date juice. It is a simpler form of the prescription Ebers 608 for easing the knee (see above).

Ebers 615—trembling of both legs

It was possible to act against the trembling of the legs using a mixture of the same amount (15 ml) of peas, pine nuts, *Anacyclus* seeds, and beef fat. The mixture was cooked and then applied on the legs for a period of four days.

Ebers 611—swollen blister

A preparation for removing a swollen blister on a leg apparently worked magically. Tadpoles from the ditch and the *wadu* plant were prepared as a mixture. They were burned and mixed in oil. The ointment was spread on the legs. The meaning of the species of the *wadu* plant is not known (Germer 2008, 50), so the effects of this mixture cannot be judged today.

Pains of the Fingers and Toes

A number of prescriptions in the preserved medical texts concerned diseases of the fingers, fingernails, toes, and toenails. Sometimes the cases are devoted to the digits or nails on the hand or foot; other times which limb is meant is specified. It is interesting that cases related to the toes are much more frequent, revealing injury of the toes or inflammation of the toenails in connection with the insufficient footwear of the population then. The majority of the common people walked in open, soft-leather shoes or barefoot, so similar injuries were not a rarity in normal walking or during work. Other times, however, it could be pain with various causes, which is not usually specified in the texts.

The cases devoted to the fingers and toes are relatively numerous in the medical texts. We find them particularly in the Hearst and Ebers Papyri, to a lesser degree also in the Berlin Papyrus and several cases have been preserved in the Ramesseum Papyri. They were mainly medicinal ointments and compresses, only rarely beverages.

Berlin 161-62—painful substances in the tips of the hand, traveling pain

This case is devoted to pains in the tips of the fingers, which was attributed to the harmful, pain-spreading substances *wekhedu*. They were pains which traveled here and there, accompanied by certain facial expressions, possibly more general manifestations in the upper part of his body (see Westendorf 1999, 332). In addition, his meat (muscles) is reminiscent of worms and shows "*Moringa* oil in the blood." The Egyptian physician labeled these symptoms, which today we can only understand with difficulty, as manifestations of the *wekhedu* substances, which could be healed. The sick person was to consume barley mash every day and avoid anything hot (Bln 161).

The following prescription describes the preparation of a mixture of the same amount (2 ml) of *Melilotus*, the *temem* and *sau* parts of dates, thyme, *shenfet* fruit, half that amount of juniper berries, and both halves of the *pesedj* fruit, a quarter of the amount of cumin and incense, 75 ml of fatty meat, 300 ml of sweet beer, and 300 ml of the strong beer *djeseret*. The mixture was left overnight to stand exposed to the dew, then was strained and given as a medicinal drink (Bln 162).

Hearst 181—finger
For an unspecified problem of the fingers, a mixture was recommended that was prepared from oil and the powder of the *tjun* plant. Its meaning is unfortunately unknown (Germer 2008, 158), so it is not possible to judge the effectiveness of this medicine today.

Ebers 616—pain of the fingers or toes
A preparation from 4 ml acacia leaves, the same amount of jujube, half the amount of the insides of a freshwater mussel, and an eighth of the amount of ocher and malachite powder was to help cool painful, apparently inflamed, fingers. The ingredients were ground, mixed, and applied on the affected place. It is worth mentioning that the ocher could act as a disinfectant, the malachite antiseptically, and the acacia leaves acted as an astringent.

Hearst 195—treatment of the finger or toe
The Hearst Papyrus pays great attention to the problems of the fingers and nails. This case refers to the treatment of the finger or toe in unspecified problems. A mixture was to help, made from the fibers of the *qaa* plant and oil, which was cooked and applied on the affected finger or toe.

Hearst 194—healing the fingers and toes, on the nails
According to this case, a preparation intended for healing fingers and toes was applied on the nail. It was a mixture of acacia leaves, resin, gum, oil, laudanum, and the ingredient called *bedet-hawret*, the amounts of which are not specified in the text.

Hearst 180—toe

Whereas the cases presented above dealt with the digits generally and could be used on the hands and feet, another group of cases was intended explicitly for the treatment of the toes. The manifestations of the disease are not usually mentioned in the text. According to this prescription, an unspecified amount of astringently acting acacia leaves was mixed with fat, and the mixture was cooked and smeared on the affected toe.

Hearst 173a and b—finger or toe

This case describes a two-part treatment of the toe or finger. In the first phase, a compress was to be applied to the digit with a remedy from red ocher, a shard of a new *hin* vessel, and the product of honey fermentation. The amounts are not given. Then a cooling ointment was to be prepared from 4 ml of acacia and the same amount of jujube leaves, half the amount of mussel, and an eight amount of ocher and malachite, which were ground and mixed. Case Hearst 173a is a parallel of the following case Ebers 621, whereas Hearst 173b is a parallel to Ebers 616, which we presented above in this section.

Ebers 620–21—a sick toe

It was possible to place on the toe a compress with a mixture prepared from 15 ml of red ocher, the same amount of a shard of a new *hin* vessel, and the same amount of the product of the fermentation of honey (Eb 621). In contrast to the prescription Hearst 173a, the precise amounts of the ingredients are stipulated.

A more complicated medicine intended for the treatment of the toe contains 15 ml each of flax seeds, starch, ocher, red ocher, natron, the great protection stone, and the *khenenu* stone "from the courtyard." The ingredients were cooked until soft and then ground. They were then mixed with honey, oil, beef fat, and marrow, until an ointment emerged, which was smeared on the affected toe (Eb 620). Ocher was added to this mixture apparently for its disinfecting effect, which could prevent a painful suppurative inflammation of the skin and subcutaneous tissue of the toe (panaritium), forming even with a slightly contaminated (infected) wound.

Hearst 175–76—an aching toe

The toe that suffered, hence apparently hurt, was treated using a combination of two ointments and compresses. First, a mixture was prepared from flax seeds, starch, ocher, red ocher, natron, the "great protection" stone, and the *khenenu* stone "from the courtyard," which were thoroughly mixed. Then were added honey, oil, fat, and marrow until a healing ointment was created, which was applied on the affected toe (H 175). It is a parallel to case Ebers 620 (see above). Another prescription contained incense, honey, oil, and fat (H 176).

Hearst 197–98—a toe
Other times, a gutted and salted salamander was applied on the toe (H 197) or the *amem* part of a frog marinated in cedar oil (H 198). According to some scholars, this could be frog brain (Hannig 1995, 141).

Hearst 200–203—swelling of the toes
A compress to help against swelling of the toes was made with honey and the *tjun* plant seeds. It is a similar remedy to the more generally formulated case Hearst 181 (see above). Other times a mixture that could help was made from peas, *Anacyclus* fruit, pine nuts, and the *tjun* plant fruit, which were ground and mixed with honey (H 201). Another prescription recommended a mixture of the carob pod, *shasha* fruit (according to Bardinet it was valerian, Bardinet 1995, 401), red ocher, and honey (H 202). Other times, a mixture of honey and the *amem* parts (perhaps the brain) of the *Clarias* catfish was applied on the toe (H 203).

Hearst 182–83—blood in the toes
To drive blood from the toe, which could refer to a bruise, finely ground acacia hulls were applied on it (H 182). Acacia has demonstrably calming effects (demulcent), so it is suitable for the treatment of minor wounds. Other times, the toes were smeared with an ointment prepared from balls of incense, which were boiled until soft in oil, and the mixture was kneaded well (H 183).

Ebers 623–24—trembling of the fingers
There were also means available to stop the trembling of the fingers, accompanying old age and noticeable especially with Parkinson's disease. According to the first prescription, 15 ml each of *tjun* plant and sycamore fruits, sea salt, milk, beef fat, and the unknown substance *seska* were mixed. The mixture was boiled and smeared on the fingers (Eb 623). Other times a mixture was prepared from the same amount (15 ml) of cumin, figs, incense, ocher, red ocher, the *netjerit* stone, the name of which means "divine," and honey. This mixture was also boiled before application (Eb 624).

Hearst 205—trembling of the fingers
According to the Hearst Papyrus, it was sufficient against trembling of the fingers to smear the fingers with oil and place compresses with watermelon on them.

Hearst 204—the disease *sut* in the finger

The name *sut* labeled a disease whose manifestations are not specified in the text. The name itself is similar to the name for wheat, so it might have been some formation reminiscent of a grain of wheat (see also Westendorf 1999, 174). A compress was to help with a mixture of myrtle, the *pesedj* plant, the unknown substance *seska*, sea salt, and honey.

Treatment of the Nails

Already from the Old Kingdom, we encounter evidence in Egyptian depictions of the care that people devoted to their body including their nails. Some scenes in tombs capturing a manicure and pedicure refer to the cleansing in connection with the purity of the funeral priests (see for instance, Strouhal et al. 2014, 81–82).

The medical papyri offer another view, namely care for damaged nails. The disease of the nails could occur as a consequence of an injury or inflammation, but the preserved prescriptions for treating the nails do not state the cause of the problem.

Ebers 618-19—means for the toenails

Generally, these prescriptions in the Ebers Papyrus are devoted to the treatment of a sick nail. The first comprised 0.45 ml of hemp, the *ibu* plant, and resin, half the amount of ocher, and 4 ml of honey. The ingredients were ground together and applied to the affected nail (Eb 618). Other times, 0.45 ml of oil, half the amount of ocher, and 4 ml of honey were mixed (Eb 619).

Hearst 185-87—treatment of the toenails

The treatment of unspecified problems of the toenails was conducted according to the Hearst Papyrus by placing a mixture of ocher with incense, fat, and honey (H 186). Other times, ocher, hematite, a copper bead, oryx fat, wax, myrtle, and red wood were mixed (H 185) or ocher, honey, oil, linen seeds, and the *wetyt* part of the sycomore (H 187).

Hearst 188-93—remedy for the toenails

The following group describes similar remedies, but this time with the precise amounts of the individual ingredients. They were sometimes very simple preparations of 0.5 ml of ocher with the same amount of oil (H 189) or 2 ml of red ocher with the same amount of honey (H 190). Other times more complex means were prepared. A mixture of 2 ml of honey and 0.45 ml of hemp, the *ibu* plant, resin, and ocher is similar to the prescription Ebers 618, but the amounts of the ingredients differ slightly (H 188). Other times, the same amount (2 ml) was mixed of each of honey, incense, and the *ibu* plant with 0.5 ml of resin and ocher (H 192). Another remedy included barley flour, 75 ml of myrrh, 2 ml of carob pod, the same amount of acacia and jujube leaves, half the amount of honey, 0.5 ml of ocher, and half the amount of incense, which were mixed together and cooked (H 191). The prescription for the preparation of a mixture of red ocher, shards of the new *hin* vessel, honey, and oil is similar to case Ebers 621 (but with the addition of the last ingredient, oil, which is not mentioned in Ebers 621), and the precise amounts are not provided (H 193).

Hearst 177–78—remedy for toenails or toes
These cases are very similar to the prescriptions of Ebers 618, Hearst 188, and Ebers 619, but the heading states a connection not only with treatment of the nail but also the toe generally. The amounts of the ingredients in the first case differ from this one, but the second case is almost a verbatim copy. It is a mixture of 0.45 ml of hemp, the *ibu* plant, and resin, half the amount of ocher, and 75 ml of honey (H 177), or from 2 ml of honey, 0.45 ml of oil, and half the amount of ocher (H 178).

Ebers 622—a toenail falling off
When the nail was so afflicted that it fell off, a medicinal mixture was to be made from equal amounts (15 ml) of natron, incense, ocher, and oil. After application on the nail, it was to be sprinkled with more natron. Ocher and natron apparently worked here as anti-inflammatory agents for prevention of an infection of the nail bed.

Hearst 179—a toenail falling off
A parallel to the previous case is a prescription for treating a nail falling off with a mixture of natron, incense, ocher, oil, and honey. The text does not present the amounts of the individual ingredients. The affected toe was also to be bandaged, but only so that the compress did not press on the nail.

Ebers 617—pain of the finger or toe, smelly liquid under the nail
In this case, serious-sounding manifestations of an illness of the finger or toe are described, when it apparently was an ongoing unpleasant inflammation of the nail bed (panaritium). These manifestations were attributed to the activity of a worm, which the physician should destroy. He did so using a medicinal mixture of 2 ml of cedar oil, a quarter of the amount of the ground *sia* stone from Upper Egypt, and the same amount of *sia* from Lower Egypt, which was

applied on the finger or toe. Cedar oil has antiseptic effects, but we do not know the medicinal effects of the ingredient *sia*.

Hearst 174—pain of the finger or toe, smelly liquid
This prescription is a parallel to the previous case, which describes the preparation of the same medicine and states in the heading that it is a medicine for extermination of the worm called *seped*.

Hearst 199—festering on the toenails
It was recommended against a festering of the nails, the cause of which is not specified, to anoint the afflicted toes with a mixture of peas, carob pod seeds, and honey. The amounts of the individual ingredients are not stated.

Hearst 184—an open wound with the toenails
If a wound has appeared at the nail with an open mouth, one proceeded in two steps following these instructions. It was first necessary to place on the wound a mixture of carob pod, acacia leaves, red ocher, sea salt, and a fermented herbal decoction. A further treatment followed with a mixture of fennel seeds, carob flour, cedar oil, wax, incense, and fat (H 184). The amounts of the individual ingredients are not specified.

Stiffness and Contortion
In the medical texts, we also find a number of remedies intended for easing stiffness, numbness, or contortion of any place of the human body. Based on the texts, however, it is not possible to decide clearly whether they are cases concerning *metu* in the meaning of tubes (blood vessels), which will be discussed in the following section, or whether they were longitudinal connective structures without a lumen, for example muscles, tendons, or ligaments that make up the motion system of the body. Although a closer determination on which structure was involved is lacking with these prescriptions, they were apparently mainly muscles and tendons, afflicted by exhaustion from strain or overload. In the texts, a localization of the problem is also lacking, which is replaced by only a neutral command "place on it," which complicates today's evaluation of the effect of the medicinal means used.

Stiffness or Soreness
Stiffness or soreness of the connective structures could happen acutely, as in shooting pain of the back nerves (lumbago), or a painful inflammation of the sciatic nerve, including sciatica, or developed over a longer period (chronically)

after an injury, as today after an operational immobilization, or in some degenerative disease. In one case, the medicine was a mixture administered orally, whereas all of the other preparations had the form of an ointment and compress on the painful place.

Ebers 630—remobilization
This prescription is intended to assure movement without a reference to a specific part of the human body. A barley cake was to help with peas and wild rue, which were mixed in the same amount of 15 ml each. This medicine was surprisingly not eaten, but was applied on the affected place.

Ebers 695—remobilization
Another preparation was recommended for assuring movement of any part of the body, or rather any limb. It comprised equal amounts (15 ml) of mint, *shasha* fruit, sculptor's clay, wax, and oil. The mixture was to be cooked, strained, and administered for four days as a medicinal beverage.

Hearst 142—remobilization of anything
This case is a parallel to the prescription Ebers 695, but it differs in the wording of the heading.

Ebers 690-92—easing
The unspecified easing was to be achieved by the placement of a mixture of equal amounts (15 ml) of cedar resin, natron, sea salt, and beer sediments. Cedar resin acts as an antiseptic, and natron with sea salt certainly had an osmotic effect (Eb 690). Other times, a cooked mixture was used of equal amounts (15 ml) of honey, oil, and fresh *tepaut* (perhaps part of the juniper?) (Eb 692), or a cooked mixture of the same amount (15 ml) of honey, sea salt, and donkey feces (Eb 691), which could be beneficial thanks to the antibacterial honey, but the admixture of donkey feces apparently acted mainly magically.

Ebers 638-41—easing
This group of cases describes the preparation of various aromatic ointments which were to help in easing of any kind of thing, hence apparently of any extremity. The first case from this group belongs rather to the easing of the blood vessels and is described in the relevant section below on page 317

For instance, a mixture of equal amounts (15 ml) of honey, fresh dates, the *wam* plant, and beef fat (Eb 641), or of honey, sediments of sweet beer, the *git* plant, and catfish meat (Eb 639) was to be applied on the affected place for four days. There was a greater number of ingredients in a medicinal mixture of equal amounts (15 ml) of carob, *Melilotus*, beans, *pesedj* fruit, the *tjun* plant, fresh seeds of an unknown plant, white oil, natron, red clay, pumice, the *khau* of copper, the *seska* substance, and the sediments of the *sedjer* drink, ibex fat, and donkey feces. The ingredients were to be thoroughly mixed and the remedy was to be used as an ointment (Eb 640). A mixture of equal amounts (15 ml) of honey, incense, natron, red ocher, the *seshu* stone, sea salt, faïence, copper beads, and ibex fat (Eb 638) was made without any plant ingredients and, like the majority of the others, was to be smeared on the body repeatedly for a period of four days.

Ebers 658—easing soreness
Another instruction for the preparation of an aromatic ointment contained 15 ml each of pork lard and fat from a tomcat, snake, mouse, and an animal called an *ibtjersu*. The usage of more types of animal fat might have been to assure the greater effectiveness of the mixture.

Ebers 635—easing soreness
According to this simple instruction, fatty beef meat was recommended to be applied on the affected place in the case of soreness of any part of the body. It was most likely more easily accessible than the types of animal fat described above.

Ebers 656—easing the stiffness of any extremity
Another prescription combines animal fats with other ingredients. They were to mix equal amounts (15 ml) of sweet myrrh, beans, honey, natron, incense, oil from the second day, and the fat of a hippopotamus, crocodile, catfish, and red mullet. The mixture was to be cooked and applied as a compress.

Ramesseum V.2—easing any kind of stiffness
We find a parallel to the previous prescription in the Ramesseum Papyri. It is a prescription for the preparation of a mixture of equal amounts (15 ml) of myrrh, beans, the *tjun* plant, honey, natron, incense, wax, white oil, and the fat of a hippopotamus, crocodile, catfish, and mullet. After cooking, this mixture was to be applied on the affected area of the patient's body until he was visibly relieved.

Ramesseum V.16—easing stiffness
Another prescription for the same problems, without specification of the affected area of the body, included 15 ml each of the *anenu* tree fruit, sweet

myrrh, and cedar resin, and the same amount of various types of oils and animal fats: white and cedar oils *(sefetj)*, goose fat, and hippopotamus, donkey, ibex, and beef fat. The ingredients were mixed and cooked, and the ointment was applied for a period of four days.

Ebers 664-69—easing the stiffness of any place of the body

In the Ebers Papyrus we also find an extensive group of prescriptions for preparations which were to help ease stiffness in various parts of the human body. They included a mixture of equal amounts (15 ml) of honey, the *git* plant, and fresh beef meat, which was smeared on the affected place (Eb 664). Other times, an ointment was used from the same amount (15 ml) of bryony, emmer wheat, peas, sea salt, and beef spleen (Eb 666), or the same amount of *Potentilla*, the *tia* plant, *Potamogeton* from Upper Egypt, and *Potamogeton* from Lower Egypt, and red ocher (Eb 669).

The basis of other mixtures comprised date purée, which was mixed with equal amounts (15 ml) of the unknown *seska* substance and beef spleen (Eb 665), carob, the *sar* plant, sea salt, honey, and wax (Eb 667), or *Melilotus*, sea salt, natron, and the unknown substance *djat* (Eb 668).

Ebers 670-74—easing the stiffness of any place of the body

Another group of prescriptions for the same problems contained a simple preparation produced from equal amounts (15 ml) of date juice, sea salt, and sediments of beer or wine, which was boiled and applied on the stiff place (Eb 674). A more complex variation was a cooked mixture of the same amount (15 ml) of date juice, figs, *Melilotus*, the seeds of an unknown plant, *shenfet* fruit, and the *seska* substance, sea salt, natron, wine sediments, beef fat, the unknown substance *djat,* and donkey feces (Eb 670), which could act predominantly magically because of the unattractive ingredient.

Other times, a mixture could be used of the same amount (15 ml) of myrtle, beans, incense, and beef fat (Eb 672), or a remedy of the same amount (15 ml) of carob, beans, the *tjun* plant, *pesedj* fruit, honey, and oil (Eb 671). Another prescription in the group was a more complicated combination of the same amount (15 ml) of carob, beans, myrtle, *pesedj* fruit, the *shepes* plant, honey, sea salt, incense, gum, red ocher, hematite, cuttlefish bones, and black flint (Eb 673). These three means were thoroughly ground and then applied on the affected place.

Ebers 675-80—easing the stiffness of any place of the body

Another possibility of compresses and ointments against stiffness was provided by a cooked mixture of equal amounts (15 ml) of carob, chaste tree, mint, juniper berries, yellow nutsedge, celery seeds, *Anacyclus* seeds, flour from the *amaa* grain, cedar resin, honey, wax, oil, incense, ocher, the *peshnet* stone, and the strong beer *djesret* (Eb 675). A simpler version without cooking was a medicine of the same amount (15 ml) of chaste tree, yellow nutsedge, celery seeds, coriander seeds, the plants *ibu* and *djesret*, camphor, malachite powder, and hippopotamus fat (Eb 677). Other times the remedy was to be cooked with 15 ml of date juice with the same amount of *shenfet* fruit, and the *seska* substance, sea salt, honey, natron, beef fat, and sediments of beer or wine (Eb 680).

It was also possible to mix the same amount (15 ml) of each of sycomore fruit, sea salt, gypsum, and sweet beer (Eb 676), or 15 ml of sycomore fruit, beans, *pesedj* fruit, the *shepes* plant, and an herbal decoction with the wings of the animal *inhennet*, which could be some type of insect or bird (Eb 678). Following another prescription, a mixture was prepared of 15 ml each of onion, sweet myrrh, *shasha* fruit, resinous balls of juniper, cedar oil, white oil, goose fat, ibex fat, and wax (Eb 679). All of these medicines were applied on the stiff place of the body.

Contortion
A contortion of the body or its part developed chronically, for example on the spine from poor posture of the body (scoliosis) or gerontic folding of the chest (kyphosis), or the influence of some diseases, such as Scheuermann's, vitamin D deficiency (rachitis, rickets), or tuberculosis of the spine (Pott's disease). Unlike the easing of stiffness, the easing or correction of contortion was hardly successful.

Ebers 689—correction of contortion and easing stiffness
This prescription was intended for easing stiffness and correcting contortion. The text does not specify the affected areas of the body or describe in more detail the manifestations and causes of these problems. A compress was to help made from the same amount (15 ml) each of date juice, wild rue, sea salt, oil, natron, and mud.

Ramesseum V.3—easing stiffness and stretching of contortion
An analogous problem can be found in the Ramesseum Papyri, but it is a much more complex prescription for a medicinal mixture of various types of oils and fats. For the remedy, the same amount (15 ml) was used of each of wax, *Moringa* oil, oil from earth almonds, white oil, and cedar oil *(sefetj)*, further the fat of a mouse, lizard, snake, donkey, hippopotamus, lion, crocodile, the

unknown animal *pertjersu,* and centipede. The mixture was to be cooked and used as an ointment every day until the complete healing of the sick person. Considering the ingredients coming from dangerous species of animals, it is a question how accessible such a medicinal mixture would have been.

Ramesseum V.4 –V.11—the same?

The following prescriptions do not have the headings preserved, but we can assume with great likelihood that they were entitled as "a different" or "another" preparation and concerned the same health problem: stiffness and contortion, but we cannot rule out that they concerned also other health problems, such as soreness. They are prescriptions whose wording has been preserved for us only partially, so that some of the names of the ingredients have been lost today.

The simple remedies included a mixture of the same amount (15 ml) each of oil, wax, and the *khentet* product of incense, which was first cooked and then applied repeatedly until the (questionable) healing of the sick person (Ram V.11). Another prescription for the preparation of a similar medicine for long-term administration included originally at least thirteen ingredients, but only a small part of them have been preserved. Besides the lost ingredients, this medicine contained 15 ml each of celery, *maa* plant seeds, the *qesenty* stone, salt, and beef fat; it was also cooked before application (Ram V.8).

Another medicinal mixture comprised sweet myrrh, onion, bryony, peas, wild rue seeds, *djabut* fruit, beef fat, wine sediment, and the *sia* stone from the north, each again in the amount of 15 ml. This mixture was first to be cooked, then applied on the affected place and exposed to the sun to be warmed (Ram V.5). This case is a parallel to cases Ebers 657 and Hearst 94.

Another cooked mixture included 15 ml each of dates, *Anacyclus* fruit, and clay and was to be applied as a compress for four days (Ram V.7). Of the other prescription, only small fragments have been preserved, mentioning the amount (15 ml) of each of the *tjun* plant, the same amount of some part of the catfish, and also a four-day application of the compress (Ram V.6).

Other times, 15 ml each of peas, the *ama* part of wheat, hematite, wax, pumice, and at least two more, lost ingredients were mixed and cooked (Ram V.9). With the last two prescriptions in this group, neither the method of preparation nor the length or frequency of the application has been preserved. They were mixtures of the same amount (15 ml) each of dates, wild rue, natron, sea salt, and beer sediments (Ram V.4), and the same amount of wheat semolina, red ocher, hematite, wax, and bull spleen (Ram V.10).

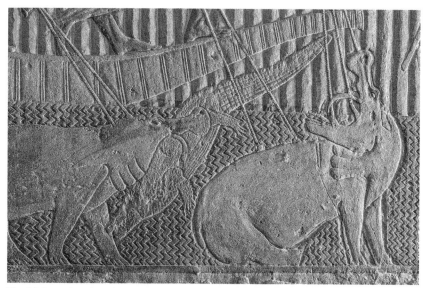

Fig. 35. In ancient times hippopotamuses and crocodiles lived in the Nile in Egypt and threatened not only the population of its banks but also one another; the reliefs in Egyptian tombs capture the dramas of the battles, with crocodiles on the lookout for hippopotamus young or, on the contrary, hippopotamuses mauling crocodiles (Fifth Dynasty, tomb of Ty in Saqqara, photo © Archive of the Czech Institute of Egyptology, Faculty of Arts, Charles University, Martin Frouz)

Ramesseum V.15—easing contortion

According to another prescription in the same text, the easing of contortion was to be made possible by a mixture of the same amount (15 ml) of each of sweet myrrh, ocher, red ocher, natron, sea salt, copper beads, honey, and ibex fat. The mixture was to be cooked and applied on the affected place, which is not specified.

Non-Arterial Blood Vessels (Veins)

Unfortunately, the term *metu* had many meanings in the anatomy of ancient Egyptian physicians. It included primarily the tube-like formations such as blood vessels, the urethras, Fallopian tubes, and ejaculatory ducts, but besides those also muscles, tendons, and ligaments. With the blood vessels, physicians then did not distinguish between arteries and veins, so that they could not work to a revelation of blood circulation. However, their knowledge that in some *metu* "the heart speaks" (Eb 854a, see also page 181) allowed us to separate them from other *metu*, along with the heart-pulsing arteries, which we dealt with above on pages 181–85. We translate the other *metu*—if they are not distinguished by context from the elongated formations without a lumen (discussed in the previous section)—with the superior term "vessels," but sometimes the context indicates that these can be considered "non-arterial" vessels, hence veins.

Prescriptions devoted to blood vessels and veins are numerously represented in the Ebers and Hearst Papyri and also in the Berlin Papyrus. We even find some in more than one papyrus.

Strengthening the State of the Veins

A number of prescriptions recorded in the medical texts are devoted to blood vessels generally, particularly their revival, strengthening, or the improvement of their condition. In these cases, the location is usually not presented, or the texts mention that they are vessels in any place in the body. The recommended medicines include predominantly compresses and aromatic ointments.

Ebers 686—strengthening of the blood vessels

The blood vessels were also to be strengthened by their being smeared with a mixture of equal amounts (15 ml) of juniper berries, bryony fruit, cumin, beef fat, incense, camphor, and wax. It was a pleasant aromatic ointment which, thanks to camphor, helped blood circulation and against possible inflammatory conditions.

Ebers 627–29—strengthening of the blood vessels, improvement of the state of the blood vessels

A group of three cases in the Ebers Papyrus was, according to its heading, a component of the "Collection of ointments" which were to benefit the blood vessels. They are prescriptions intended for the improvement of the state of the blood vessels generally, without stipulating a certain bodily region or indication. The first medicinal remedy comprised the equal amount (15 ml) of tomcat fat, petrified wood, and resin of the *ikeru* tree (Eb 627). Another prescription recommended a mixture of the same amount of coriander seeds, the unknown *seska* substance, and the leather for the production of sandals, which had to be thoroughly ground and then mixed (Eb 628). According to the last prescription, it was enough to smear a certain place with 15 ml of snake fat (Eb 629). All of these means acted most likely magically, although snake fat is sometimes recommended for improvement of the condition of skin for its supposed regenerative characteristics.

Hearst 96–98—improvement of the state of the blood vessels

This group of prescriptions contains parallels to the cases Ebers 627 and 628, but their wording is not entirely identical and they are listed under a joint heading, which includes them among the means for the improvement of the state of the blood vessels.

Ebers 651 and 653—improvement of the state of the blood vessels
Generally, a preparation was used for the improvement of the state of the blood vessels made from the same amount (15 ml) of each of the chaste tree, pine nuts, honey, wax, beef fat, galenite, cuttlefish bones, and mud. Before application of the mixture, the determined place wherever on the body was to be first smeared with myrrh (Eb 651). Another ointment for the same purpose comprised a mixture of the same amount (15 ml) of coriander and *tenti* plant seeds, laudanum, and the highest quality incense. It was intended for long-term use, literally for "many and many days" (Eb 653).

Hearst 102-103—improvement of the state of the blood vessels
A prescription for a medicine generally beneficial to vessels describes a mixture of the twigs of tamarisk and the *wam* plant in equal amounts (15 ml), which was to be applied on the blood vessels (H 102). A more complicated mixture was made from the same amount (15 ml) of dates and the *hemu* part of *Ricinus*, further 1 ml of honey, 2 ml of incense, and 600 ml of juniper berries. The amount of juniper is striking and it is possible that the scribe here erroneously wrote down 1/16 of a measure instead of 1/16 *ro*, which would correspond to 2 ml of this spice. This mixture was also applied on a stipulated place after mixing (H 103).

Hearst 237—improvement of the state of the blood vessels
According to another prescription for the improvement of the state of the blood vessels, a suitable remedy was made from equal amounts (15 ml) of sweet myrrh, garlic, bryony fruit, leek fruit, wine sediments, fat, fresh incense, the *sia* stone from the south, and the soot removed from the wall. The ingredients were mixed and boiled; the mixture was then applied to the appropriate blood vessel.

Hearst 228-31—improvement of the state of the blood vessels in any extremity
Another group for blood vessels in any limb or even part of the body included some more prescriptions. They were medicines from equal amounts of myrtle, bryony, yellow nutsedge, pine nuts, coriander seeds, the *sar* plant fruit, camphor, galenite, wax, and fat. The mixture was to be cooked and applied on the specified place, which was smeared with myrrh first (H 228). Another prescription included 15 ml each of myrrh, fine myrrh oil, wild mint, incense, galenite, calamine, wax, goose fat, red clay, and honey. It was recommended that this

aromatic ointment be cooked and applied repeatedly until healing was complete (H 229).

A simpler variation of the medicinal ointment contained 15 ml each of sorghum, camphor, natron, incense, and honey, which after cooking was spread on the sick vessel (H 230). Such a mixture could act osmotically, support the blood supply, and ease an inflammation. Another medicinal ointment cooked from the same amount (15 ml) of myrrh, wild mint, incense, galenite, wax, fat, and hematite was used for a period of four days (H 231).

Berlin 51—improvement and perfection of the condition of the blood vessels

According to the Berlin Papyrus, a common means for blood vessels was a mixture of myrtle, myrrh, garlic, a powder from the *bay* fruit, sweet *Moringa* oil, honey, and incense, which was mixed in wine. This medicinal ointment was to be applied to the vessels for a period of four days. The text does not state the precise amounts and ratio of the ingredients.

Hearst 122—revival of the blood vessels

To revive the blood vessels, a mixture was used made from myrrh, pine nuts, the unknown *shabet* plant, and incense. The ingredients, whose recommended amounts are not listed in the text, were mixed and applied to the stipulated place of the body.

Ebers 652—revival and revitalization of the blood vessels

A mixture serving for the revival and revitalization of the blood vessels was made from the same amount (15 ml) each of coriander seeds, sawdust of the camphor and cedar trees, cedar oil, wax, resin, incense, and pork lard and beef fat. The mixture first had to be cooked and then applied to the affected place after a previous smearing of the veins with myrrh.

Hearst 101—revival and refreshing of the blood vessels

This case in the Hearst Papyrus is a parallel to case Ebers 652 and contains a prescription for a remedy which included coriander seeds, sawdust of the camphor and cedar trees, cedar oil, wax, resin, incense, and beef fat. The method of preparation and method of application remained the same, but the amounts of the ingredients used are not presented in this version, and the scribe left out pork lard.

Ebers 642–43—preparation for the blood vessels to accept a medicine

According to the heading, these prescriptions are intended to help the blood vessels accept the medicinal mixture. The specified place could be smeared with a mixture of date purée and beer sediments (Eb 643). A more sophisticated method required the application of sour human milk. It was to be the milk of the mother of a male offspring, which is left to stand and curdle in a new *hin* vessel. Such a medicine worked on any painful place of the body (Eb 642). It was a magical remedy, which most likely referred to the milk of the goddess Isis, mother of Horus.

Hearst 111–12—preparation for the blood vessels to accept a medicine

These prescriptions are a parallel of the previous cases Ebers 642 and 643. It recommends mixing the milk of a mother of a male offspring with sea salt and leaving it overnight to curdle in a new *hin* vessel (H 111). Other times, the product *pekhekh* of date purée was mixed with beer sediment (H 112). Both remedies could be used on any painful place of the body.

Overall Diseases of the Veins

Ebers 687—easing of the blood vessels

For the general calming of the blood vessels, an ointment was prepared from equal amounts (15 ml) of dried myrrh, sweet *Moringa* oil, camphor, wax, incense, galenite, and beef fat. It was intended to be applied for a period of four days. This mixture could act antiseptically and as an anti-inflammatory, help the blood supply, and assist in rheumatic problems.

Ebers 637—easing of the blood vessels

In the group of prescriptions for the easing "of everything," which was described above on pages 308–309, a remedy was also included from the same amount (15 ml) each of myrrh, ocher, red clay, gum, wax, and beef fat. The mixture was to be applied to vessels heated by the sun (Eb 637). The specific method of application suggests that it was a prescription intended for curing the blood vessels.

Ebers 649—easing of the blood vessels

A prescription in the Ebers Papyrus for a general, further unspecified easing of the blood vessels, apparently improving their condition, comprised equal amounts (15 ml) of myrtle, yellow nutsedge, pine nuts, coriander and bryony seeds, *sar* plant seeds, fresh incense, wax, galenite, and beef fat. After cooking, it could be applied to the blood vessel, which was smeared with myrrh before that. This preparation is very similar to the prescription in Hearst 228 for improvement of the state of the blood vessels (see above, page 315), but it is not identical to it.

Ebers 657—easing of the blood vessels

Another preparation for the same problems comprised equal amounts (15 ml) of myrrh, onion, peas, bryony fruit, wild rue seeds, the *sia* stone from Upper Egypt, incense, beef fat, wine sediments, and soot from the wall. The last-mentioned ingredient apparently acted magically. The mixture was to be smeared on the relevant part of the body, which was warmed in the sun before that.

Hearst 94—easing of the blood vessels, improvement of pain

This case is a parallel to the previous prescription, but its heading is more informative. Case Ramesseum V.5 is also similar, which belongs to the entire group of prescriptions for pain (page 312).

Ebers 688—easing of the blood vessels

Another remedy for smearing comprised equal amounts (15 ml) of sweet myrrh, date flour, cedar sawdust, and oil, which was used by a spinner (of yarn, cloth). After cooking, this mixture was applied to the sick vessel for a period of four days.

Hearst 232—easing of the blood vessels in any extremity

In the Hearst Papyrus, we find another remedy for which were used 15 ml each of sweet myrrh, dried myrrh, yellow nutsedge, incense, wax, galenite, hematite, and goose fat. This cooked mixture was spread on the affected place for a period of four days.

Hearst 100 and 104–109—quietening of the blood vessels

Another group of prescriptions was intended for quietening of the blood vessels. Neither the symptoms of the disease nor their cause is explained in the texts. Only one case from this group stipulates the amount of the ingredients, namely a prescription for a mixture of equal amounts (15 ml) of the fruits of the sycamore, bryony, the *ibu* plant, and sea salt, which were mashed with an unspecified amount of wheat flour (H 100).

The other cases do not present the amounts of the ingredients. A coating with a cooked mixture of sorghum, wheat flour, and six-row barley (H 105) or sweet myrrh, wild mint, wax, incense, hematite, galenite, and beef fat could help (H 109).

Other times, a mixture was used of myrrh, wild mint, *pesedj* fruit, honey, oil, incense, calamine, and red clay, which was applied on the intended place (H 104). The other mixtures contained sorghum with honey, camphor, incense, and sea salt (H 108), or cumin, the "great protection" stone, and the unknown substance *seska* (H 106). An ointment from myrtle, yellow nutsedge, coriander seeds, and bryony fruit, pine nuts, wax, fresh incense, and galenite was applied after a previous coating of the relevant place with myrrh (H 107).

Special Diseases of the Veins
Ebers 644–46—protruding blood vessel
The heading of this group of cases refers to a blood vessel which protruded on whatever place of the body. It was apparently the surfacing of an expanded vein from under the skin or the emergence of a varicose vein (varix) on the lower leg (crus). Their result could be the emergence of leg ulcers (ulcus cruris). Egyptian physicians treated them by smearing with a mixture prepared from the same amount (15 ml) each of the product of honey fermentation, the *tjun* plant, and the *khesau* part of the *ima* tree (Eb 644). Our lack of knowledge of the meanings of these plants does not allow us to judge the effectiveness of this medicine. Other times, the same amount (15 ml) of *Moringa* oil, laudanum, honey, incense, beef meat, sea salt, and the unknown *seska* substance (Eb 646) were mixed, or the same amount of wheat semolina, ibex fat, beef meat, and brain or innards, sea salt, and hematite (Eb 645).

Hearst 99—protruding blood vessel
It is a parallel to case Ebers 644. The wording of the prescription is not entirely the same; moreover, in the conclusion the painfulness of the protruding veins is indicated.

Ebers 681–83—protruding blood vessel on any place of the body
This group of cases comprised prescriptions intended for a protruding blood vessel anywhere on the body, according to which compresses were prepared. It was recommended, for instance, to place a heated lump of pomace and a fermented herbal decoction on the affected place (Eb 681). Other times, a medicinal mixture was cooked from equal amounts (15 ml) of the sediments of sweet beer and sycomore fruit (Eb 683). It was more complicated to prepare a mixture of the same amount (15 ml) of celery, yellow nutsedge, bryony fruit, the *hepat* plant, starch from barley malt, cedar resin, incense, the unknown substance *seska,* and the unknown *nehet* stone. The mixture was to be cooked and applied as a compress (Eb 682).

Ramesseum V.17—easing a knotted blood vessel
For easing a knotted blood vessel (which we can evidently interpret as contorted varicose veins), a medicinal mixture was prescribed in one of the

Ramesseum Papyri made from the same amount (15 ml) each of beans, the *tjun* plant, *pesedj* fruit, gum, red ocher, hematite, black flint, sea salt, and honey. The ingredients were thoroughly crushed and mixed; the mixture was to be applied for a period of four days.

Ramesseum V.18—easing blood vessels
This case follows the previous one, but its heading does not mention whether it is again a knotted vein (which is likely), where it refers to "easing." Moreover, the composition differs significantly. It was a mixture of equal amounts (15 ml) of date seeds, emmer wheat, incense, beef fat, tongue, spleen, and marrow. The mixture was applied to the relevant blood vessel for four days.

Hearst 113—driving away swelling of the blood vessel
In several texts, we find a group of remedies against venous swelling. Such swelling is created either against the flow of the deoxygenated venous blood (distally) under the expanded veins (varices), or as a consequence of the weakening power of the right half of the heart during venous return, first around the ankles and progressively upwards along the calf. The medicinal mixtures were applied by coating or placement on the affected place. The Hearst Papyrus recommends smearing the sick vein with a mixture of oil and celery.

Ebers 659-61—easing the swelling of a blood vessel
In contrast, the Ebers Papyrus refers to a more complicated healing ointment on venous swelling called *shut*. Here, we find a medicine from the same amount (15 ml) each of myrtle, beans, incense, beef spleen, and fat (Eb 659). Other times, a part (15 ml) each of carob, onion, watermelon, the substance *seska*, honey, sea salt, ibex fat, beef meat, and hematite were mixed (Eb 660), or the same share of coriander seeds, dates, and "male" clay (Eb 661).

Berlin 49—easing a blood vessel (?)
A parallel to the above-presented case Ebers 659 is this case from the Berlin Papyrus. It has been preserved only incompletely, and a part of its heading and a part of the prescription itself have been damaged. The preserved ingredients include myrtle, beans, incense, and beef spleen, from which the compress was to be prepared after cooking.

Ebers 662—mitigating the tremor of a blood vessel
This case is devoted to the tremor of a vein. The tremor or shaking of the vein

is not a commonly observable symptom; rather it could be an internal feeling or idea. For calming such a tremor, the Ebers Papyrus recommended a mixture of the same amount (15 ml) each of dried date juice, sea salt, sediments of sweet beer, and freshwater mussels called *djat*.

Hearst 120—calming the tremor of a blood vessel
We find a parallel in the Hearst Papyrus, but the wording of the cases is not entirely the same. The amounts and ratios of the ingredients here are not specified, and the recommended mixture contains also six-row barley, which does not appear in the version from the Ebers Papyrus.

Berlin 174–78—quivering of the blood vessel, pain when walking, painful substances
There is an interesting group of cases related to pain when walking, which are put into the context with the quivering of the blood vessel and the painful substances *wekhedu*. According to the Berlin Papyrus, the means against these problems were applied in the form of an enema. That could indicate that they were blood vessels directly in the rectum, and it can be noticed that the ingredients presented in the medicinal mixtures in this case are somewhat similar to those that we find in the prescriptions for treating the rectum (see pages 248–63).

According to one instruction, two types of enema were to be prepared. First, an enema was applied for four days made from 75 ml of *Moringa* oil and the same amount of oil and sweet beer with 1.2 l of honey, and 1 ml sea salt. The next four days, the sick person was to continue with a simpler mixture in a different ratio of 1.2 l of *Moringa* oil and honey with 75 ml of sweet beer (Bln 174). Another remedy contained 112.5 ml of fennel water solution, 75 ml of sweet beer, and 37.5 ml each of honey and *Moringa* oil, which were mixed into a smooth concoction and applied for four days (Bln 175). Other times, 150 ml of carob juice was mixed with the same amount of sweet beer and 37.5 ml of honey (Bln 176), or 2 ml of *Moringa* oil, twice the amount of honey and sea salt, and 225 ml of the *debyt* beverage from a sweet date mash (Bln 177). All these medicinal enemas were to be used for four days.

Ebers 693—cooling of the blood vessels
A number of means with indications for the cooling of the blood vessels could be related to an acute inflammation of the surface veins. It could be relieved by an ointment prepared from equal amounts (15 ml) of peas, bryony, *pesedj* fruit, sea salt, and beef, and donkey and ram fats (Eb 693).

Hearst 121—cooling of the blood vessels

A parallel to the previous prescription is a preparation recommended in the Hearst Papyrus. However, ram fat is missing in the list of ingredients, and the amounts of the ingredients used are not specified.

Hearst 95 and 238—cooling of the blood vessels (in any extremity)

The Hearst Papyrus also recommends applying a plant remedy for four days made from a share (15 ml) of acacia, willow, and jujube leaves, leek, and sea salt. According to the heading, this remedy was suitable for application on any limb of the sick person (H 238). Another prescription contains a similar mixture from the same amount of acacia, willow, and jujube leaves, wild rue, garlic, and sea salt (H 95).

Hearst 249-51—cooling of the blood vessels

Another group of cases presents more means intended for the cooling of the blood vessels, but these parts of the text are poorly preserved. Several ingredients or instructions for the preparation and application have not been preserved. They were ointments containing equal parts (15 ml) of acacia leaves, flour from the *amam* grain, and other ingredients lost today (H 249), 15 ml each of date seeds, coriander seeds, sycomore leaves, and *ihy* tree leaves, natron, and the substance called *shebet* (H 250), or a mixture of the *tjun* plant, parts of the sycomore, fat, sweet beer, and salt (H 251).

Ramesseum V.12-13—cooling of the blood vessels and strengthening a weakness

Similar prescriptions in the Ramesseum Papyri recommend preparing an ointment from the same amount (15 ml) of acacia and jujube leaves and honey (Ram V.12), or from the same amount of acacia leaves, cedar sawdust, and beef fat (Ram V.13). Both remedies were mixed and applied as an ointment for a period of four days.

Ebers 694—stiffened blood vessel

A very simple preparation for a stiffened blood vessel contained 15 ml each of *Potamogeton* and the *niania* plant. This mixture was applied on the relevant place of the body. A stiff blood vessel could most likely be an artery affected by arteriosclerosis (see pages 199–200).

Hearst 110—stiffened blood vessel

We find a parallel to the previous prescription in the Hearst Papyrus. Both texts are copied almost word for word, with only slight differences. However, we do find in addition here a note that the application is to be repeated until the sick person is relieved.

Ebers 663—softening of the blood vessel

One of the longest prescriptions captured in the Ebers Papyrus is a prescription for a remedy intended for softening of the blood vessel (arteries rather than veins). For its preparation, more than thirty ingredients were necessary: myrrh, carob, fennel, beans, onion, watermelon, the *amaa* grain, the *tiu* and *ineb* plants, the *ibu* plant from the Delta, pine nuts, flax seeds, *sheny-ta* fruits, *shasha* and *pesedj* fruits, *ima* tree fruit, offshoots of the *git* plant, sawdust of cedar, willow, jujube, juniper, and fig, leaves of acacia, jujube, sycomore, and *ima* tree, white oil, goose fat, beef fat, pig feces, ocher, and red ocher, natron, and sea and mountain salts. This mixture is reminiscent of a list of the curative ingredients from the inventory of all the available medicines, which along with the inclusion of pig feces (!) reveals its magical character.

Hearst 37—against the bursting of blood vessels

This prescription describes a curative mixture which was to help against bursting of the blood vessels, explicitly in all the extremities of a man or woman. They were likely small hematomas from injured veins or capillaries in the subcutis from the influence of injuries or exertions. It was an ointment from crushed resin cooked in oil until soft.

Localized Diseases of the Veins

Some cases are related to blood vessels in some specific part of the body, which is then named in the text. We find here problems dedicated to the shoulder, knee, calf, and toes, but it remains an open question how to understand the problems of the blood vessels in these areas today and whether it really was about veins or in several cases rather about ligaments or tendons.

Ebers 650—calming of the blood vessels in the shoulder

The problems which the sick person suffered from in the shoulder are not explained in the text, but a mixture to improve the condition of his blood vessel was prepared from equal parts (15 ml) of sweet myrrh, yellow nutsedge, chaste tree, dill seeds, and the *ibu* plant seeds, *ished* fruits, cedar sawdust, starch from barley malt, incense, the unknown substance *seska,* and a heavy (literally male) herbal decoction, which was applied on the affected shoulder.

Ebers 634—easing the blood vessels in the knee

A prescription for blood vessels in the knee was significantly different. It contained the same amount (15 ml) each of celery, onion, the *heny-ta* plant, honey, oil, sea salt, beef and ibex fat, incense, natron, zinc, copper grains, and the *nehdet* stone. All of the ingredients were thoroughly ground, mixed, and applied on the knee.

Berlin 122—correction of the blood vessels of the calf and driving away swelling

The means against the swelling of the calf, which according to the physicians then had a relation with the blood vessels, was a mixture of carob flour, date juice, and honey. The amounts of the individual ingredients are not presented in the text. The mixture was applied on the sick person's calf.

Ebers 647—calming of the blood vessels of the toes

Other cases in the medical texts are associated with the blood vessels in the toes. It is, for instance, a remedy which needed the same amount (15 ml) of carob flour, powder from the *tjun* plant, powder from gum, acacia leaves, *Cynodon* root, wax, amber, beef fat, and honey. After cooking, the mixture was applied to the affected toes.

Hearst 116–19—improvement of the condition of the blood vessels of the toes

This group of cases was also related to the blood vessels of the toes. The first of these prescriptions is a parallel to case Ebers 647, but it records only a part and moreover without the amounts of the ingredients (H 116). The second two prescriptions are parallels to cases Ebers 660–61, which are, however, dedicated to easing swelling according to their heading, and we discuss them on page 000. They are mixtures of carob pod, watermelon, the substance *seska*, sea salt, hematite, beef meat, and ibex fat (H 117–18) and dates, coriander seeds, and "male" clay (H 119).

Berlin 50—the same?

It might be a parallel to cases Ebers 660 and Hearst 117 (Grapow 1958, 59). However, only the beginning is preserved from the text, mentioning onions as the first of the ingredients of the prescription; the following ingredients can be reconstructed (see also Westendorf 1999, 305).

Ebers 648—easing of the blood vessels of the toes

Besides the cases for improving the condition of the blood vessels, we also find a prescription for their easing. It was a preparation from equal amounts

(15 ml) of *amaa* grain of emmer and barley, which was scalded in 15 ml of oil. After cooking, the mixture was left to cool to body temperature and then was applied on the sick toes. According to the final note, this medicinal ointment was very effective, but our lack of knowledge of the *amaa* grains prevents us from judging its effectiveness.

Unknown Venous Diseases

Hearst 114–15—the *shut* disease of the blood vessels

According to the Hearst Papyrus, it was possible to ease the unknown venous disease called *shut* in Egyptian using a mixture prepared from wheat semolina, hematite, beef spleen, beef brain, and ibex fat (H 114). Other times, incense, sea salt, honey, the wings and body of the scarab beetle, and the unknown substance *seska* were used (H 115). The amount or ratio of the ingredients used is not stipulated in either prescription.

Ramesseum V.14, V.19–20—the venous *shut* disease

We find other means for the same problem in the fragments of the Ramesseum Papyri. It is recommended to mix the same amount (15 ml) of mint, sorghum, honey, wax, oil, and beef, goat, and sheep fat. This mixture was cooked and then applied on the sick blood vessel (Ram V.14). Other times, it was possible to use a curative ointment from the same amount (15 ml) of dates, onion, *pesedj* fruit, laudanum, incense, sea salt, goose fat, ibex fat, and other ingredients, which have not been preserved in the text (Ram V.19). The following case does not have a preserved heading, so it is not entirely clear whether it was another prescription for the same problem or a different type of medicine. It is a mixture of the same amount of carob, honey, wax, incense, beef fat, copper grains, and black flint (Ram V.20), which was cooked and applied on the body.

Ebers 684–85—the venous *shepet* disease

Another unknown venous disease was called *shepet*. It seems that it was not too severe, because the recommended means are rather simple. According to one set of instructions, it was sufficient to eat and properly chew yellow nutsedge and while doing so place the egg yolk of the pintail duck in the rectum (Eb 684). Other times, a mixture was applied of wild carrot, wax, and honey. The precise place of this application is, unfortunately, not listed in the text, just like the symptoms of the disease (Eb 685). The application of these means by mouth, rectum, and surface could indicate that the *shepet* disease was related to the final segment of the digestive tract.

Ramesseum III.B, I. 8–10—the *tepau* disease

The case of another unknown disease, *tepau*, was countered by applying on the body of the sick person, on the places of the manifestations of the disease, a salamander that was chopped and cooked in oil until soft. First, the medicine was applied only to one *tepa*, which indicated that it was some kind of manifesting center; it might have been scabs (Westendorf 1999, 142–43). If this *tepa* reacts to the medicine with heat, nothing more is to be done, and, if not, the medicine is to be applied also on the other *tepau*, namely repeatedly and in the long term. At the same time it was also recommended to fumigate the sick person. In this case, it was apparently an inflammatory disease, as is indicated by the mention of the heat of the *tepau* in reaction to the medicine given. Other authors present this case in connection with a general or unknown disease of the head (Westendorf 1999, 142–43).

Pain (Unlocalized) and an Illness (Unspecified)

We encountered pain as a frequent accompaniment of various closely specified or categorized illnesses in a number of the cases discussed. The pains are attributed here to the *wekhedu*, harmful substances, which according to the conceptions of that time caused painful conditions in the body. We encountered these substances above in the sections dedicated to various parts of the body, and we find them everywhere that the cause of the pain was not known to the Egyptian physicians. For the sake of completeness, pain without giving the places that hurt must be discussed with the recommendation of the means to alleviate or eliminate it. Some of these medicinal mixtures were applied as ointments or compresses, whereas others as medicinal beverages or enemas. It indicates that even in these general, unspecified cases, they were both external and internal problems.

Ebers 131—incantation of the substances causing pain

This lengthy treatise was to work against the substances causing pain, which supposedly were created from swelling. Although the medical texts contain a wide range of prescriptions for the preparation of medicines against the substances *wekhedu*, which are discussed above in the relevant sections, in this case the treatment is purely magical. The text contains not only the incantation itself, but also the instructions concerning how often it is necessary to recite which part of the text. The first part must be recited twice. It refers to a scroll with the text, which the author of the papyrus assures that he has not changed. It is thus apparently a text of a powerful magical nature, which was to help to relieve the sick person. The second part contains the incantation itself, which promises that until the sick person is better, the rituals will not be conducted in one of the most important cult centers of ancient Egypt, Abydos, and also the significant cult places of Mendes and Busiris will be destroyed. On the contrary, once the sick person is better, the exorcism is to be finished. The causes of the problems are not directly described in the text, but they are ascribed to all possible originators, including the gods, deceased people, evil demons, and evil substances, which are found in the body of the sick person. After the fourth recitation, the healer was to spit on the painful place. The efficacy of this method was claimed to have been proven a million times, which was certainly to increase the credibility of this incantation.

Ebers 121, 124, and 129—painful substances
In the Ebers Papyrus, a medicinal ointment is presented for the removal of the substances causing pain prepared from the same amount (15 ml) of sorghum, resin, laudanum, the unknown substance *seska*, honey, and fat, gum, balsam, ocher, and red ocher (Eb 121). Other times, a mixture was recommended made from the same amount (15 ml) of fresh *Moringa* oil, cedar oil, natron, and tortoise shell. This unguent was to be heated and applied still warm on the painful place (Eb 124). Another prescription recommended preparing a mixture of the same amount (15 ml) of wheat, barley, and sorghum flours, myrtle, and honey, which was also applied to the painful place (Eb 129).

Berlin 168—painful substances
Even in this case, the center of the pain is not specified, but the medicine was to be applied to the rectum as an enema for a period of four days. It could thus be problems connected with a disease of the abdomen, digestive, or excretory tracts (see pages 223–29 and 255–57). The recommended medicine was composed of the same amount (2 ml) each of fresh *Moringa* oil, honey, myrtle, and jujube leaves, a little bit of acacia leaves, and 375 ml of sweet beer. This mixture could act as an anti-inflammatory, antibacterial, and antiseptic agent.

Ebers 126-27—manifestations of the painful substances
Other means had the aim of removing the presumed seeds of the substances causing pain, which might have been weak or initial pains. Among these medicines we find a mixture containing 2 ml each of figs and *ished* fruit, and a quarter of the amount of wheat flat cakes and ocher, which were mixed in 375 ml of water. The mixture was then left overnight to stand exposed to the dew. It was used as a curative drink for a period of four days (Eb 126). Other

times, the same amount (15 ml) of carob, acacia leaves, and *aru* tree leaves, *shenfet* and *shasha* fruit, cow's milk, and ocher were mixed. This mixture was cooked and drunk for a period of four days. The method of the administration of these medicinal mixtures indicates that the seeds of the painful substances acted inside the body.

Ebers 584—painful substances in all extremities
In the case of the substances causing pain which were developed in all the limbs of a person, it could be unbounded pains. According to the Ebers Papyrus, a remedy was to help, whose composition reveals that it was a magical medicine. The mixture included the myrrh fruit, the *shamu* sediments, and disgusting dog and crocodile dung. Its application on the painful place, which is not stated in the text, was to remove the pain, which was accompanied apparently by swelling.

Hearst 41—painful substances in all extremities
We find a parallel to the previous case in the Hearst Papyrus. The wording of the two cases significantly differs overall, but the contents are the same.

Berlin 74—painful substances and all pains
The Berlin Papyrus recommended fumigation of pains of all types, namely with a mixture from myrtle and lichen (Bln 74). It is possible that this treatment was combined with other types of remedies recommended in other, more specifically aimed prescriptions.

Ramesseum III.A, l. 27—painful substances [. . .]
Of this case, only a small part of the heading written in red has been preserved. It was a prescription or incantation against the painful substances, but the place of the body where these substances plagued the person is not preserved in the text.

Besides unspecified pains, we also encounter in the preserved medical texts cases of an unspecified disease, possibly one whose meaning we do not know how to determine today.

Ebers 301—a disease in any place of the body
A preparation for the removal of further unidentified diseases, which could be found in any place of the human body, comprised a mixture of an infused and fermented herbal decoction. This medicine was to be applied on the affected place as an ointment or compress.

Ebers 625-26—quivering in any limb

These two cases follow after the prescriptions against the tremor of the fingers (se epages 301–305), but here the tremor affects any part of the body. However, the causes are not presented. Both prescriptions are accompanied by a call for the physician not to place a hand on the treated place and the medicines that covered them. That might have been from magical (or practical?) reasons. They were a mixture of the same amount (15 ml) each of sorghum, resin, verdigris, honey, and greyhound feces (Eb 625), and a cooked mixture from the same amount (15 ml) of sorghum, carob, and malachite (Eb 626). Both medicines were used for external application and their efficacy is difficult to judge, because the text does not reveal to us which problems the sick person suffered from.

Ebers 326-35—the extermination of the *gehu* disease

According to the heading of the first of these cases, a relatively lengthy part of the Ebers Papyrus is a "Collection of remedies for extermination of the *gehu* disease." Unfortunately, the meaning of this Egyptian expression is not known and the texts do not reveal anything on the nature of this illness or its manifestations or symptoms. It is therefore very difficult to compare the *gehu* disease with today's diagnostics. The group follows immediately after the means against a cough, but differs quite a lot from them. Specialists interpret the *gehu* disease diversely, for instance, as asthma (Ebbell 1924, 147–48; Westendorf 1999, 342) or a parasitic illness (Bardinet 1995, 178), but more often the expression is left untranslated as an unknown internal complaint, weakness, limpness, and tiredness (Westendorf 1999, 607–608; Hannig 1995, 905).

The prescriptions included the commonly prescribed ingredients of a plant origin, to which were added also animal fats (goose fat) and mineral raw materials. We do not know a large part of the ingredients because the meaning of the relevant Egyptian expressions is unclear, which further complicates the understanding of the given disease. The medicinal mixtures also contained solvents such as oil, wine, or beer. Some ingredients, such as the feces of animals or rotting meat, could work on the magical level.

The remedy against the *gehu* disease was prepared from 2 ml of *Moringa* oil, to which half the amount of freshwater mussels, the *hemut* stone, the feces of the *idu* bird, and unknown ingredients called in translation "divine falcon" were added. The ingredients were mixed with 75 ml of sweet beer (Eb 326). Another prescription contained equal amounts (2 ml) of figs, ripe sycomore fruits, grapes, *ished* fruit, and goose fat, half the amount of juniper berries, and an eighth of the amount of incense and cumin. All the ingredients were ground, mixed with 75 ml of beer, and half that amount of wine, and the resultant mixture was strained (Eb 327). Another case contains the instructions for the preparation of a mixture of 37.5 ml of fresh bread, 75 ml of oil, and the unknown *amau* fruits, 4 ml of sea salt, half the amount of juniper berries, and an eighth of the amount of ocher. It was all mixed and strained (Eb 328). In another prescription, we find a remedy from the same amount (2 ml) of onion, goose fat, the unknown *sheny-ta* fruit, the *tia* plant, the *hemut* stone, half that amount of strong beer, and 75 ml of rotting meat. The ingredients were simmered together and strained (Eb 330). It could be mixed also with equal amounts (1 ml) of wine, sea salt, ocher, and a stone which was called in translation "great protection," with 75 ml of strong beer. The mixture was to be strained (Eb 332).

Another preparation was to be made from equal amounts (2 ml) of celery, *sheny-ta* fruit, and the *pekhet-aa* fruit, half the amount of green reed, fresh bread, juniper berries, figs, and grapes, and an eighth of the amount of cumin. Then, 375 ml of strong beer and 37.5 ml of wine were added to that and the mixture was strained after a thorough mixing (Eb 334). For the same illness, the papyrus also recommended a mixture of 2 ml of juncus (reed), 0.5 ml of carob, and half the amount of incense, which were mixed in 75 ml of wine. The mixture was to be simmered and strained (Eb 329). All of these medicinal mixtures were to be used for a period of four days.

According to the recorded instructions, the other preparations included in this group were used for a shorter period. One such case describes the same mixture as the previous case Ebers 329. The recommended amounts of the individual ingredients are also identical except the different amount of wine, which was to be twice as much as the juncus (reed). The method of preparation remained the same, but the use was recommended for only one day (Eb 331). Beer, this time sweet, could be mixed with the feces of a crocodile and *wedja* part of the date, where each of these ingredients was to be used in the same amount (75 ml) (Eb 333). The admixture of crocodile dung was apparently a magically acting substance. A simple medicinal mixture could be prepared from 5 ml of wine with 4 ml of the strong beer *djesret* and 0.5 ml of honey, which was strained before use (Eb 335). Both of these remedies were to be used for only one day.

5

CONCLUSION

The internal cases from ancient Egyptian medical papyri as well as from two ostraca have provided insight into the medical theory and practice of the earliest medical system recorded in the literature. Unlike the almost entirely rational contents of the Edwin Smith Surgical Papyrus and several cases of "knife treatment" in the Ebers Papyrus (see Strouhal et al. 2014, 84–90), ancient Egyptian internal medicine can be considered a precursor to the empirical creation of a comprehensive compendium intended for the treatment of common as well as rare diseases. We are aware of the positives and negatives of the extant medical texts.

Physicians in ancient Egypt had not explored the inside of the human body enough to known the function of healthy organs, just like embalmers, who could not and did not want to deal with it in their coarse handiwork. The physicians could only infer human anatomy and physiology from the entrails of eviscerated animals and apply them to humans, mammals similar to the other mammals, of which ancient Egyptians were well aware (Strouhal 1994a, 117–18).

In many respects, the internal cases are incomplete, although only a few of them have been damaged over time. The headings of particular cases and prescriptions or their groups are brief, not always entirely clear, and only to a lesser extent diagnostic. They contain rather vague terms such as the removal of the symptoms of the disease (most likely the cure), relief (the improvement of the condition?), rectification (removal?), hotness which must be cooled (probably inflammation), or the shifting of the pain from one place to another in the body. The efforts to strengthen an organ, improve its function, or relieve pain seem to be more understandable. This unusual or metaphorical-sounding terminology used in Egyptian originals has not always been clearly deciphered. The cases contain only very few actual descriptions of symptoms, frequently only mere hints. The part of the body or organ to be treated is not always specified, so that numerous cases must be considered generally valid, especially in the cases where the heading is missing. Other times, there might have been confusions that make our understanding even more difficult, for instance between prescriptions for the treatment of heart and gastrointestinal tract diseases, which are sometimes surprisingly similar. Most of the cases of internal medicine that have been preserved in the Egyptian texts consist of only a prescription for the preparation of a medicinal remedy without any further explanation. This severely limits our understanding of the ideas and medical possibilities of the time.

The index of predominantly herbal remedies is extensive, but it does not show specific indications for particular groups of organs or disease symptoms. Their healing properties will be discussed in detail in the forthcoming third volume in this series. At this point, it can be stated that the remedies described in this volume in relation to internal medicine mirror the great empirical experience of ancient Egyptian physicians. On the one hand, the physicians obviously did not use chemical drugs and did not and could not know the cause of many internal problems, but among all the prescriptions directly concerning internal medicine, there are only very few of those that are purely magical. Incantations as such are not very frequent and definitely are not predominant in the texts, although they undoubtedly played a vital supportive role in the application of various medicines during the treatment.

It is remarkable that many recipes list very precise amounts of the ingredients used and their ratios. The mixtures were prepared exactly by weighing and measuring, and it was of utmost importance to observe the amount of ingredients, especially in the cases of the dangerous ones, such as henbane or bryony. The preparation of medicinal remedies was sometimes simple and the ingredients were only to be mixed and applied. Other times, however, the preparation required more steps, when the mixture was to be cooked first and then allowed to stand, and also strained or sieved if needed. Several cases demonstrate some procedures when one method was tried and then another step followed depending on whether the patient's condition had improved or not.

Our understanding and the possibility of evaluating the medicines are largely limited by the fact that there are numerous Egyptians names of ingredients that we cannot translate now. Therefore, it is impossible to determine the effectiveness of many of the mentioned mixtures. The benefits of some ingredients are indisputable, as in the cases of carob for digestion, camphor in medicinal ointments, various antiseptic or antibacterial ingredients, and many others. Even rather common food was frequently used—it could have significantly affected human health and the functioning of the internal organs. Even now, this issue is taken into account by many alternative methods of treatment, which often complement Western, rational medicine.

The presence of magically active ingredients from the *Dreckapotheke* ("filth pharmacy") sometimes discredits the rationality of the entire recipe. In many cases, however, it is not clear whether these names are to be taken literally or they could have designated some specific substances or herbal ingredients in the popular language. A severe deficiency is also the occurrence of too many disease symptoms and medicines that cannot be translated yet and thus contain still unrevealed secrets.

When we realize that the papyri (or their models) were composed four to five thousand years ago, their internal cases provide, despite all the objections expressed, unique evidence for the history of the creation of rational medicine, which grew empirically through the thorny path of discoveries and mistakes.

Egyptian medical papyri undoubtedly belong among rare, ancient literary texts on the verge of belles-lettres. They rightly deserve even this modern edition not only as scientific documents but also as literary forms. At the time when they were created and copied, the only competition they had was in the clay tablets with medical texts of the Mesopotamian physicians (for Mesopotamian medicine, see for instance Haussperger 2012).

BRIEF CHRONOLOGY
OF ANCIENT EGYPT

T he history of ancient Egypt today is divided into several periods that reflect the greater or lesser stability of the state. For each dynasty we present the brief characteristics and selected monuments. These dates are only approximate, with only events dating back to the first millennium BC being certain (Verner et al. 2007).

Predynastic Period (about 4500–3150 BC)
Early, Middle, and Late
Dynasty 0: process of unifying Egypt

Archaic Period (about 3150–2700 BC)
First Dynasty (about 3150–2930 BC)
Second Dynasty (about 2930–2700 BC)

Old Kingdom (about 2700–2180 BC)
Third Dynasty (about 2700–2630 BC): step pyramids (Djoser in Saqqara)
Fourth Dynasty (about 2630–2510 BC): centralized state, large pyramids in Meidum, Dahshur, Giza
Fifth Dynasty (about 2510–2365 BC): more modest pyramids in Abusir and Saqqara, sun temples
Sixth Dynasty (about 2365–2180 BC): pyramids in Saqqara, Pyramid Texts, gradual disintegration of the state structure

First Intermediate Period (about 2180–1994 BC)

Seventh Dynasty (about 2180–2170 BC): weakening of central power, development of local traditions

Eighth Dynasty (about 2170–2160 BC): development of local traditions

Ninth and Tenth Dynasties (about 2160–2137 BC): rulers based in Heracleopolis

Eleventh Dynasty (about 2137–1994 BC): rulers based in Thebes, unification of Egypt

Middle Kingdom (about 1994–1797 BC)

Twelfth Dynasty (about 1994–1797 BC): pyramids in Saqqara, Dahshur, Lisht, Lahun, Hawara

Second Intermediate Period (about 1797–1534 BC)

Thirteenth Dynasty (about 1797–1634 BC): gradual decline of central power

Fourteenth Dynasty: less important sovereigns ruling in the Delta

Fifteenth Dynasty (about 1634–1526 BC): Hyksos sovereigns ruling in the northern parts of the land

Sixteenth Dynasty: vassals of the Hyksos

Seventeenth Dynasty (about 1634–1543 BC): sovereigns based in Thebes and ruling in the southern parts of the land, unification of Egypt and expulsion of the Hyksos

New Kingdom (about 1543–1078 BC)

Eighteenth Dynasty (about 1543–1292 BC): expansive politics and the boom of diplomacy, rock-cut tombs in the Valley of the Kings, large temple complexes

Nineteenth Dynasty (about 1292–1186 BC): military expeditions, extensive construction activity

Twentieth Dynasty (about 1188–1078 BC): gradual decline of central power

Third Intermediate Period (about 1078–715 BC)

Twenty-first Dynasty (about 1078–945 BC): division of power between the rulers and high priests

Twenty-second Dynasty (945–715 BC): rulers of Libyan origin in Tanis and Bubastis

Twenty-third Dynasty (818–715 BC): rulers of Libyan origin in Leontopolis

Twenty-fourth Dynasty (728/727–720 BC): independent rulers in the western part of the Delta

Late Period (715–305 BC)

Twenty-fifth Dynasty (745–664 BC): rulers from Nubia

Twenty-sixth Dynasty (665–525 BC): return to Egyptian traditions, the so-called Saite Renaissance, Greek communities in Egypt

Twenty-seventh Dynasty (525–404 BC): first Persian rule

Twenty-eighth Dynasty (404–399 BC): the short reign of Pharaoh Amyrtaeus

Twenty-ninth Dynasty (399–380 BC): the shorter reigns of rulers, originally military commanders

Thirtieth Dynasty (380–343 BC): prosperity of the land, building on the traditions from the time of the Persian rulers, battles for the independence of Egypt

Thirty-first Dynasty (343–332 BC): second Persian rule

Alexander the Great and other Greek rulers, Wars of the Diadochi (332–305 BC)

Ptolemaic Period (305–30 BC)

Great influence of Greece on Egyptian culture, Alexandria as the center of education

Roman Period (30 BC–AD 395)

Byzantine Period (AD 395–640)

AD 640 conquest of Egypt by the Arabs

BIBLIOGRAPHY

el-Abbadi, M. 1992. *Life and Fate of the Ancient Library of Alexandria.* 2nd ed., Paris: UNESCO.

Abdelfattah, Alia, A.H. Allam, S. Wann, R.C Thompson, G. Abdel-Maksoud, I. Badr, H.A. Amer, A. Nur el-Din, C.E. Finch, M.I. Miyamoto, L. Sutherland, J.D. Sutherland, and G.S. Thomas. 2013. "Atheriosclerotic Cardiovascular Disease in Egyptian Women: 1570 BCE–2011 CE." *International Journal of Cardiology* 167/2: 570–74.

Allam, A.H., R.C. Thompson, L.S. Wann, M.I. Miyamoto, A. Nur el-Din, G.A. El-Maksoud, M.T. Soliman, I. Badr, H.A. Amer, M.L. Sutherland, J.D. Sutherland, G.S. Thomas. 2011. "Atherosclerosis in Ancient Egyptian Mummies. The Horus Study." *JACC: Cardiovascular Imaging* 4/4: 315–27.

Allen, J.P. 2005. *The Art of Medicine in Ancient Egypt.* New York: The Metropolitan Museum of Art.

Arias Kytnarová, K. 2017. "Social Dynamics in the Material Culture: Pottery of the Late Old Kingdom from the Complex of Princess Sheretnebty at Abusir South." PhD dissertation, Charles University.

———. Forthcoming. "Ceramic Finds." In M. Bárta and B. Vachala, *Abusir XXI. The Tomb of Inti.* Prague: Charles University, Faculty of Arts.

Bardinet, T. 1995. *Les papyrus médicaux de l'Égypte pharaonique.* Lyon: Fayard.

Bareš, L., K. Smoláriková, with contributions by R. Landgráfová, J. Janák, J. Dušek, J. Mynářová, J. Beneš. 2011. *Abusir XXV. The Shaft Tomb of Menekhibnekau I. Archaeology.* Prague: Charles University, Faculty of Arts.

Barns, W.B. 1956. *Five Ramesseum Papyri*. Oxford: Oxford University Press.

Birch, S. 1871. "Medical Papyrus (Brit.Mus. 10059) with the Name of Cheops." *Zeitschrift für ägyptische Sprache und Altertumskunde* 9: 61–64.

Borghouts, J.F. 1978. *Ancient Egyptian Magical Texts*. Religious Texts Translation Series NISABA 9. Leiden: Brill.

Breasted, J.H. 1930. *The Edwin Smith Surgical Papyrus*. Chicago: University of Chicago Press.

Brothwell, D.R. 1972. *Digging up Bones*. 2nd ed., London: British Museum Press.

Brugsch, H. 1862. *Recueil des monuments égyptiens. Deuxième partie*. Leipzig: J.C. Hinrichs.

———. 1863. *Notice raisonnée d'un traité médical datant du XIVme siècle avant notre ère et contenu dans un papyrus hiératique du Musée Royal (département des antiquités égyptiennes) de Berlin*. Leipzig: J.C. Hinrichs.

Bryan, C.P. 1930. *The Papyrus Ebers*. London: Geoffrey Bless.

Cockburn, A., R.A. Barraco, and T.A. Reyman. 1975. "Autopsy of an Egyptian Mummy." *Science* 187: 1155–60.

Cockburn, A., E. Cockburn, and T.A. Reyman. 1998. *Mummies, Disease and Ancient Cultures*. 2nd edition, Cambridge: Cambridge University Press.

Cockitt, J. and R. David (eds.) 2010. *Pharmacy and Medicine in Ancient Egypt. Proceedings of the Conferences Held in Cairo (2007) and Manchester (2008)*. BAR International Series 2114. Oxford: Archaeopress.

Contis, G. and R. David. 1996. "The Epidemiology of Bilharzia in Ancient Egypt: 5000 Years of Schistosomiasis." *Parasitology Today* 12/7: 253–55.

Dabernat, H. and É. Crubézy. 2010. "Multiple Bone Tuberculosis in a Child from Predynastic Upper Egypt (3200 BC)." *International Journal of Osteoarchaeology* 20: 719–30.

David, R., A. Kershaw, and A. Heagerty. 2010. "Atherosclerosis and Diet in Ancient Egypt." *The Lancet* 375/9716: 718–19.

Dawson, R.D. 1935. "Studies in the Egyptian Medical Texts V." *Journal of Egyptian Archaeology* 21: 37–40.

von Deines, H. and H. Grapow. 1959. *Wörterbuch der ägyptischen Drogennamen*. Grundriss der Medizin der alten Ägypter VI. Berlin: Akademie Verlag.

von Deines, H., H. Grapow, and W. Westendorf. 1958. *Übersetzung der medizinischen Texte*. Grundriss der Medizin der alten Ägypter IV/1–2. Berlin: Akademie Verlag.

von Deines, H. and W. Westendorf. 1957. *Zur ägyptischen Wortforschung V. Proben aus den Wörterbüchern zu den medizinischen Texten*. Abhandlungen der Deutschen Akademie der Wissenschaften zu Berlin. Berlin: Akademie Verlag.

————. 1961. *Wörterbuch der medizinischen Texte*. Grundriss der Medizin der alten Ägypter VII/1–2. Berlin: Akademie Verlag.

————. 1962. *Grammatik der medizinischen Texte*. Grundriss der Medizin der alten Ägypter VIII. Berlin: Akademie Verlag.

Diodorus of Sicily. 1933. *The Library of History, Book I–II*. London: William Heinemann Ltd..

Donoghue, H.D., O.Y.-C. Lee, D.E. Minnikin, G.S. Besra, J.H. Taylor, and M. Spigelman. 2010. "Tuberculosis in Dr Granville's Mummy: A Molecular Re-examination of the Earliest Known Egyptian Mummy to Be Scientifically Examined and Given a Medical Diagnosis." *Proceedings of the Royal Society B: Biological Sciences* 277: 51–56.

Dreyer, G. 1998. *Umm el-Qaab: Das prädynastische Königsgrab U-j und seine frühen Schriftzeugnisse*. Mainz: Philipp von Zabern.

Ebbell, B. 1924. "Die ägyptischen Krankheitsnamen I." *Zeitschrift für ägyptische Sprache und Altertumskunde* 59: 144–49.

————. 1927. "Die ägyptischen Krankheitsnamen IX. Epilepsie." *Zeitschrift für ägyptische Sprache und Altertumskunde* 62: 13–20.

————. 1937. *The Papyrus Ebers. The Greatest Egyptian Medical Document*. Copenhagen: Levin & Munksgaard.

————. 1939. *Die altägyptische Chirurgie. Die chirugische Abschnitte der Papyrus E. Smith und Papyrus Ebers*. Skrifter utgitt av Det Norske Videnkaps-Akademi i Oslo. II Hist.-Filos. Klasse No.2. Oslo: Dybward.

Ebers, G.M. 1875. *Papyros Ebers: Das hermetische Buch über die Arzneimittel der alten Ägypter in hieratischer Schrift I–II*. Leipzig: Engelmann.

Erman, A. 1890. *Die Märchen des Papyrus Westcar I–II*, Mitteilungen aus den Orientalistischen Sammlungen VI. Berlin: W. Spermann.

————. 1899. *Aus den Papyrus der Königlichen Museen*. Berlin: W. Spermann.

Erman, A. and H. Grapow. 1926–61. *Wörterbuch der aegyptischen Sprache*. Berlin: Akademie Verlag.

Fischer-Elfert, H.-W. 2005. *Papyrus Ebers und die antike Heilkunde. Akten der Tagung vom 15.–16. März 2002 in der Albertina /UB der Universität Leipzig*. Philippika 7. Wiesbaden: Harrassowitz.

Fukagawa, S. 2011. *Investigation into Dynamics of Ancient Egyptian Pharmacology: A Statistical Analysis of Papyrus Ebers and Cross-cultural Medical Thinking*. BAR International Series 2272. Oxford: Archaeopress.

Gardiner, A.H. 1935. *Hieratic Papyri in the British Museum III. Chester Beatty Gift*. London, British Museum Press.

————. 1955. *The Ramesseum Papyri*. Oxford: Oxford University Press.

————. 1957. *Egyptian Grammar Being an Introduction to the Study of Hieroglyphs*. 3rd ed., Oxford, London: Griffith Institute.

Germer, R. 1979. "Untersuchung über Arzneimittelpflanzen im Alten Ägypten." PhD diss., Hamburg University.

————. 1989. *Die Pflanzenmaterialien aus dem Grab des Tutanchamun*. Hildesheimer ägyptologische Beiträge 28. Hildesheim: Gerstenberg Verlag.

————. 1985. *Flora des pharaonischen Ägypten*. Deutsches archäologisches Institut Abteilung Kairo, Sonderschrift 14. Mainz am Rhein: Philipp von Zabern.

————. 2002. *Die Heilpflanzen der Ägypter*. Düsseldorf, Zürich: Artemis & Winkler.

————. 2008. *Handbuch der altägyptischen Heilpflanzen*. Philippika. Marburger altertumskundliche Abhandlungen 21. Wiesbaden: Harrassowitz.

Ghalioungui, P. 1987. *The Ebers Papyrus. A New English Translation, Commentaries and Glossaries*. Cairo: Academy of Scientific Research and Technology.

Goedicke, H. 1986. "Symbolische Zahlen." In *Lexikon der Ägyptologie IV*, edited by W. Helck and E. Otto, 128–29. Wiesbaden: Harrassowitz.

Granville, A.B. 1825. "An Essay on Egyptian Mummies, with Observations on the Art of Embalming amongst Ancient Egyptians." *Philosophical Transactions of the Royal Society* 115: 269–316.

Grapow, H. 1958. *Die medizinische Texte in hieroglyphischer Umschreibung autographiert*. Grundriss der Medizin der alten Ägypter V. Berlin: Akademie-Verlag.

Halioua, B. 2004. *Medicína v době faraonů. Lékaři, léčitelé, mágové a balzamovači*. Prague: Brána.

Hannig, R. 1995. *Großes Handwörterbuch Ägyptisch-Deutsch: die Sprache der Pharaonen (2800–950 v. Chr.)*. Mainz: Zabern.

Hannig, R., P. Vomberg, and O. Wittkuhn (eds.) 2007. *Marburger Treffen zur altägyptischen Medizin. Vorträge und Ergebrisse des 1.–5. Treffens 2002–2007*. Göttingen: Seminar für Ägyptologie und Koptologie.

Hart, G.D., N.B. Millet, D.F. Rideout, J.W. Scott, G.E. Lynn, T.A. Reyman, U. de Boni, R.A. Barraco, M.R. Zimmerman, P.K. Lewin, and P.D. Horne. 1977. "Autopsy of an Egyptian Mummy (Nakht-ROM I)." *Canadian Medical Association Journal* 117: 461–76.

Haussperger, M. 2012. *Die mesopotamische Medizin aus ärztlicher Sicht*. Baden-Baden: Deutscher Wissenschafts-Verlag (DWV).

Herodotus. 1972. *Dějiny aneb devět knih nazvaných Múzy I* (The Histories), translated by J. Šonka. Prague: Odeon.

Hibbs, A.C., W.E. Secor, D. Van Gerven, and G. Armelagos. 2011. "Irrigation and Infection: The Immunoepidemiology of Schistosomiasis in Ancient Nubia." *American Journal of Physical Anthropology* 145: 290–98.

Horne, P.D. 2002. "First Evidence of Enterobiasis in Ancient Egypt." *The Journal of Parasitology* 88: 1019–21.

Janák, J. 2005. *Brána nebes: bohové a démoni starého Egypta* [Gate of heaven: gods and demons of ancient Egypt]. Prague: Libri.

———. 2009. *Staroegyptské náboženství 1. Bohové na zemi a v nebesích* [Ancient Egyptian religion I: gods on earth and in the heavens]. Prague: OIKOYMENH.

———. 2012. *Staroegyptské náboženství 2. Život a úděl člověka* [Ancient Egyptian religion II: life and lot of a man]. Prague: OIKOYMENH.

Jírovec, O. 1954. *Parasitologie pro lékaře* [Parasitology for the physicians]. Prague: Státní zdravotnické nakladatelství.

Joachim, H. 1890. *Papyros Ebers: das älteste Buch über Heilkunde*, Berlin: Georg Reimer.

Jonckheere, F. 1944. *Une maladie égyptienne. L'hématurie parasitaire*. Brussels: Fondation Égyptologique Reine Élizabeth.

Jonckheere, F. 1947. *Le papyrus médical Chester Beatty*. Brussels: Fondation Égyptologique Reine Élizabeth.

Jonckheere, F. 1954. "Prescriptions médicales sur ostraca hiératiques." *Chronique d'Égypte* 29: 46–61.

Junker, H. 1928. "Die Stele des Hofarztes Irj." *Zeitschrift für ägyptische Sprache und Altertumskunde* 63: 53–70.

Korbelář, J. 1990. *Naše rostliny v lékařství* [Our plants in medicine]. Prague: Avicenum.

Kosack, W. 2011. *Der medizinische Papyrus Edwin Smith. The New York Academy of Medicine, Inv. 217. Neu in Hieroglyphen übertragen, übersetzt und bearbeitet*. Berlin: Christoph Brunner Verlag.

Krejčí, J. and D. Magdolen. 2005. *Zajímavosti ze země pyramid aneb 100 NEJ ze starého Egypta* [Interesting things from the land of the pyramids or 100 BEST from ancient Egypt]. Prague: Libri.

Leake, Ch.D. 1952. *The Old Egyptian Medical Papyri*. Lawrence: University of Kansas Press.

Lefebvre, G. 1956. *Essai sur la médecine égyptienne de l'époque pharaonique*, Paris: Presses Universitaires de France.

Leitz, Ch. 1999. *Hieratic Papyri in the British Museum VII. Magical and Medical Papyri of the New Kingdom*, London: British Museum Press.

Lexa, F. and A. Jirásek. 1941. "Papyrus Edwina Smitha" [The Edwin Smith Papyrus]. *Rozhledy v chirurgii* 20: 79–82, 107–109, 145–47, 169–72, 227–28, 286–90.

Manniche, L.1989. *An Ancient Egyptian Herbal*. rev. ed. London: British Museum Press.

———. 2000. *Starověký egyptský herbář* [An ancient Egyptian herbal]. Prague: Volvox Globator.

Massart, A. 1954. *The Leiden Magical Papyrus I 343 + I 345*. OMRO Supplement 34. Leiden: E.J. Brill.

Meyerhof, M. 1931. "Über den „Papyrus Edwin Smith", das älteste Chirurgiebuch der Welt." *Deutsche Zeitschrift für Chirurgie* 231: 645–90.

Miller, R.L. 1989. "*Dqr*, Spinning and Treatment of Guinea Worm in P. Ebers 875." *Journal of Egyptian Archaeology* 75: 249–54.

Miller, R.L., G.J. Armelagos, S. Ikram, N. Dejonge, F.W. Krijger, and A.M. Deelder. 1992. "Palaeoepidemiology of Schistosoma Infection in Mummies." *British Medical Journal* 304: 555–56.

Miller, R.L. 1994. "Ḏaajs, Peganum harmala L." *Bulletin de l'Institut français d'archéologie orientale* 94: 349–57.

Miller, R.L. and R.K. Ritner. 1994. "'Radiating' Symptoms of Gallstone Disease in Ancient Egypt." *Göttinger Miszellen* 141: 71–76.

Nunn, J.F. 1996. *Ancient Egyptian Medicine*. London: British Museum Press.

Nunn, J.F. and E. Tapp. 2000. "Tropical Diseases in Ancient Egypt." *Transactions of the Royal Society of Tropical Medicine and Hygiene* 94: 147–53.

Petrie, W.M.F. and J.E. Quibell. 1896. *Naqada and Ballas*. London: Quaritch.

Pinch, G. 1994. *Magic in Ancient Egypt*. London: British Museum Press.

———. 2010. *Magie ve starém Egyptě* [Magic in ancient Egypt]. Prague: Mladá fronta.

Pommerening, T. 2005. *Die altägyptischen Hohlmaße*. Studien zur altägyptischen Kultur. Beihefte 10. Hamburg: Helmut Buske Verlag.

———. 2010. "Von Impotenz und Migräne. Eine kritische Auseinandersetzung mit Übersetzungen des Papyrus Ebers." In *Writings of Early Scholars in the Ancient Near East, Egypt, Rome, and Greece. Translating Ancient Scientific Texts*, edited by A. Imhausen and A. Pommerening, 153–74. Beiträge zum Altertumskunde 286. Berlin and NewYork: De Gruyter.

Posener, G. 1938. *Catalogue des ostraca hiératiques littéraires de Deir el-Médineh, I.3*. Cairo: Institut francais d'archéologie orientale.

———. 1976. *L'enseignement loyaliste. Sagesse égyptienne du Moyen Empire*. Haut Études Orientales 5. Geneva: Droz.

Reisner, G. 1905. *The Hearst Medical Papyrus*. Leipzig: J.C. Hinrichs.

Riedel, M. 2009. *Dějiny kardiologie* [History of Cardiology]. Prague: Galén.

Rochholz, M. 2002. *Schöpfung, Feindvernichtung, Regeneration. Untersuchung zum Symbolgehalt der machtgeladenen Zahl 7 im alten Ägypten*. Ägypten und Altes Testament 56. Wiesbaden: Harrassowitz.

Ruffer, M.A. 1910. "Note on the Presence of Bilharzia haematobium in Egyptian Mummies of Twentieth Dynasty (1250–1000 BC)." *British Medical Journal* 1: 16.

Sanchez, G.M. and E.S. Meltzer. 2012. *The Edwin Smith Papyrus. Updated Translation of the Trauma Treatise and Modern Medical Commentaries*. Atlanta: Lockwood Press.

Sandison, A.T. 1972. "Evidence of Infective Disease." *Journal of Human Evolution* 1, no. 2: 213–24.

Schultz, M., B. Gessler-Löhr, and J. Kollath. 1995. "The First Evidence of Microfilariasis in an Old Egyptian Mummy." *Proceedings of the First World Congress on Mummy Studies*, 317–20. Santa Cruz: Archaeological and Ethnographical Museum of Tenerife.

Smith, G.E. and W.R. Dawson. 1924. *Egyptian Mummies*. London: George Allen and Unwin.

Smoláriková, K. 2009. "Embalmers' Deposits of the Saite Tombs at Abusir." *Göttinger Miszellen* 223: 79–88.

———. 2010. "Embalmers' Caches in the Shaft Tombs at Abu Sir." *Egyptian Archaeology* 36: 33–35.

Sobotková, V. 2012. "Diagnostika ve staré Mezopotámii" [Diagnostics in ancient Mesopotamia]. *Acta Fakulty filozofické Západočeské univerzity v Plzni* 2: 75–92.

Stephan, J. 2001. "Ordnungssysteme in der Altägyptischen Medizin und ihre Überlieferungen in den Europaischen Kulturkreis." PhD diss., Hamburg University.

———. 2011. *Die altägyptische Medizin und ihre Spuren in der abendländischen Medizingeschichte*. Berlin: LIT.

Strouhal, E. 1994a. *Život starých Egypťanů* [The Life of Ancient Egyptians]. 3rd ed., London: Opus Publ.

———. 1994b. "Tod und Mummifikation der alten Ägypter." *Mitteilungen der Berliner Gesellschaft für Anthropologie, Ethnologie und Urgeschichte* 15: 15–23.

———. 1995. "Secular Changes of Embalming Methods in Ancient Egypt." In *Proceedings of the First World Congress on Mummy Studies*, 859–66. Santa Cruz: Archaeological and Ethnographical Museum of Tenerife.

————. 2006. "Old Egypt a tuberkulóza" [Ancient Egypt and Tuberculosis]. *Zdravotnické noviny* 55/43: 17.

Strouhal, E., B. Vachala, and H. Vymazalová. 2010. *Lékařství starých Egypťanů I. Staroegyptská chirurgie. Péče o matku a dítě* [The Medicine of the Ancient Egyptians I: Surgery, Gynecology, Obstetrics, and Pediatrics]. 1st edition, Prague: Academia.

————. 2014. *The Medicine of the Ancient Egyptians I: Surgery, Gynecology, Obstetrics, and Pediatrics.* Cairo and New York: The American University in Cairo Press.

Tapp, E. 1979a. "The Unwrapping of a Mummy." In *Manchester Museum Mummy Project*, edited by A.R. David, 83–94. Manchester: Manchester University Press.

————. 1979b. "Disease in the Manchester Mummies." In *Manchester Museum Mummy Project*, edited by A.R. David, 95–102. Manchester: Manchester University Press.

————.1986. "Histology and Histopathology of the Manchester Mummies." In *Science in Egyptology. Proceedings of the Science in Egyptology Symposia*, edited by: A.R. David, 347–50. Manchester: Manchester University Press, Manchester.

Tapp, E. and K. Wildsmith. 1986. "Endoscopy of Egyptian Mummies." In *Science in Egyptology. Proceedings of the Science in Egyptology Symposia*, edited by: A.R. David, 351–59.

————. 1992. "The Autopsy and Endoscopy of the Leeds Mummy." In *The Mummy's Tale*, edited by A.R. David and E. Tapp, 132–53. London: Michael O'Mara Books.

Thompson, P., P.G. Lynch, and E. Tapp. 1986. "Neuropathological Studies of the Manchester Mummies." In *Science in Egyptology. Proceedings of the Science in Egyptology Symposia*, edited by: A.R. David, 375–78. Manchester: Manchester University Press.

Vachala, B. 2014. "Včely a med ve starém Egyptě. Dary slunečního boha Rea" [Bees and honey in Ancient Egypt: gifts of the sun god Re]. *Vesmír* 93: 234–37.

Verner, M., L. Bareš, B. Vachala. 2007. *Encyklopedie starověkého Egypta* [Encyclopedia of ancient Egypt]. Prague: Libri.

Vymazalová, H. and F. Coppens. 2010. "Medicine, Mathematics and Magic Unite in a Scene from the Temple of Kom Ombo (KO 950)." *Anthropologie* 47/2: 127–31.

————. 2011. *Moudrost svitků boha Thovta. Vědecké poznání za vlády faraonů* [The wisdom of the scrolls of the god Thoth: scientific knowledge from the time of the pharaohs]. Prague: Univerzita Karlova v Praze, Filozofická fakulta.

Weeks, K.R. 1970. "The Anatomical Knowledge of the Ancient Egyptians and the Representation of the Human Figure in Egyptian Art." PhD diss., University of Yale.

Westendorf, W. 1966. *Papyrus Edwin Smith. Ein medizinisches Lehrbuch aus dem Alten Aegypten. Wund- und Unfallchirurgie, Zaubersprüche gegen Seuchen, verschiedene Rezepte*, Bern and Stuttgart: Hans Huber.

————. 1992. *Erwachen der Heilkunst. Die Medizin im Alten Ägypten.* Zürich: Artemis and Winkler.

————. 1999. *Handbuch der altägyptischer Medizin*, Handbuch der Orientalistik 36. Leiden, Boston, and Köln: Brill.

Wilkinson, R.H. 1999. *Symbol and Magic in Egyptian Art*. London: Thames and Hudson.

Wissenschaft im Alten Ägypten. http://sae.saw-leipzig.de/liste/wissensbereich/heilkunde-medizin-und-heilende-magie/

Wreszinski, W. 1909. *Der grosse medizinische Papyrus des berliner Museums (Pap. Berl. 3038) in Facsimile und Umschrift mit Übersetzung, Kommentar und Glossar*. Leipzig: J.C. Hinrichs.

————. 1912. *Der londoner medizinische Papyrus (Brit. Museum Nr. 10059) und der Papyrus Hearst in Transcription, Übersetzung und Kommentar*. Leipzig: J.C. Hinrichs.

————. 1913. *Der Papyrus Ebers, Umschrift, Übersetzung und Kommentar I–II*. Leipzig: J.C. Hinrichs.

Zink, A.R., C. Sola, U. Reischl, U., W. Grabner, N. Rastogi, H. Wolf, and A.G. Nerlich. 2004. "Molecular Identification and Characterization of Mycobacterium Complex in Ancient Egyptian Mummies." *International Journal of Osteoarchaeology* 14: 404–13.

Ziskind, B. 2009. "La Bilharziose urinaire en ancienne Égypte." *Nephrologie et Thérapeutique* 5/7: 658–61.

Ziskind, B. and B. Halioua. 2007. "La tuberculose en ancienne Égypte." *Revue des Maladies Respiratoires* 24/10: 1277–83.

INDEX

Ruffer M.A. 284

Sakhmet 86, 138
Sais 13, 171
Schistosoma haematobium 284, 287
schistosomiasis 169, 284–85
scoliosis 311
Sekhemu *see* Letopolis
Selket 3, 223, 225
Senedj 131, 183
Seth 1, 14, 118, 138, 139, 148, 171, 172,
　　173, 176, 177, 260, 296
Sokar 137, 173
stomatology 153
stricture of the urethra 266
Strongyloides stercoralis 287
subileus 241
symptoms, symptomatology 1, 7, 9, 46,
　　47, 57, 88, 89, 125, 130, 152, 153,
　　154, 169, 170, 182, 186, 189, 190,
　　200, 202, 204, 210, 213, 214, 215,
　　230, 231, 233, 234, 240, 241, 246,
　　259, 262, 263, 270, 273, 274, 276,
　　284, 288, 290, 292, 294, 302, 318,
　　320, 325, 329, 331, 332, 333
syndromes 152, 202, 222, 295

tapeworm 25, 26, 27, 28, 29, 93, 116,
　　119, 277–81, 287
Tefnut 56, 103, 138, 173, 174
Thoth 14, 118, 131, 148, 171, 172, 260, 296
thrombosis 187, 295
tracheitis 204
Trichinella spiralis 287
tuberculosis 204, 210, 311; spine
　　(Pott's disease) 311
tumor 247, 248, 283; malignant
　　248
Tutankhamun 160

ulcus cruris 319; pepticum 218;
　　ventriculi 218
urethrolithiasis 265
urocystitis 265, 267
urology 153

Valley of the Kings 198, 203
Valley of the Queens 2, 225, 288
varicose veins 295, 319

Wadi Halfa 285
Wepwawet 116
Westendorf, W. 10, 202, 218